Begun during a time of disability rights crisis in the early 1970s, this book will remain a basic touchstone about the horrors of Willowbrook, a clear commentary on the fundamentals of deinstitutionalization and a classic about conscience, economic interests and public policy. Dr. William Bronston's and other photo journalist's camera speed were set at 1/300th second. The 82 images captured at Willowbrook were all taken in less than 1 second but will last 100 years. The crimes against humanity here are vivid. Systems change is much slower with Americans with developmental disabilities and our society's older citizens still living with segregated models that have crossed three Centuries. We are an impatient people and this outdated dehumanizing mindset must end.

Colleen Wieck, PhD
Executive Director, Minnesota Governor's Council on Developmental Disabilities

The sad images of inhumanity captured at Willowbrook confirm the words of Justice Ruth Bader Ginsburg in *Olmstead Ruling* when she stated:

> "…[C]onfinement in an institution severely diminishes the everyday life activities of individuals, including family relations, social contacts, work options, economic independence, educational advancement, and cultural enrichment."

In every chapter, the message in his book is that segregation of individuals with disabilities must end, which is consistent with the constitutional promise to bring equal justice to all. Or, in the words of Aristotle, "life in the community is a necessary condition for a person's complete flourishing as a human being."

Donovan W. Frank
United States District Judge United States District Court for the District of Minnesota

"Under the guidance of Bronston and his colleagues and allies, a societal change as profound as any, ever, has fundamentally altered the status of the disabled in society. Hundreds of thousands across the country have been freed of their institutional prisons and given a new lease on a more decent life. Their friends and families have similarly had their lives positively impacted. Challenges abound. Much remains to be done and the issues are constant. Many of them are chronicled in this fine book, but Bronston and company have already changed the destinies of millions."

Geraldo Rivera, Fox News

The shocking horrors of Willowbrook State School have been exposed and will never be forgotten. In Doctor William Bronston's defining book, Public Hostage Public Ransom: Ending Institutional America, he takes on all of America's institutions, the segregated nursing home industry, that have not learned the lesson of the tragedy of Willowbrook. His muckraking efforts remind one of a latter-day Lincoln Steffens, Ida Tarbell, or Jacob Riis. His book is a scathing reminder of all we still have to do to build a sympathetic and just world for the many who are unable to find it for themselves.

Jonathan Sanger
American Film Producer
The Elephant Man

I met Dr. Bronston (Bill) in 1972 and we have been profound friends and colleagues since then. He exposed me to the hell hole called Willowbrook State. School. *Public Hostage* should make you outraged. The mistreatment of disabled people in Willowbrook and the mistreatment today of disabled people living in institutions must be understood and together we must fight to provide people the supports they need to live their lives integrated in our communities with dignity and respect. We as a society are responsible for these atrocities if we remain silent.

Judith E. Heumann
International Disability Rights Advocate

☆—CRITICS REPORT—☆

PUBLIC HOSTAGE PUBLIC RANSOM: ENDING INSTITUTIONAL AMERICA

BY: WILLIAM BRONSTON, M.D.

SCORE:

Plot/Idea: 10 out of 10
Originality: 10 out of 10
Prose: 9 out of 10
Character/Execution: 9 out of 10
Overall: 9.50 out of 10

booklife
PRIZE

Public Hostage, Public Ransom:
ENDING INSTITUTIONAL AMERICA

William Bronston, M.D.

ISBN: 978-1684569090
Language: English
Pages: 384

ASSESSMENT:

Plot/Idea: Bronston forcibly advocates for people with special needs, arguing that institutionalizing those populations is harmful and, in many cases, abusive. He draws from his professional experience as a physician in the early 1970s at Willowbrook State School, a New York state facility, to explain the horrific conditions suffered in such spaces; the subject matter is painful and shocking to read, but a powerful call-to-action for reform.

Prose: Bronston is brutally honest with the information he presents, sharing real-life examples of individuals institutionalized at Willowbrook that will stun and outrage readers. His prose is matter-of-fact but electric, as he delves into his contributions to ending the institutionalization of special populations and calls instead for compassionate support of human rights.

Originality: This is a compelling exposé of the inhumane treatment individuals with special needs receive when institutionalized for care.

Character/Execution: Bronston's succinct writing and inclusion of photographs, news clippings, and other artifacts reveals the devastating abuse and mistreatment of a population in desperate need of empathy and protection. His role in the ensuing class action lawsuit against New York state is riveting and unfolds against a backdrop of corruption, oppression, and cruelty.

DATE SUBMITTED: January 31, 2025

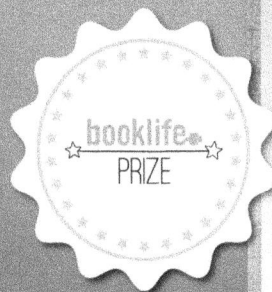

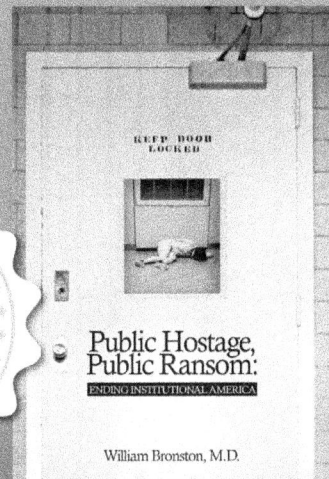

HOLLYWOOD BOOK REVIEWS

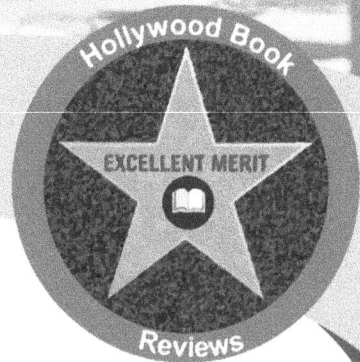

EXCELLENT MERIT

Hollywood Book Reviews

PUBLIC HOSTAGE, PUBLIC RANSOM
Ending Institutional America

BY WILLIAM BRONSTON, M. D.

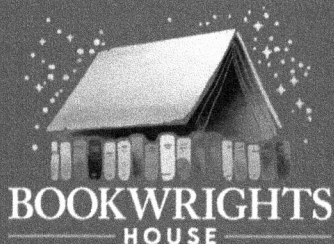

BOOKWRIGHTS
HOUSE

Reviewed by: David Allen

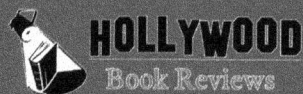

HOLLYWOOD
Book Reviews

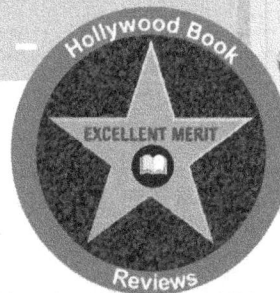

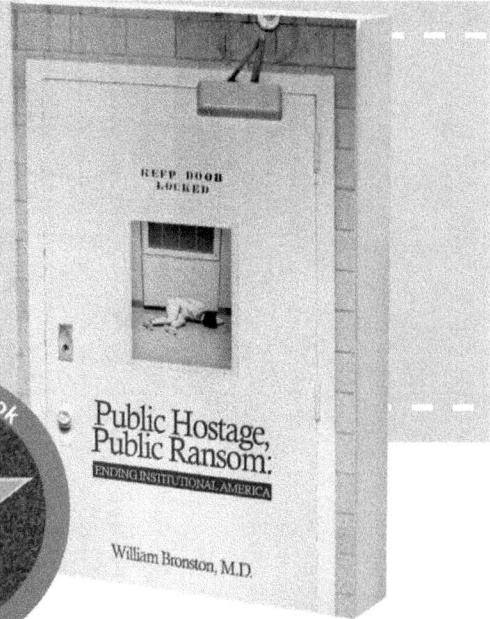

Public Hostage,
Public Ransom:
ENDING INSTITUTIONAL AMERICA

William Bronston, M.D.

PUBLIC HOSTAGE, PUBLIC RANSOM
Ending Institutional America
by William Bronston, M. D.

'Institutional America' includes but is not necessarily limited to 'hospitals' and 'schools' for the mentally retarded, the disabled, and the elderly. According to author Dr. William Bronston, who spent a consciousness-raising and harrowing three years as physician and psychiatrist at Willowbrook School in Staten Island, New York, institutions are NOT the way for America to go. (Willowbrook became the iconic locus of the public deinstitutionalization debate in this country in the 1970s.)

His message in *Public Hostage, Public Ransom: Ending Institutional America*, could not appear at a more opportune moment, when funding for necessities like healthcare and education are getting strangled at the source. Bronston's book persuasively argues that a single payer system needs to replace Medicaid-based 'specialty' funding for individuals with developmental disabilities and for seniors currently in nursing homes. Bronston argues with great force that community-based solutions, such as local housing and placement, serve not only the disabled but the surrounding community as well, and better.

There is a long and aggrieved history to the struggle. In the 1970s in America, deinstitutionalization became a rallying cry for increasing awareness of human rights abuses in institutions such as Willowbrook. Bronston, who had the intestinal fortitude not only to stick it out there but to apply himself and his colleagues passionately to lobbying, to writing memos, to educating the legislature and public, is an activist whose writing, whose appeal for humane treatment and common sense in our treatment of the most fragile, is a clarion call for further ongoing action.

The warehousing of human flesh is a dreadful thing to behold. Mental hospitals and nursing homes are usually built out of the public eye, away from the thoroughfare, for good reason: cosmetize the unwanted, hide them away in blockhouses behind the service road of the expressway. *Public Hostage, Public Ransom's* 80-plus photographs, many of them stark black and white, provide a visual documentary to the narrative of forced custody and depredation that accompanies. Bronston is one of those masterfully articulate champions who gets right in there and rubs it in our collective face. When you see the human debris, the living skeletons, that once populated Willowbrook and sister institutions across the land, the blasted denizens of this nether world whose daily routine is limited to 'three cots and a hot' and heavy-duty meds and kicks and punches and blows...you will certainly agree, that something must be done.

Thanks to the unstinting efforts of Dr. Bronston, and of like-minded heroes roused to positive action by his and others' muckraking humanitarian efforts, courts and legislatures closed down Willowbrook in the early 1970s. To his greater credit, the author of this testament to human suffering, waste, and occasional reparation relates changes at Willowbrook to parallel events and progress across the land. *Public Hostage, Public Ransom* is an extraordinary narrative and photo documentary of one doctor's quest to make things better.

This book will challenge readers to rethink the structures that govern care for society's most vulnerable and propels for a future that prioritizes human rights over institutional convenience.

Reviewed by: David Allen

HOLLYWOOD
Book Reviews

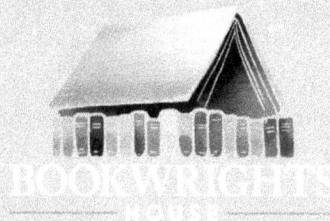

BOOKWRIGHTS
HOUSE

Public Hostage Public Ransom:

Ending Institutional America

WILLIAM BRONSTON, M.D.

978-1-965552-68-1 (Paperback)
978-1-965552-67-4 (Hardback)

Library of Congress Control Number: 2026903263

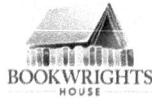

BOOKWRIGHTS
HOUSE

admin@bookwrightshouse.com
☎ (213) 286 6700

Dedicated to
my towering teachers …
My child development medical
genius Richard Koch M.D.
and
My fiery, prophetic, Nobel quality,
worldly 'change agent'
Wolf Wolfensberger Ph.D.

CONTENTS

Part II: Public Ransom

PREFACE

THIS WORK IS MOSTLY about an institution in Staten Island, New York, called Willowbrook State School. Willowbrook was one of thirty such facilities in New York State for people labeled as mentally retarded. The New York State Department of Mental Hygiene, a gigantic bureau with a politically appointed psychiatrist as commissioner, operated the institutional system in the state for people labeled both mentally retarded and mentally ill.

The core of this work covers the three years during which I worked at Willowbrook as a physician and a subsequent two years during which I was on "educational leave" (with pay) in a postdoctoral fellowship at Syracuse University, away from the institution.

During this five-year span, an immense national struggle developed in relation to the rights of people with mental, developmental, and physical disabilities. It was a turning point in the effort of many citizens with special needs and their families to address the inhumane violations inflicted upon them by Willowbrook and by other identical institutions around the United States and Canada.

In 1971 and 1972, constitutional lawsuits were filed against the states of Alabama, Massachusetts, and Pennsylvania on behalf of citizens labeled as retarded, in order to enforce the right to quality public education; the right to treatment and appropriate services to enhance their abilities and achievements; the right to freedom from abuses; and the right to those processes ensuring life, liberty, and the pursuit of happiness guaranteed all citizens by the US Constitution. This ultimately expanded to class action suits in thirty-seven states.

Willowbrook, the largest institution of its kind in the nation and the place where these human rights violations were piled up the highest, became the symbol of public abuse against powerless citizens. To this day, I have been part of the movement to bring all Willowbrook's and the Medicaid Title 19 invented and funded institutional system in America to account.

This book is a personal documentary. I was not an outsider at any time, although it would have been easier that way. It would have been easier not to have lived for three years inside the buildings of Willowbrook, wrestling with the institutional decay, the cynicism, corruption, deprivation, disease, and violence within the bureaucracy that took their relentless toll on the residents and workers. For three years, I was filled with apprehension and turmoil at the bestial conditions on the wards, the lurching struggle of the employees against their own helplessness and imposed collusion.

My background never prepared me to be objective, impartial, uninvolved. All of my training had instilled in me the ability to identify and care. I completed both my premedical requirements and a major in modern history at the University of California at Los Angeles in 1961. I went to the University of Southern California School of Medicine afterward, a school linked with the Los Angeles County General Hospital, which was one of the largest medical facilities serving poor people in the United States. One could not help but see the massive unmet needs of people, the wretched oppression caused by poverty. I became outspoken, turning to my fellow medical students as well as those colleagues in nursing and dental schools, to organize and become involved in community service and enrich our sterile and antisocial professional school curricula.

Between medical school semesters and during summers, it was customary to get a job, a fellowship. Searching for health-related work, I was hired my first summer and thereafter by Dr. Richard Koch, the director of a special service for children with suspected disabilities or delayed development, at the Child Development Clinic in Children's Hospital of Los Angeles.

Hundreds of families were seen in this clinic every year. Each feared the worst—that their child was "retarded," that in place of a name would be substituted a feared label. Dr. Koch's department would carefully evaluate each child from every clinical aspect and decide if, in fact, there was some abnormality in typical growth and why. One-fifth of the children were found to be within normative limits of development. The others received a diagnosis, a label, and were provided ongoing services by the members of the multi-professional team of the clinic.

In retrospect, one must be critical of the traditional medical approach to labeling that was carried on. At that time, though, the immense respect and positive concern which animated all the staff, as well as their tremendous hope and confidence in the future which they transmitted to the families seeking help, was something I just took for granted and allowed to soften my judgment.

Dr. Koch, even then, was in constant battles with the interests in the state that upheld institutionalization as an appropriate solution for children labeled retarded. This struggle between a community-based approach to service and an institutional approach had been going on for decades. Historically, the institution proponents have held sway everywhere. It has been a simple, all-inclusive panacea for dealing with devalued persons.

Despite this traditional reliance on institutions, the community service advocates, though a small voice, gained ground slowly but surely. It was among this group nationally that I was nurtured and my scientific values fashioned. Then, I was ignorant of what the institution was as a national economic and political system. I just didn't give it any thought at the time and felt very good seeing and sharing in the dignified care given at Children's Hospital.

The years of my subsequent medical school training preoccupied me. I completed my internship in pediatrics in Los Angeles, and a two-year residency in psychiatry at Menninger School of Psychiatry in Topeka, Kansas, after which I moved to New York. The opening existed there to become a member of the staff at Willowbrook State School. It looked to me like a good opportunity to continue my familiar work serving people with special needs. When I arrived at Willowbrook in the spring of 1970, I was genuinely looking forward to finding the same spirit of caring and hopefulness for which my training had prepared me. I was utterly not expecting the trauma of what I experienced.

Five years later and far from the tortured reality of Willowbrook, when the first telling of this narrative was in progress, it was still an overwhelming ordeal to set down the full story apart from my feelings of the anger, sadness, frustration, angst, and pathos that had literally become a part of my personal architecture and perspectives. Remarkably, the story had never yet been told from the inside. I have pulled together reams of paper and photos that I have used as the backbone of this documentary. Here is the essence of what it was like as a health worker, citizen, and organizer inside Willowbrook that reveal and interpret the profound drama.

Families allegedly "decide" and seek help to place their disabled or elderly relatives into large or small institutions. Theoretically, they have the option not to institutionalize them, and also the right to freely take them back home again. The law, Title 19 of the Social Security Act of 1965, Medicaid, provides a massive funding stream for these institutions and all out-of-home placement. Institutions are mostly financed by multi-billions of tax monies, public grants, Medicare, Medicaid, and social security funds (as are all public and most voluntary "nonprofit" human services agencies). The budgets and fees are ceded to legitimate public bureaucracies. In fact, the public in New York and the majority of our states had no solution other than the institutions for the care of their disabled relatives if care at home was not feasible. In fact, emancipation from the institution is overwhelmingly difficult. In fact, the unimaginable amount of public resources that are chained to the operation of the institutional system does not serve those institutionalized toward their eventual return and integration to society, nor are these funds spent, in large part, on meaningful habilitation or rehabilitation services of any kind. Instead, the public tax dollars flow into the hands of the bureaucracies and their administrators who run the system, for interests other than the public welfare. In every state, violations of human rights—systematic crimes against humanity—are being perpetrated daily at the highest levels of the bureaucracy and human services delivery system. Our disabled brethren and the elderly are hostages in our institutional culture. We continuously pour out our tax-derived payments as "ransom" for their care and eventual release—return to open society. Our expectation for their deliverance is incredibly naive.

The central purpose of this document is a unitary one: to provide help in understanding the evil of our segregated and congregate residential institutional system in such a way as to fashion stepping-stones for public policy to foreclose on this system of profit from out-of-home services forever. It is my deep conviction as a professional in the public service of people with special needs that there is not a single justification for institutionalizing people who need health, educational, or social supports to enhance the quality, social status, and competency of their lives.

So overwhelming is the evidence of the scientific, social, and economic harm done by residential institutions in this nation that it warrants the utter vilification and rapid phasing out of the entire institutional system.

The issue at hand is political. Unless the institutional system is exposed and shown in its bankrupt, immoral reality, profound alternatives to institutions will never have a chance to grow. Healthy tissue and cells in living things can be overwhelmed by cancerous cells. Cancer presents itself as super life, growing exuberantly, young in appearance, but fundamentally too simple and monotonous to do the complicated and adaptive things required by living organisms. It ultimately competes for vital blood supply and space in the body needed for adaptive life. It kills by exhausting its own host.

So, too, institutional out-of-home residential placement is a cancer eating up our precious social resources. It offers a simple, rigid answer, multiplying from its own size, leaving no strength or a healthy alternative able to sustain real growth. Segregated institutions, like cancer, kill! They must be treated exactly the same way: with radical surgery, obliteration. They must be equally feared and rejected by the public who must bear the responsibility for demanding an end to both diseases—the one socioeconomic, the other physiological.

Willowbrook was but a giant example of this societal cancer in our community. It stood as a symbol, as a general case, representing the majority of instances, notwithstanding the few so-called good institutions that are sold to the public as a light to guide the institutional system forward. Such token good institutions are a futile and cruel facade to confound us about the true nature of the sanctioned warehousing in this country, where New York State is far and away the leader in backwardness and human abuse. We must understand who controls, who benefits, who pays, who suffers, what is true, and what is illusion—in short, the politics of human abuse, not just that human abuse abounds.

The first part of this work, "Public Hostage," describes the personal part about Willowbrook. It is meant for the reader to touch, feel, see, and vicariously smell. It is a case in point upon which a greater body of fact and understanding about institutions in America can then be established.

The second part of this work, "Public Ransom," is to offer a broader analysis of the conditions that support and nourish our current out-of-home placement policies and institutions and prevent the development and success of full inclusion and individualization for such services for devalued people in our society. The philosophical and economic underpinnings of segregating and removing people, elders, and those with disabilities, who are different and devalued from our society, and the economic consequences of such ideological underdevelopment will be made plain. It is only with a national paradigm shift to end Medicaid, Title 19, "long-term care" and replace it with "lifetime care," birth-to-end-of-life individual planning and care, within a "universal health care as a right" system, a single-payer system, that we can end our public hostage, institutional culture. Without such a grasp of conditions, no successful strategies for change, a paradigm shift can be forged—and forged it must be!

PART I

PUBLIC HOSTAGE

KEEP DOOR

LOCKED

CHAPTER 1

Lillian

LET ME TELL A short story about a typical situation of a typical girl inside Willowbrook. Such daily facts of life relentlessly directed my efforts to challenge this atrocity.

Lillian was nine years old when she was admitted to Willowbrook. It was not an unusual course. The road to the institution was well-worn, inevitable, and relentless for most children like Lillian. She was born in Brooklyn. Her family was just another struggling family, victims of innocence about children that grow differently. Brooklyn is a large place, at the time, the fifth largest "city" by population in the world. With its largeness, there was barrenness when it came to help for children with special needs.

Lillian couldn't talk when she was at the age that other children could. She had difficulties taking care of herself the way typical five-year-olds could. There are no records of exactly what happened, but Lillian was labeled as mentally retarded. Her family moved to Pennsylvania, where the girl was placed in a special class for children with retarded mental development. It was predictable that this move to a station of little value for the girl would more likely than not accelerate her chances for further exclusion and set low expectation from those around her. Her classroom—undoubtedly overburdened, generally staffed with teachers who accepted and expected Lillian's low performance, in a state that excluded massive numbers of its children from school due to the deficiencies in the school system—would be easily defeated by Lillian's special needs.

Ordinary people confronted with a united and unaccountable professional front of teachers, doctors, social workers, psychologists tend to do what is expected of them. It takes little imagination to penetrate the agony and helplessness of Lillian's family confronted with a professional system that really didn't want the child, a community with token resources, and a cultural tradition of institutionalizing those it did not like or couldn't serve successfully. It is only in the most recent history that institutionalization has been challenged as the universal recommendation to families. I don't know exactly what helps families resist this sentence when they do. I know that every family somehow resists for a while, sometimes privately, sometimes openly, always painfully. But families, ordinary people, are fragile. Most families ultimately surrender to the pressure. Staten Island's Willowbrook became the destination for this youngster.

Lillian's records at age nine, when she entered the institution, labeled her as autistic. This means that she was seen as basically having a severe cognitive and behavioral disorder. The reason this is important is that although mental retardation can legitimately flow from autism disturbances, Willowbrook was never set up to serve people with such developmental disturbances. It never had the trained people, the supportive settings, and the concern for the individual to put into practice what has been known for a long time about treatment.

Everyone who came to Willowbrook had to be labeled with mental retardation by law. But on admission, Lillian still retained the label of autism, that, under normal circumstances, would have made her eligible for a psychiatric children's facility, that shows how clear her problem was at that time despite her misplacement, which the institution ignored. Regardless of this, the child was given an IQ test, and in four lines a "senior clinical psychologist" summed up what the IQ test was meant to do—designate the hopelessness of the situation and permit the institution to ignore her condition, justify keeping her in a mental retardation warehouse, and proceed on to the next case. Lillian was not formally tested again until eight years later, when she was seventeen. No description of the young woman's performance was to be found. No recommendations were noted on the IQ test, and the tester decided that nothing had changed. Thus, at the points where real changes could have been instituted, the opportunity was dropped. Lillian was just like so many—a captive, an institution ward, in actuality another of New York State's Medicaid-funded hostages.

The Record

When I had a chance to review her records, soon after first seeing her, I was moved by the monotonous and concise descriptions by which Lillian's identity had been bleached away. Notation after notation, placed in the record as a matter of minimal effort and bureaucratic regulations, were like a litany over a lost soul, another commodity with a female name. The headings in the summary sheet were capitalized, followed by a short paragraph essentially reaffirming the headings. One either had to turn off and just read, or risk seeing through the unscientific, rhetorical code that had become so familiar to me in reading every chart.

> Admission Note: Underdeveloped and undernourished negro female 1964: Adjusting slowly, hyperactive, withdrawn; feeds herself with coaxing, grabs things and holds tightly
>
> 1965: Entaemeba Histolytica (a mild form of amoebic dysentery)
>
> 1966: Gets along with others, on Thorazine treatment, talks in sentences, functions on a moron level 1967: Overactive, masturbates alone
>
> 1968: Prefers to stay alone, hard to manage, self-abusive, kept in a straitjacket; disturbed, confused, attacks others. Consider transferring as mentally ill
>
> 1969: Abusive to herself and others, on phenobarbital and Nembutal yet walks around day and night talking to herself
>
> Transfer to Building 23 (adult female building for disturbed women) for observation for 6 weeks. Placed on Thorazine 600 mg.
>
> 1970: Easily disturbed in straitjacket for long periods of time because she hits others. Abusive and needs supervision.

There were no details in the voluminous chart. Instead, it was filled with required forms recording her continuous confinement in the straitjacket; the nurses' massive check-off reports of administered medications day in and day out; the almost illegible yellow forms with their carbon scribbles by other physicians, logging accident after accident where Lillian had incurred injuries.

A lot of correspondence between the institution and the family filled up much of the back part of the chart. "Your relative is being transferred to the hospital ward for (this or that) injury or illness." "Your relative is being transferred to another building for administrative reasons." "Yes, you can visit." "Yes, you can take your daughter home on weekends." "Yes, you can take your daughter home for the holiday." Even though Lillian was systematically being extinguished, the family visited religiously.

Family

Lillian's family continued to commute from Harrisburg twice a month. Lillian's grandmother was along in years. She was a great, stout woman who, despite her obvious strength, always had the most terrible look on her face when she visited. It was like she was just arriving at the scene of a severe auto accident searching for her loved one and terrified at what she would find—what mutilation, what destruction, what loss. The expression of anxiety and apprehension was fixed on her face and in her sad eyes. Reverend Reynolds always came with Lillian's grandmother. He did most of the talking. "We never can find anybody to talk with or ask how our Lillian is doing. She looks so awful, she's lost so much. You know, she used to talk and wear a dress. She's lost so much weight. Doctor, what's happening to our girl? What can we do? Doctor, please help us! Why does she have so many accidents and look so bad? We'll do anything you say."

Downhill Road

What could I say? I had been at Willowbrook for two years. I knew why Lillian was going downhill. I knew why. There was so much piled up over so long that was taking the life out of the child who had been entrusted to Willowbrook to revive. I began meeting with the family more as Lillian's condition worsened. I had come very late indeed to witness the spectacle. Lillian was one of thousands. Willowbrook was full of Lillians, people who were slowly dying, robbed of their basic humaneness. The important difference with this girl was that she was fighting back against the forces pitted against her. What was so tough was how grotesquely the struggle marked her.

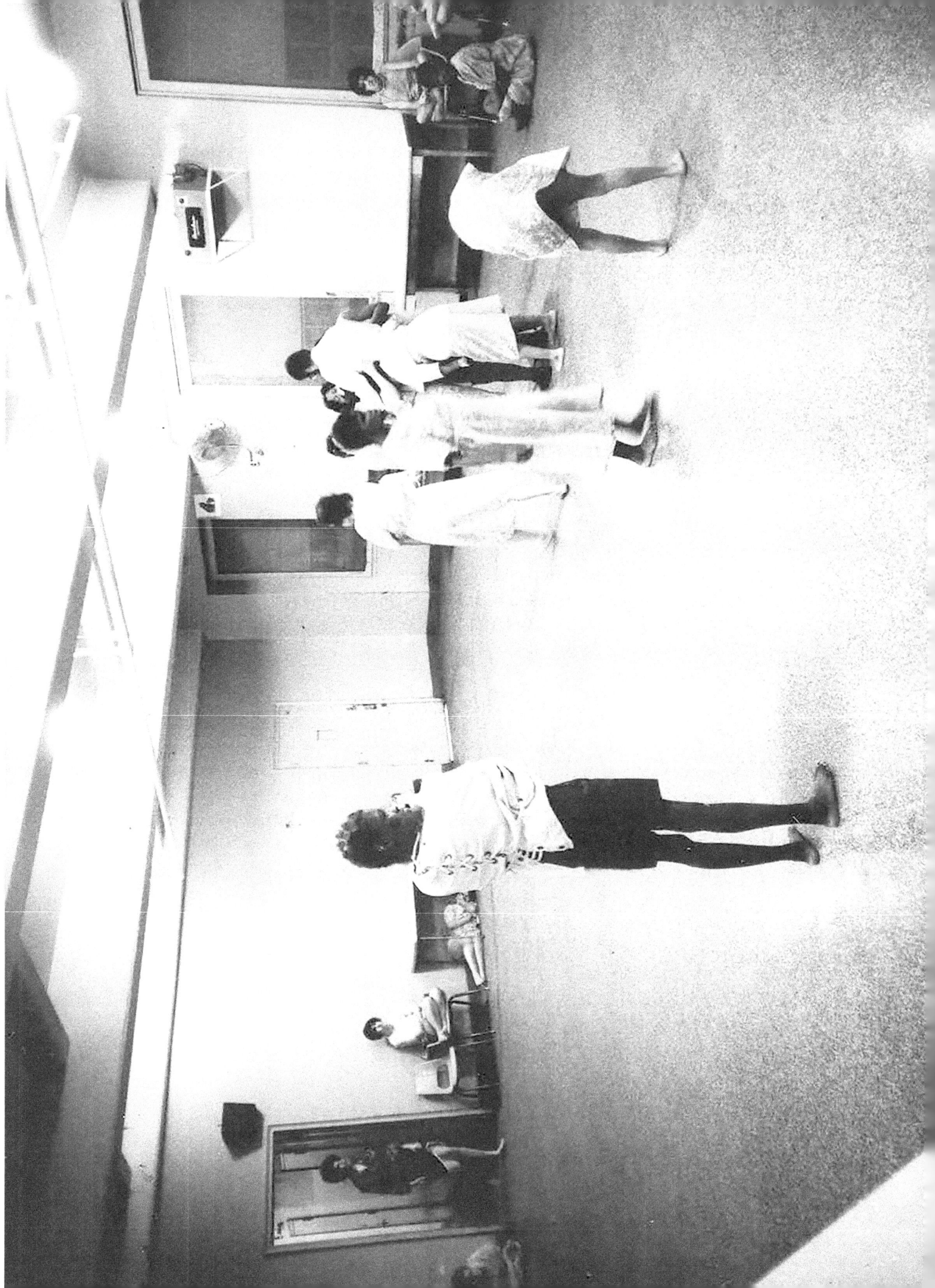

Control

Lillian was on a combination of two essentially identical tranquilizing drugs in massive amounts, in addition to being daily confined in a straitjacket. She was continually reported for head banging against the floors and stone walls by the workers, who had clearly come to expect violent behavior from the girl; thus, the demand to further drug her to ease the "management" problems she posed on the ward. Only by kicking, biting, and head banging could Lillian attract attention. Her voice was reduced to an incoherent croak that defied understanding. Laced into the heavy canvas camisole, Lillian alternately crouched near a wall or lay heaped asleep on the stone floor or dashed about the ward menacing everybody like a great wingless bird. She was a creature whose years in the institution had converted her into a specter of scrawny dishevelment. Always alone, watching, moaning, drifting here and there, searching for something—broken lips, disfigured nose, matted hair, bare feet, coarse institution pullover dress protruding from below the white canvas and brass-ringed restraint.

But Lillian was only one of twenty-two women in Building 23 where I had been newly consigned, who were in continuous camisole restraints when I was introduced to the duty of signing the daily slip that continued this practice. I had really not seen the straitjacket before in the children's buildings. I had been cloistered. It was clear that I was at the bottom, the gut center of Willowbrook. I had been assigned to the job that only the most trusted or the most hated had seen.

There was no right decision that could be made in Lillian's case. She was just an ordinary victim. There were no places that might provide sanctuary, let alone minimum treatment in the institution. What complicated the problem was that the ward workers held her fate in their hands. If they could not be convinced of what was needed and helped to accept their true service role, then things would go from bad to worse.

I held some keys, but I was new in the building. My heart was still not in this insane situation into which I had been thrust to oversee such an ocean of adult misery and deprivation. The danger of advocating for any of the residents, given the utter hopelessness of the conditions for the workers, threatened to backfire and sow resentment, as I had already learned from my last assignment in the children's Building 76.

If there was to be change, the first was to change how Lillian was perceived by all the people around her. She had become seen as an animal, rather than a deeply suffering young woman who desperately needed help. As long as she was on the massive amounts of tranquilizing drugs and wore the camisole, there was no hope. The power of these personal facts and her assignment on a ward that was known as hyperactive because of the behavior of women assigned there made the expectation of Lillian's wild behavior overwhelming and self-fulfilling.

Damage Done

One thing helped. A cluster of the workers on the day shift recognized the girl's profound deterioration and were fearful for her to the point of continually pushing that something be done. After I arrived, within one month, I was able to wean the girl off tranquilizers and out of the straitjacket. Shortly thereafter I was summoned to assess her situation. She had been found with massive swelling of both eyelids. It was obvious to anyone that either the girl had suffered a severe injury or that some major malfunction in her chemical system was occurring. In such a condition, she must be carefully evaluated by a specialist.

I had very rapidly come to learn that the Willowbrook environment caused conditions not seen outside of the institution that occurred commonly within it. Whether Lillian's condition was malnutrition, kidney disease, intoxication from something, trauma, or a combination of all these things had to be determined. Even though the quality of care in Building 2 (the so-called Medical and Surgical Building where people were sent for more intensive care) was far below minimum standard, but, compared with what could be done in the residential building, 23, it was a relative paradise.

Before seeking to transfer Lillian, I carefully examined her. Sure enough, a sickening finding. Virtually half of her scalp, instead of feeling firm and taut over her head, sponged in nearly a finger's width at my touch. I had never seen such an extensive edematous bruise. The softness was due to free fluid that had collected under the scalp. Undoubtedly, the swelling of her eyelids came from the extension of the fluid under her scalp into areas where there was the least tissue resistance. The possibility that she might have a fractured skull, let alone her obviously severe injury, warranted close scrutiny and medical supervision.

The Role of the Medical and Surgical Building 2

Many times in the past, conflicts had erupted when I had moved people with medical-care problems to Building 2. What was defined as acceptable basis for moving a resident into the Medical and Surgical Building varied significantly. At the heart of the matter was whether one accepted what Willowbrook routinely did to people, or whether one wanted to utilize what resources that were available and hope to treat and alleviate individual suffering. Unfortunately, the extent of pathology that was tolerated by staff physicians usually defined the criteria for admission to Building 2. What was missing was the empathy, the ability to identify each person as a possible relative having the common right to quality medical care and freedom from pain and suffering. But the day was too hectic for me to stop and worry whether or not I would have to fight with the admitting medical officer in Building 2 over Lillian's need.

Yet, forty-eight hours after sending her to Building 2 for assessment and serious medical care, Lillian was returned in my building. Moreover, she was delivered again in a straitjacket, pathetically disfigured, still—croaking, wild-eyed. I was thunderstruck at the attitude of my colleagues. I knew, intellectually, where they were coming from. But each time the lack of pity, the arrogance, and the inhumanity caused the anger to well in me and I was frozen, not knowing how to deal with such practices. I didn't have to phone them. I knew what I would be told: "She wrecked the ward. You know we don't have enough staff here to deal with one like that, and besides, what the hell did you send her here for when you could have taken just as good care of her over there?"

It was through such collisions in the past that my course had become clear to me. It was essential that each instance such as Lillian's be carefully logged and documented. The Willowbrook staff professionals were simply incapable of responding to the human needs of others. Only if something threatened their professional status and security would they move to benefit the residents. The staff professional had become more retarded than the most "retarded" person in the institution. Fear was the only way to mobilize the precious few resources and opportunities for survival of the warehoused and forgotten.

The workers on the wards were deeply humiliated daily by the staff physicians' attitudes. Basically, the workers had to be made to see that their fate and working conditions were as desperate as the residents, whom they were "trained" to tend. As long as the residents could be ignored and abused, the workers would receive the same treatment by those above them. To educate and win the trust of my coworkers in the building, I had to walk a tightrope every day. No mistakes would be tolerated, no slips. I had to avoid any tone of blame in my voice, be careful not to shrug off a worker's observation, nor ignore looking at each of the residents every day.

On the active side, I had to oppose each and every administrative and professional transgression openly. Taking risks to urge common action and pride among the ward workers and nursing assistants became the cement of our relationship. More than medications and bandages, it was the healing of torn and disfigured attitudes and replacing these—grafting however small, wherever possible—the respect for the residents and one another. Here was the treatment program that would slowly bring about what Lillian and all residents needed to survive.

How slow this effort was, and how constant the repetition of crises each day, for so many of our women. We could barely escape one tragedy when another would crash in and demand attention. The relentlessness of such things takes its toll on everybody who is there to experience them.

What to Do?

Lillian kept deteriorating before our very eyes. She became thinner and thinner despite the efforts of the ward workers to feed her. She would lie on the floor in the back of the ward, rigid and shrieking in what was left of her torn voice. Then, in driven outbursts, she would speed about the ward babbling, indifferent to the peers whom she scattered in her trajectory. The ceaseless din, the echo in the stone ward chamber defied description and added to the mad atmosphere.

All of us were becoming more frightened and more defeated, seeing such a bizarre decline. Nothing other than the persistent massive scalp swelling showed. I racked my mind for an answer, where to look. Certainly, the whole cause was the ward—the emptiness, the crowding, the violence of everyday life, being treated like an animal. But what if this was another medical condition, not just major trauma, a disease that we just had not been able to find? Lillian had to go back to Building 2 and somehow be seen by a real specialist from outside the institution. The admitting physician in the Medical and Surgical Building had already rejected her first admission. This time, each issue would have to be spelled out: The patient had been deteriorating since June. Head banging, loss of appetite, bizarre behavior, loss of ability to communicate, weight loss, all pointing to the possibility of a tumor or other growing lesion in Lillian's head. She had to be tested. She had to be thoroughly examined and x-rayed. She had to have a brain wave test. She had to be observed outside of Willowbrook. The reasons were all there, but so was the opposition's power. They kept her for one day and then returned her with a note from a top administrator:

> The policy of Willowbrook with reference to working-up of residents with suspected illness or lesions is that the physician in the patient's residential building will order whatever procedures he thinks are necessary to be carried out from the home building. This includes consultations, etc. Acute medical surgical conditions will be transferred to Building 2 after provision is made with the physician in charge of Building 2. Lillian might well come under the non-emergency status where most procedures could emanate from the building of residence.

That's how things worked—delay, rules, red tape, delay. But the crux of the matter was the fact that Lillian's condition was serious, regardless of whether her injury was medically caused in origin or stemmed from the deprivation and trauma of her environment. Though every subterfuge, every reasonable-sounding memo would eat away time—Lillian's time—pressure had to be unrelenting.

Breakthrough

Finally, the consultants from the institution capitulated to my emergency demand to have the girl moved to Bellevue Hospital in Manhattan. Fourteen days later, we overcame seemingly intransigent bureaucratic blockade, and Lillian went to a real hospital. For six weeks, she remained out of Willowbrook. Bellevue didn't do their job; Lillian came from Willowbrook, and "there is only so much you do for one of those."

But for six weeks, she was out of the institution in a clean bed with clean food. We all knew she would be back, but all of us breathed easier during those rushing days.

It was the beginning of the new year of 1972. Willowbrook had become a volcano of scandal. All of New York and much of the nation had seen the Willowbrook exposé on the television sets and had begun to realize what had been going on with public money. But things that have gone on for so long don't change that fast, and Lillian came back to her building. She was better than I had ever seen her. She talked!

Her voice was raspy, but it was a human voice, a woman's voice. She smiled! I had never seen her smile over the four months before her transfer; I didn't think that it was possible. When a person like Lillian smiles and there is recognition in her eye—well, it's hard to say what that does to you inside. I couldn't believe the change.

I read the report from Bellevue. It was nasty, cold, and explained why most of the tests had not been done. However, a neurologist had seen her and, to the best of his ability, could not find anything that indicated a fracture or medical cause. They had to send Lillian back because they just couldn't handle her. Who could be convinced that six weeks on a medical ward in Bellevue could have so rejuvenated a tormented soul from Willowbrook Building 23? I was really moved. After all, it was our ward that had taken its toll and for all intents and purposes had mimicked a physical problem.

Misfire: An Endless End

I explained to Lillian's grandmother what had happened. They had to get Lillian out somehow, but there was nowhere but home. The solution had to recognize Lillian's special needs. Nothing could be as bad as the institution, but the family needed concrete help. Things had begun to change, ever so slowly. The class action lawsuit was on the federal court docket on behalf of each and every resident of the institution, charging that the institution was heinously authoring gross human abuse through neglect, incompetence, deprivation, and violation of every conceivable human right. Whereas previously there had been no social workers to move people out and gain needed community services for them, a dribble of such workers were being hired under the pressure of the media and impending court action. The greatest threat to the institution was the charge that they kept scores of people in locked isolation rooms for years on end and trussed in straitjackets with no due process nor recourse on the part of the residents or their families to challenge such commonplace practices.

It was so ironic. Our efforts to get Lillian—and many others in Buildings 22 and 23—out of the straitjacket resulted in the loss of opportunity for these women to be moved into a small unit which the administration had quickly fashioned to take the heat off the charge of flagrant abuses. Only those still in continuous confinement were considered "eligible" for that unit.

The first eight months of 1972 passed. During this time, despite so much having happened, nothing of real consequence changed for Lillian. Gradually, the smile stopped. She talked less and less, and the flat, empty look returned. Watching this happen, and being powerless to change the brutalizing environment, destroys the spirit as surely as abuse. Lillian was only one of the many that we watched sink further into the abyss.

Around us were the publicity, lawyers, and a weak effort on the part of the institution to try to cut down the staggering overcrowding. Yet, the food was still awful; the meager, one-piece dresses issued by the state continued to be the mainstay when there were real clothes to be had. No new workers on the wards arrived. The institutions continued to destroy its inhabitant—residents and employees alike.

The story about Lillian is a very painful one to share. I never know if she was still there—inside Willowbrook—with no advocate. One year after the filing of the federal class action suit, Lillian developed cataracts in both eyes which had not been there six months before. At the end, we fought for surgery to remove the blockade of her vision. The loss of sight had come so fast, so irrationally, it drove Lillian back further into herself.

Lillian was one of five thousand, but her destruction was a battle she never surrendered. She would not stop suffering out loud. I can only hope she is still fighting. It is highly likely that her family is still being brutalized by the New York State Department of Mental Hygiene. When I left, Lillian was nineteen.

CHAPTER 2

Framework

ENGAGE, AMERICA! WE ARE confronted with a catastrophic, dehumanizing terminus. Not death through disease or long life, but a status, artificially imposed by public policy and law that establishes a set of conditions for our commoditized management that benefit the few. It is a national system that currently tyrannizes us all and institutionalizes unspeakable sorrow, suffering and ignominy upon all as we wrestle with terribly challenging and inevitable human dependency needs that ultimately arise in our lives and those of our loved ones. It is framed within the policies, practices, and financing of Medicaid, Title 19, of the federal Social Security system aimed at selectively funding a system to deal with the elderly poor, blind, and disabled Americans.

Here, our national system's architects, the presidents beginning in the 1960s and '70s, and Congress, at the behest of their grand masters, the ever-shrinking corporate elite, have gradually constructed a socioeconomic, publicly funded tyranny, a "service delivery" paradigm. This American reality pays for and channels us all into a wretched, machined, institutional ending—human warehouses, concentration centers, segregated assisted living complexes, "nursing" homes, hospitals, assisted living and hospices— all, staggeringly costly. This out-of-natural-home spectrum of residential facilities is the principal publically funded solution to end-of-life management. Its system-wide beginning was enshrined in the origin of the federal Medicaid's malignant core that was the invention of a river of tax dollars and incentives to pay for housing and services to those eligible under the law for only out-of-home placement, in effect creating a massive *domestic refugee* population of citizens who are devalued, perceived, labeled, and marketed as deviants in the society, that is, different in a negative way from the mainstream norm.

The justification and validation for managing this population of America was confirmed and legitimized by imposing medical labels, a socially acceptable status that not so subtly robbed those within its scope of first-class, individualized, and human social identity. In its place were woven stereotypes that permanently embedded variations of pity, helplessness, sick, eternal child, menace, holy innocence, charity, and animal imagery. This well-understood alchemy of identity then allows a range of socially acceptable dehumanizing practices, controls, perceptions, and expectations that become self-fulfilling norms. The carving away of human rights, freedoms, individuality, and social norms that existed prior to Title 19 has now become the contemporary default, an easy shift for the most devalued of us.

The calculated social analogue that led to the "final solution" in Nazi Germany began similarly with the change of language describing people with mental illness and retardation as "mental deadness," engineered by a social worker and a psychologist, and became the Third Reich's rail to introduce mass euthanasia as humane and reasonable. Gray window-darkened buses evacuated all the major institutions of both people labeled as mentally ill and mentally retarded, and transported their residents to their state-imposed extermination. Without this planned change of human identities, instilled among the mainstream population by professional labeling and public relations, the stark mass murder that resulted would have been unthinkable. Once tested, the expansion of new dehumanizing language and new laws eroded the status of bloc after bloc of Hitler's unwanted populations, ethnic and national minorities, targeted religions, and organized labor and leftists, in the narrow interests of the economic elites of the Axis alliance to "make Germany great again."

So, in the tumult of our transforming twentieth- and twenty-first-century society, people with special needs become the necessary object of legislated essential "benevolent care and support." First and easiest to address are elders and those with major disabilities for which no system of entitlement preexisted the Social Security Act, apart from our society's traditions of voluntary largesse, social inclusion, and identification. The ingenious policy that had to be newly devised was to both reduce the economic and social burdens on individuals and family members, but, perversely then, to conflate how to make that profitable for the establishment as our America's policy opportunity. Meeting public demands for family relief for caregiving of dependent members in the ever-isolating urbanization of society, and, thus freeing the power elite of primary responsibility and drag on their profits for such support. This demanded an acceptable unitary public policy solution. The paradigm had to be acceptable to the public, rely on the bulwark of unfunded or supported care volunteers. It had to be predicated on expanding private enterprise. It had to be supported by public taxes rather than corporate profits, and not change the balance of reliance on the nation's poorest people to staff the almost limitless need.

Such social solutions had always depended on the willingness of ordinary people to fend for themselves. As urban society matured, local, regional, and then state governments gradually became the providers of last public support to handle the gamut of human dependencies. Finally, the federal government was compelled to weigh in but with strict prohibitions of delicately taxing the states in the solution's funding. States had, and have, enormous latitude in solving their poor and dependent population's needs able to opt in or sidestep federal mandates. When Medicaid was federally legislated in 1965, it provided a dollar-for-dollar match that required and regarded states buy in for its four designated categorical beneficiaries—the elderly poor, people with disabilities, the blind, and finally dependent children with disabilities.

What was diabolical was the new Title 19 Medicaid, until very recently, channeled federal funding not to individuals or directly to families to support their dependent members in the family home or community, but to an intermediary industry of residential service providers, facilities tasked with providing the support to eligible individuals. Thus, a growing population was progressively exiled from their homes and communities in order to get funding for care. A massive and growing administration was simultaneously invented, de novo, to manage the funds and oversee the implementation of minimally defined subsidized services.

Large institutions that had preexisted the new national Medicaid entitlement suddenly found themselves flooded with first-time federal money to expand in number and size the preferred and historically familiar destination for deviant and unwanted populations. Introducing a medical management legitimization and intermediary managerial oversight by doctors sanitized the operations, shielding them from layman's challenges. It imposed an administrative leadership able to sanction and define managed life or premature death. "Doctors know best" and the closed system of doctor-patient privacy was an ideal insulation for the political strategy of such an initially undemocratic and unaccountable solution. Once admitted to any such residential, congregate setting, funded by required doctor-signed annual certifications submitted to Medicaid of continued need, a stream of dollars reinforced the unwillingness of institutions to release their residents who perforce become veritable hostages.

Here the equation of never-to-be-released "public hostages," held for "public ransom," for the promise of some betterment, grew and grew as corruption of the system, adverse to habilitated emancipation for its societally unwanted and institutionally placed, and incarcerated residents became the norm within every state. First, millions, then billions, then trillions of dollars cascaded down the Title 19 sluice to fuel this "domestic refugee"-generating managerial administration. First, almost any person defined as significantly disabled was justified as segregated placements, but as more and more dependent elders join the national population of people indistinguishable from those with physical, mental, medical, sensory, and social disabilities, the strategy made any distinction between people with disabilities and the aged merely cosmetic.

In the Special Committee on Aging of the United States Senate Long Term Care Report, June 2002, the scope of the problems facing the 77 million baby boomers (14 million over 85 years old by 2040, of which 58 percent of those over 80 have severe disabilities) about to enter the Medicare/Medicaid-eligible population is concisely and dramatically described. The facts are moving. Medicaid is the primary source of funding, exceeding 45 percent and Medicare 14 percent, spent for long-term care in the country. One-third of the costs are borne by individuals out of pocket. Government projections developed by the Lewin Group predict long-term costs will reach $207 billion by 2020, $346 billion by 2040, and $379 billion by 2050. Seventy-two and a half percent of Medicaid dollars are spent on institutional care, and 27.5 percent for home and community-based services. Health-care inflation rates grow on average 13 to 15 percent, and prescription drug inflation 18 percent annually. The average cost of nursing home care today is $50,000 per year, projected to reach $190,600 annually by 2030! Unremunerated is the vast army of Americans, 80 percent women, the senate report documents, who currently alter their lives, reduce or end their workdays, invest their life time on demand, to cope with the needs of children with disabilities or aging family members at home, forfeiting a saving to the national system of an estimated $196 billion, annually, for unfunded caregiving work, lost pensions, and Social Security income.

This staggering aggregate treasure accrues to the 1 percent wealthiest in America directly or indirectly and is paid for by the 99 percent directly or indirectly through taxes and long-term care coverage of this contrived economy. The unprecedented common interests of Big Pharma, consolidating insurance and hospital corporations, medical long-term care residential and assisted-living cartels, the organized medical establishment, and even the human service worker unions, whose members staff the public and private delivery systems, join politically to reap the almost limitless benefits of the "ransom" paid by American taxpayers.

Exploited to the extreme are the public and private human service workers on whom the whole system depends to accept low wages, long hours, lack of professional opportunities for advancement, system-wide understaffing, lack of workers' compensation for inevitable injuries, and assured emotional duress and trauma. Worst is the enforced complicity demanded among the majority of human service workers in this dead-end work to keep secrets, witness and often engage in violent and sexual abuses, theft, alienated cruelty, and studied neglect. All this from the compelling expectations dictated by their orientation to not seeing their patients, residents, clients as whole or valued other than as hopeless diagnostic objects. Instead, out-of-home placement is the alchemy for people becoming income-based commodities to their agencies, negatively stereotyped in every way reinforced by the co-opted professionals that surround them in their jobs and, often including the family and individual themselves, all who have bought into the conscious and unconscious roles they are forced to accept.

In 2000, I was invited to attend and speak at the twenty-fifth anniversary of the federal court-ordered agreement, called the Consent Decree, on the part of the state of New York who had been successfully sued to move all the residents of Willowbrook State School out, by the then euphemistically renamed Staten Island Developmental Center. The three New York governors whose tenure had framed the struggle and had administered the Consent Decree spoke. In the audience sat over two hundred people, the parents who had once collectively organized to challenge the inhumanity and illegality of Willowbrook, and scores of people who had been emancipated from their institutional lives. It seemed that the victory over what were so clearly crimes against humanity was to be memorialized. However, the forty to fifty families of the 1970s, twenty-five years later, were now in their late sixties, seventies, and older, and themselves facing institutionalization due to advanced age! And, their children, now also aging, were again at the precipice of re-institutionalization, not for their disabilities. The cosmic irony of the situation was suffocating as the trillion-dollar out-of-home institutional system that had grown as an insatiable carnivore of every elderly American unable to personally afford a king's ransom, individualized home care, or better, buyout.

This is the context, the crisis, the drama, the framework of my story. The US federal court and the general public found an unmitigated antisocial horror, violation of constitutional rights to care, education, due process, and freedom from cruel and unusual punishment, and had ordered Willowbrook State School to close its operation and move the entirety of its incarcerated nearly six-thousand-person developmentally disabled, special needs population into individual home and community-based small residences.

Willowbrook is now the harbinger of what lies ahead for the entire US population. Once exclusively seen as a crime against people with disabilities, Willowbrook State School is a blueprint, the inevitable functional end point of our existing national legislated policy and financing system that will draw the majority of Americans into being dehumanized, segregated, congregated, and the status of becoming a profit-driven hostage, in an out-of-home, professional staff facilities.

This true story aims to sound a profound alarm and reminder of this threat to our democracy, humanity, society, and the imperative to immediately face, address, and fix the problem with a single central policy antidote and permanent correction. This is to establish a provision for expanded and improved Medicare for all; single-payer, universal, single-quality tier of health care; and rightful coverage for all Americans. This will establish a true health-care system that will eliminate all private medical insurances; vet planning for comprehensive regional and neighborhood services in citizens' hands; dissolve the need for the charity industry; and fund all medical research, prevention services, and health professional education as the basic core of benefits from that policy.

Until this essential mandate is sought and won by the American people, we will live in the barbarous and relentless reality of the story that I will tell here.

CHAPTER 3

Social Control: Origins

Who hates

Who causes war

Who destroys cities

Who sells its young

And who ends a man's days before his turn

Who plunders for gain

Who is slothful

Who pollutes

Who is greedy

Who is false

Who tells tales

And who spins intrigue

Not the fools you call fools

But your kings and princes

—Burton Blatt

IN 1938, THE NEW York State Legislature recognized a need for additional accommodations for people labeled mentally retarded. At that time, the greater New York area was being served by one institution, Letchworth Village, located well north of the city in the woods of Rockland County. Despite World War II, $12,000,000 was spent to build a new institution on Staten Island, which was completed in 1942.

The needs of wartime required that the new institution be used by the Veterans Administration as a general hospital and prisoner-of-war setting. Thus, Willowbrook was first named Halloran General Hospital until 1947, when the intended purpose to house the retarded was restored; ten people from Letchworth and ten people from Wassaic State Schools in New York were transferred to begin the geometric expansion of Willowbrook

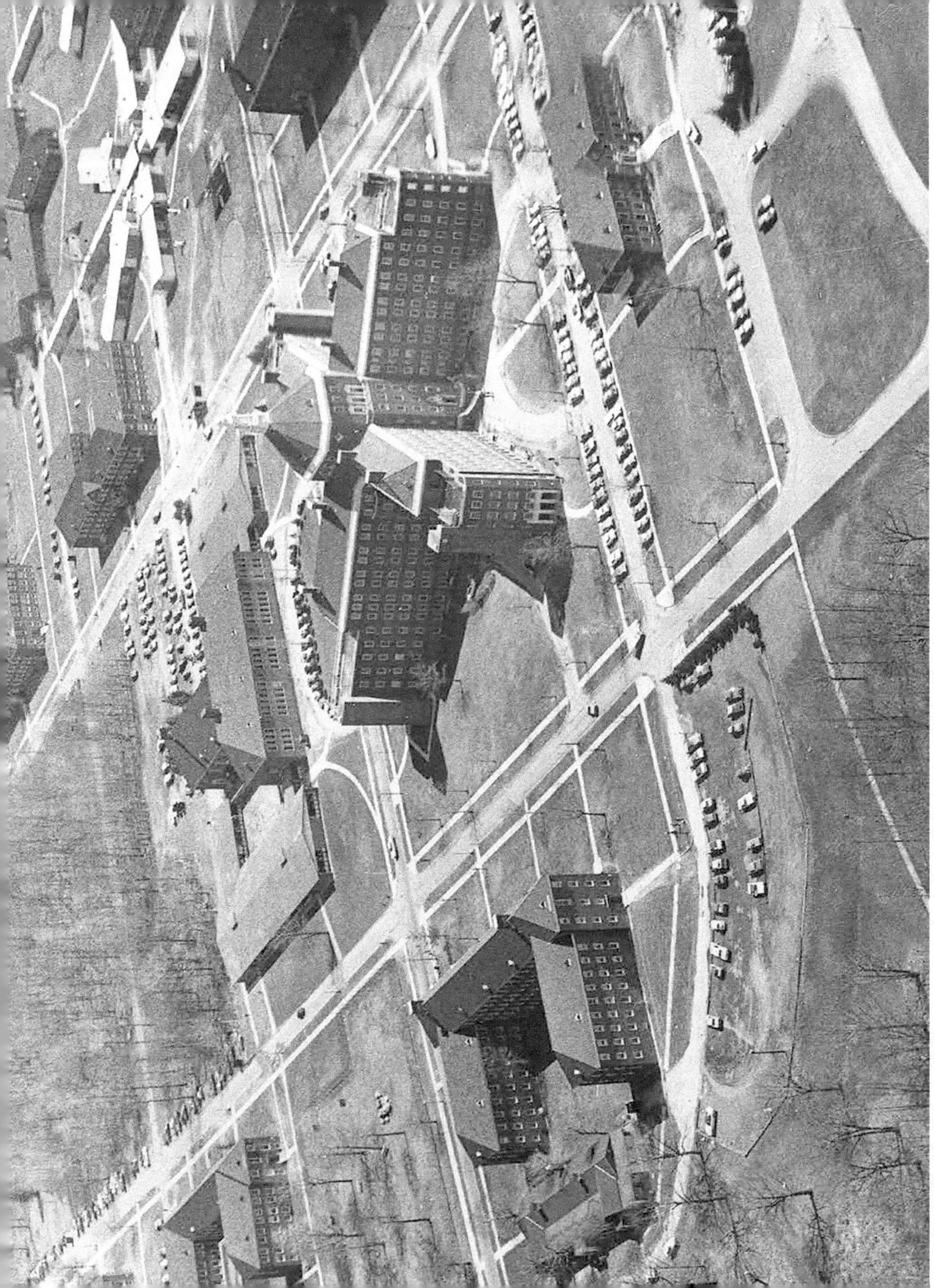

There were over sixty buildings built on the grounds: two-story brick rectangles, each with four wards; seven one-story brick buildings, also with four compartments; a six-story, giant X-shaped building slated to be the hospital (in the future, twenty-seven buildings in all would house residents.) The rest included supply and logistics service buildings and eighteen elegant homes for the doctors and top administrators, comfortably spread over gently rolling hills with a street allowing them exit and entry in the back—away from the visibility of the residents' buildings.

As the VA phased out its operations, Willowbrook expanded until April 1951, when it took over the entire facility. Located 12 miles from Manhattan and occupying 382 acres of suburban Staten Island, Willowbrook was the first "school" planned to accept and treat placed children, under five, as well as older people labeled retarded. The first two infants were admitted in July 1948.

It was the sixth state school opened in the state of New York, with the existing schools already 40 percent overcrowded. The 1949 per-person maintenance cost was $834 per year. By 1965, this cost had risen to $1,800. By 1975, it was just under $17,000 per person.

Willowbrook's first superintendent and director was Dr. Harold Berman, appointed in 1949. The years 1947 through 1951 were formative ones during which Willowbrook was staffed, organized, equipped, and programmed to serve some 3,000 persons. The essential clinical, educational, and support facilities were initiated.

By 1952, admissions began to outnumber transfers. The population continued to increase rapidly. In 1954, Willowbrook was first counted in the "overcrowded" column, where it still remains. (Also in 1954, a school building was activated. This "educational" facility accommodated fewer than 200 youngsters.)

In the face of this expansion, the state Department of Mental Hygiene gradually increased the number of "allowable" residents, with the effect that the apparent number of excess people reported was misleading. From 1954 on, the overcrowding officially varied from 406 to 1,811 people, but this was over and above the expanded tolerable ceiling that had reached 4,726 by 1971, from the early 3,000 figure.

In fact, during the ten years between 1954 and 1964, Willowbrook continued to admit residents until 6,084 persons, a high-water mark, was reached in 1963. The staggering overcrowding led to a public health crisis. Hepatitis, the deadly viral liver disease, was epidemic, as were a dozen other tropical parasitic diseases and illnesses directly related to the environmental and overcrowded conditions.

It was during this period that Dr. Saul Krugman, of New York University School of Medicine, entered the scene to take advantage of the situation to do "research" on hepatitis. Arrangements to obtain Army money to carry on the work were carefully made, so as to sidestep the stringent requirements set up to safeguard against abuses in human experimentation. As a result of the terrible conditions, the disease research, and the toll they both were taking, the situation became explosive.

Dr. Berman stepped down under public pressure, and Dr. Jack Hammond became Willowbrook's second superintendent and director in July 1964. Hammond had been groomed for directorship at Rose State School, a similarly glutted institution in upstate New York. The political pressure was on to reduce the population and to bring some reforms.

The physical plant was expanded with a 200-bed infirmary, a "children's" complex for 1,000 residents, and a small physical rehabilitation unit for people with physical disabilities. A federal demonstration grant was obtained to erect two prefab complexes for 300 more children. Admissions were stopped for a short time and then opened to any family willing to submit their child to hepatitis research as a means of circumventing the waiting list*.

Despite all these efforts, the lid blew off the following year in a media exposé. Senator Robert Kennedy visited on September 1, 1965. He came, briefly saw "the good and the bad," and propelled Willowbrook into national prominence and visibility. Some staff were added, notably in the occupational and recreation therapy departments. But things quickly went back to business as usual, since there was no community organization or even a solid alternative ideology to institutionalization in existence.

It was clear that the special needs of those labeled severely retarded and those with multiple handicaps, particularly children under ten years of age, were simply not being met. As the admission rate declined, the population within grew older, and the deaths, coupled with the less than 1 percent trickle of persons somehow leaving the institution, caused a slow decline in the rolls. By 1971, there remained over 5,200 residents.

At no time did the total employee complement exceed 3,200. The highest direct-care ward staff figure, excluding administrative and nonclinical employees, was officially reported at 2,196, in early 1971, to cover the 27 resident-care buildings over three eight-hour shifts. The real figures, of people actually on duty, were not recorded until the advent of the federal class action lawsuit in 1972–'73, when it was documented that a 20 percent discrepancy existed between the administration's paper estimate and the warm bodies actually present.

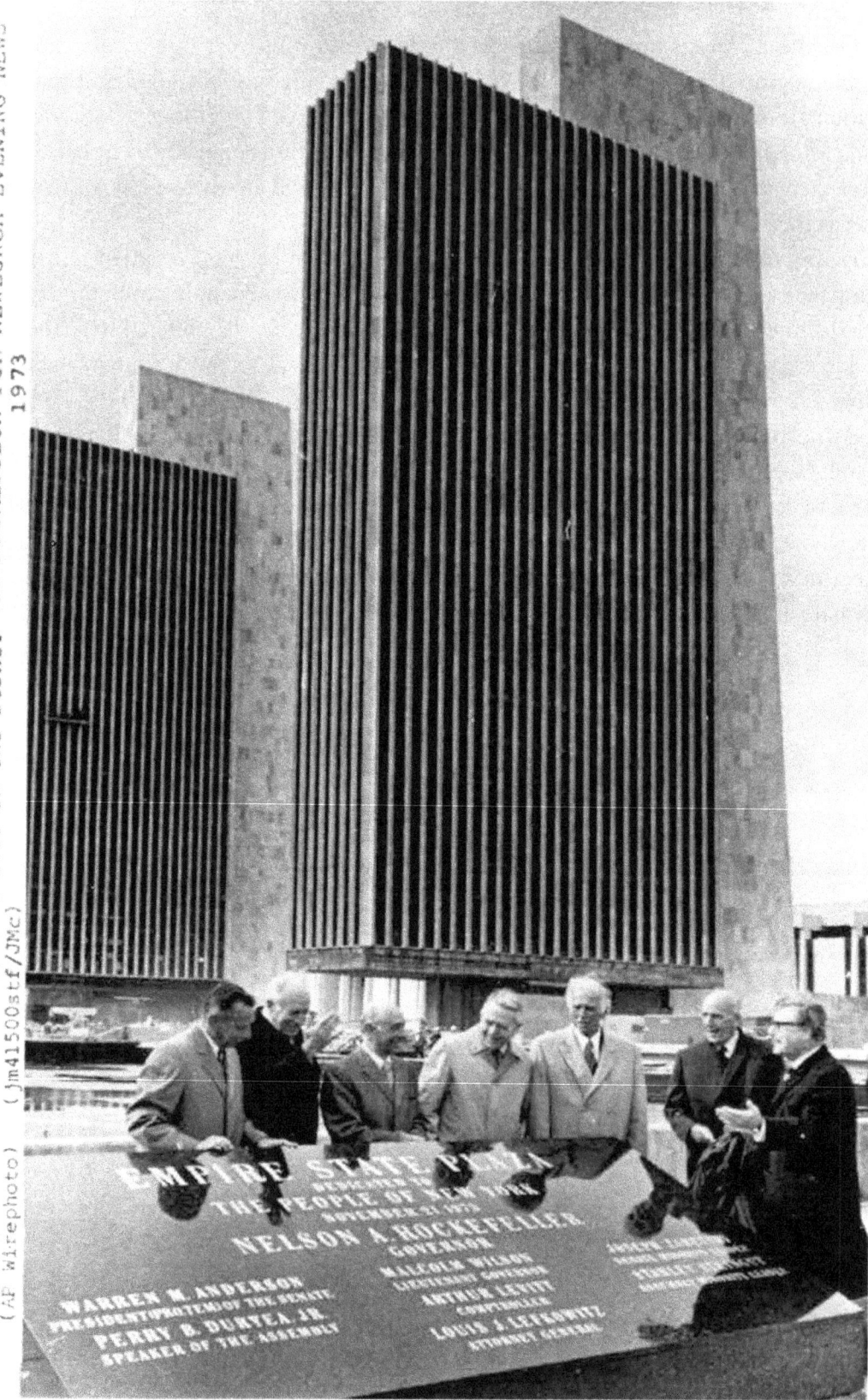

(A49)ALBANY, N.Y., Nov. 21--CHANGING THE NAME OF THE SOUTH MALL--New York State Governor Nelson A. Rockefeller, right, offers apologies to Albany's mayor, Erastus Corning II, second from left, because Corning's name was not on the plaque at Wednesday's dedication of the Empire State Plaza, formally known as the South Mall project of state office buildings. Joseph Zaretzki, senate minority leader, whose name is located on the stone below the governor had his name misspelled. Zaretzki's name appears on the stone as "Zaretski". The letters were painted on in gold but the finished stone will have the names carved in the stone. RETRANSMISSION FOR NEWBURGH EVENING NEWS (AP Wirephoto)   (jm41500stf/JMc)   1973

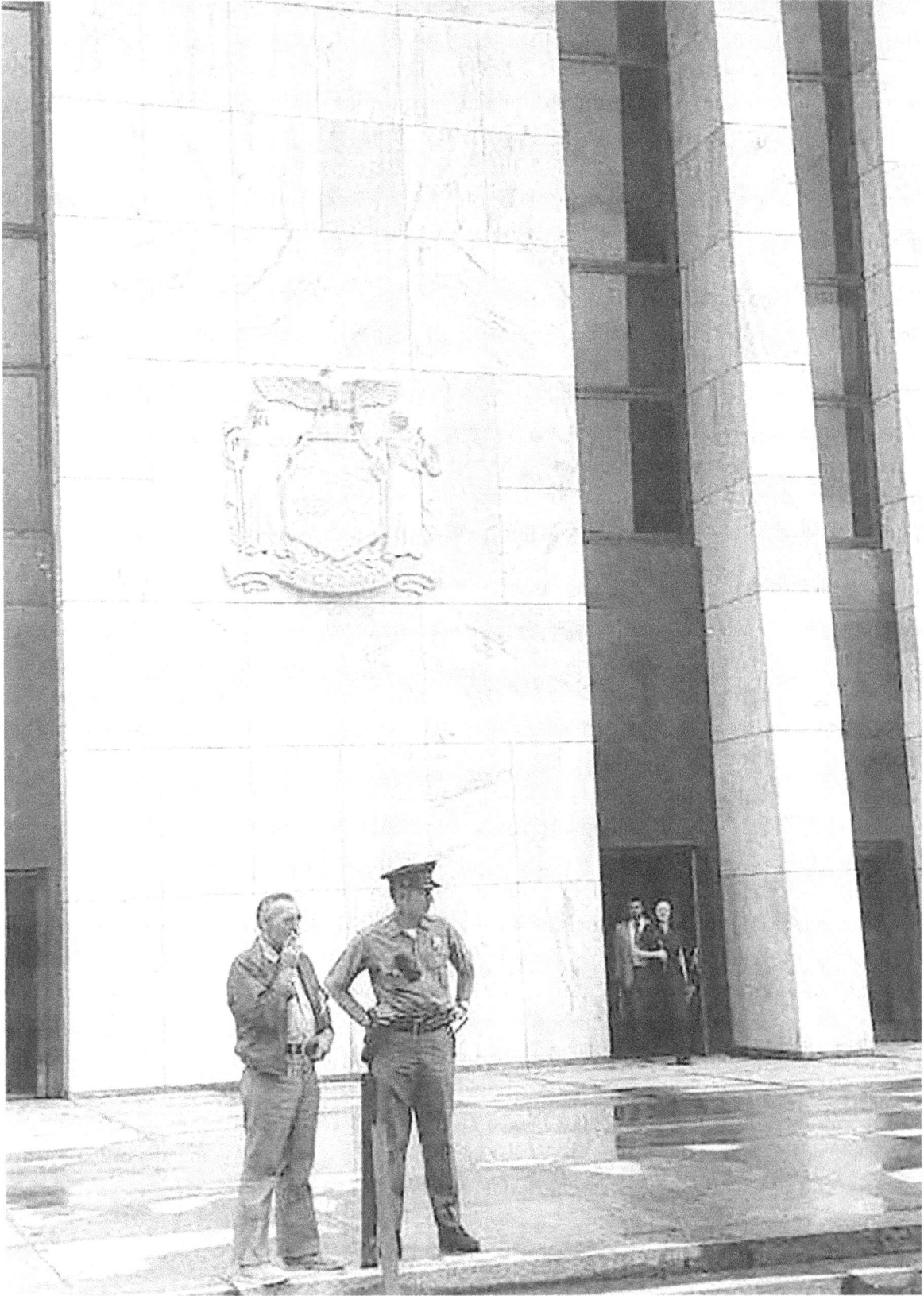

A job and budget freeze imposed by the governor to save the state money, the exact mount that was used to build his new Albany State Capital marble and gold offices, came on December 7, 1970. All hiring, promotions, and new programs in the state were stopped. No losses by attrition were to be replaced. One year later, there were 683 fewer employees at Willowbrook. Actually, 1,000 jobs were unfilled, representing a full one-third reduction in workers, most of whom had been doing the ward work. In practice, this meant a staff-to-client ratio that varied from 1:18 to 1:60 people. Such a critical depletion of staff, both in clinical and support services, resulted in increasing problems of low morale, minimum ward coverage, and inadequate equipment, supplies, food, and clothing. All of this and more caused an unimaginable deterioration in what had been, at best, a holding action in custodial resident care.

In an official report, the Department of Mental Hygiene described two basic problems when it was called to account during the 1971 TV exposé by the New York media community: "overcrowding and understaffing." In relation to understaffing, the department stated, "The problems here have included a constant shortage of dollars and positions; the non-availability of staff, mostly ward service people, earlier in Willowbrook's history; and, most recently, a sharp rise in chronic absenteeism which averages about 100 unscheduled absences daily, with as many as 130 to 140 out on weekends, as well as excessively high staff turnover. The job freeze most seriously compounded all of Willowbrook's problems. Finally, it is almost redundant to point out the management difficulties in a facility the size of Willowbrook."

If one accepts the basic assumptions that the department knew how to run such giant enclaves, in themselves much like small cities, and that institutionalization was an appropriate and effective model to serve the needs of the public, then one could succumb to the calls of the Department of Mental Hygiene for more money, qualified staff, and less responsibility. At the heart of the situation issue are some economic facts which must be understood to illuminate what is, in fact, the real political dynamic of the institutional system.

In order to stay in business, the Division of Mental Retardation, within the New York State Department of Mental Hygiene, had to serve a population that nobody else wanted or felt they could serve. Funds tended to be tied to how hard the job of caring for these societal "deviants" could be made to look. Thus, widespread agreement among the professional leadership of the division in defining the describing the massive disabilities among the institutionalized population was a given.

The hopelessness of rehabilitation was a second myth floated by the bureaucracy, so that the legislature had to continually concede increasing sums of money and, thereby, power to the department. From only six institutions in 1942, New York funded and constructed thirty mass institutional settings housing over twenty-four thousand people. The number of institutions and the population continue to expand. For every year that these persons are held in institutions, the Medicaid Title 19 matching funds, the "public ransom" for them, continue to grow.

The rhetoric of the state implies the eventual return of its institutionalized population to the community through such images and service labels as "state school," "developmental center," "occupational and vocational therapy," "rehabilitation," and "medical care." Yet, like some desert mirage always receding, the promise is unfulfilled, and the public is further extorted for more and more ransom.

The irony is that the public fortune conceded to the department is now independent of the number of residents held and continues to multiply because of the increasing momentum of a self-perpetuating system. More importantly, with such a large population crammed into what, in effect, were concentration centers, control becomes the overriding consideration.

"It did not matter who or what the retardate was, whether young or old; whether borderline or profoundly retarded; whether physically handicapped or physically sound; whether deaf or blind; whether rural or urban; whether from the local town or from 500 miles away; whether well-behaved or ill-behaved. We took them all, by the thousands, 5,000 and 6,000 in some institutions. We had all the answers in one place, using the same facilities, the same personnel, the same attitudes, and largely, the same treatment. And, if our guest did not fit, we made him fit."[1]

In anticipation of extensive documentation of abuses of the situation, some of the public ransom paid to the captors (the chiefs of the Department of Mental Hygiene) does, in fact, go to keeping the hostages alive—just barely. Some go for public relations directly, so that periodic glowing propaganda can be put into the mass media. Some go for public relations indirectly—into the maintenance of a subdued and poorly trained medical and nursing community within the walls, to give the appearance of protection and legitimate care. However, the 1975–'76 proposed budget earmarked $17.1 million ($82 million—2020) for what is described as "executive management." These are people who never set foot on the grounds of the state schools but are justified because of the scope of the system to push paper.

---

[1]   *On the Nature and Origins of Our Institutional Models;* Wolfensberger, W.; 1959

DEPARTMENT OF
MENTAL HYGIENE

OFFICES OF: FL

ADMINISTRATION & FISCAL MGNT.
- ADMINISTRATION   8
- BUSINESS OFFICE   6
- CENTRAL SERVICES   1
- INST. SERVICES GROUP
  - ADMINISTRATION   8
  - EQUIPMENT SVCS   6
  - INST. RETAIL SVCS   4
  - LAUNDRY SVCS   6
  - NUTRITION SVCS   4
  - INST. ENGINEERING SVCS.   6
  - SAFETY SVCS   6
  - SUPPLY SUPPORT SVCS.   5
- BUDGET & FINANCE   8
- COST ANALYSIS   6
- MANAGEMENT IMPROVEMENT   2
- PATIENT RESOURCES   2

FACILITIES & CAPITAL SERVICES
- ADMINISTRATION   5
- CAPITAL MANAGEMENT BUR.   5
- CAPITAL IMPROVEMENT BUR.   5
- LAND MANAGEMENT BUR.   5
- COMMUNITY FACILITIES BUR.   7

COMMITTEE FOR CHILDREN   8

EXECUTIVE COORDINATION
- COMMUNICATIONS
  - ADMINISTRATION   8
  - OPERATIONS   6
  - CONSULATION & TRAINING   6
  - LIBRARY   6
  - PHOTOMEDIA SVCS   4
  - PSYCHIATRIC QUARTERLY   4
- COUNSEL   8
- INTERGROUP RELATIONS   8
- LEGISLATIVE RELATIONS   8
- OFFICE OF CITIZEN
  - PARTICIPATION   8

MANPOWER, EMPLOYEE RELATIONS
& TRAINING
- ADMINISTRATION   8
- CLASSROOMS   6
- EDUCATION & TRAINING   6
- EMPLOYEE RELATIONS   7
- PERSONNEL   7
- VOLUNTEER SERVICES   4

OFFICES OF: FL

STAT. & CLINICAL INF. SYSTEMS   8
- DIRECTOR   8
- ADMINISTRATION   2
- CENTRAL FILES   2
- DATA PROCESSING   2
- STAT. & MEDICAL RECORDS   2

DIVISIONS OF: 1 & 7
- ALCOHOLISM
- MENTAL HEALTH
  - ADMINISTRATION   8
  - FORENSIC PYCHIATRY   8
  - FUNCTIONAL PROGRAMMING   7
  - PROGRAM ANALYSIS   7
  - SERVICES TO THE AGED   8
- MENTAL RETARDATION
  - ADMINISTRATION   8
  - CHILDREN SERVICES   8
  - EDUCATION   7
  - FUNCTIONAL PROGRAMMING   7
  - HEALTH SVCS & STANDARDS   8
  - PROGRAM OPERATIONS   7

DIVISIONS OF:
- RESEARCH   6 & 8
- UNIFIED SVCS MANAGEMENT   8
- STANDARDS, INSPECTIONS
  - & PROGRAM EVALUATION   7

REGIONAL OFFICE
- ALBANY   1

But this is small potatoes. It was estimated by experts that the department spent $1 billion during Rockefeller's administration (1959–1973), or $8,545,345,000 in 2019 value, to maintain and expand construction alone of the state's institutional system. The provision of scores of thousands of jobs often represents the core of the economy in many lesser-populated places of the state. But although wages represent the largest fraction of fixed costs, the financial plums are in the contracts for laundry, food, drugs, trucking and transportation, clothing, and equipment. Those bonanzas invariably go to "friendly" and politically loyal agents.

The central bureaucracy decides who will get the bid. Quality control—against the padding of bids—is never performed by anyone, let alone the department that derives its patronage power from its freedom to award such lucrative contracts. But most of all, the construction of the sprawling institutions is the real pot of gold. Here is where the fast buck times 100 million is made and why institutions remain so politically impregnable. The cost to build the warehouses ranges between $30,000 ($144,000—2020) and $1,000,000 ($4.84 million—2020) per bed, just in capital expense alone.

CHAPTER 4

The Heritage of Caregiving

I HAD NO CLEAR idea of facts about New York or Willowbrook when I arrived in 1970, but I had belief in myself as a caregiver, enough to do some good in the most difficult setting. But to say that I was green about what I walked into is the understatement of all time!

People see what they want to and block out what they don't. I did not want to see evil, abuse, incompetency, tyranny, aggrandizement. It took a while to adjust, to feel the nerve center and heart of Willowbrook. It has been said that a person cannot know the essence of a thing until he has tried to change the thing. Beyond its mere appearance, the only way to know what coffee is like is to drink some. It was through the slow and truly painful effort to stand by basic, good medical practice and public health principles (and work to get the institution to adopt them) that I came to know the essence of Willowbrook the essence of the institutional system, wherever it exists. I tried to see everybody in my care at least daily, doing the things I had been taught that were required for minimal professional scientific and compassionate care, keeping some semblance of true records and expressing concern about the amazing medical and administrative malpractice that existed.

Many months, then a year, passed in my adjustment. I spent my whole day on the wards among the children and workers touching, questioning, teaching, writing, and helping. I was thunderstruck at what I was doing. In my first assignment in a building for the youngest children in Willowbrook (ages three through eighteen), I had two hundred individuals to care for! Children's Hospital of Los Angeles, one of the most opulent and massively staffed centers of its kinds in the country, had only two hundred beds served by over four hundred physicians! Here, I was alone, with two hundred significantly disabled kids! Why was that? How could they, whoever "they" were in my mind at that time, think that one doctor and three nurses could serve, with any effectiveness at all, this community of children who had every possible sort of medical, social, and educational need? I was just upset and confounded enough to keep asking the superintendent and my fellow physicians such questions. I felt strongly compelled, morally bound to work very, very hard.

None of the children's records were intelligible to me. Medical diagnoses were inaccurate, workups, the laboratory and physical evaluations that I thought were just customary were absent. Psychological reports were shocking in their brevity. Instead of the meticulous four-and five-page reports rich with observations and program recommendations which I had come to expect, tiny one-paragraph, repetitive, contentless, long-outdated reports were to be found in every Willowbrook chart. There was simply no area that didn't require complete review and reorganization for each and every child. I became totally engrossed in the "trees" and only vaguely aware of the "forest" of negligence all about. I threw myself into the work at hand, feeling my way and grappling with the incredible problems.

I came to know the children well, hundreds of them over the months. I came to know the ward workers, feel their plight, sense their lack of adequate preparation for what they were expected to do. I came to know parents, a few at first and then a score, then hundreds.

Like a giant puzzle, far bigger than I was able to grasp at first, pieces began to fall together. Patterns began to emerge. The almost-stereotyped situation existed for each child, each family, each worker, all filled with horror, mismanagement, underdevelopment, victimization, and routine violence in every form. Yet, I still did not know what to make of what I was seeing and what I was called on to do every day at work. I blamed myself when there was work left undone. I felt guilty when I had to suppress crying with parents whose humiliation and pain, through years of trying to shield their children, had become overwhelming tragedies. The tragedies were created by professionals who held the power to define and control all possible resources, bludgeoning families with advice to surrender their children to the institution. I felt in conflict when workers, incredibly overworked, heroic in what they undertook in the face of impossible conditions and no training, turned to me for help or asked why things were this way. I could only say that their employees' union or the administration simply was not doing the job to establish the supports needed to do good work.

I turned repeatedly to the administration with my observations, reports of conditions, asking for help and clarification about this or that. I was in the director's office at least once a week trying to see what could be done. Was there a more effective way to do the job? Why didn't people among the medical staff talk with one another? Why were there not regular published internal reports of all illnesses in the institution? Why, when people died, was there not a case review to try to improve the collective problem-solving strength of the staff? Why was there no in-service education for the medical and nursing staff?

I went so far as to send away for training films and began regular training operations in one of the buildings where I was assigned. I thought a solution was as close at hand as cooperation and good, basic medical practice. That would have solved at least the rampant preventable diseases that mushroomed everywhere in Willowbrook.

Slowly, very slowly, and only after repeated rebuffs, indolence, empty promises, rhetoric, excuses, did the seriousness of the situation begin to strike home. Something general was going on from the top down to the wards—a general lack of resolve; a general disregard of modern medical practices; and a general acceptance, even defense, of underdevelopment and ignorance among the workers, the doctors, and the administration. I was plagued with whys. Vaguely at first, then the questions became sharper, more recurrent. The "forest" began to take shape. I began to see a benefit, a perverse explanation beyond cruelty, that had to exist for the system and its leaders. Otherwise the situation, so intransigent, so stubbornly unyielding, would be totally irrational.

I began, reflexively, to push harder for administrative and medical attention to the situation. From my questions came assertions. The assertions became demands. I became locked into trying to solve the situation. The tension with the administration began to build. The issues began to emerge, and the foundation for sticking it out became firmer and firmer. I became deeply involved in the lives of many, many people and always held the abiding conviction that the power to change Willowbrook resided within those workers and families, though I did not know how to inspire this at first.

The adults associated with the institution, the family members, the workers—each in their own way, each as a part of a special group—had a vital stake: survival. I believed in their capacity to change the situation if given help, knowledge, encouragement, friendship, tenderness, and love. My fulfillment came from knowing and sharing in that struggle. I was not alone, though I often felt I was, and truly frightened at the awesome job that was before us.

In Willowbrook, in the institutions, it is a fight for the right of life, the right of people to be respected, nurtured, and elevated. One is never really alone in that kind of pursuit. One can never really ultimately lose that struggle, for the alternative is basically unacceptable to people, to the public. Holding on to that intuitive overview with its inherent optimism shored me up every day. I had to prepare every day—every day—with a reminder to myself of what this work was all about.

CHAPTER 5

Replacement

HUMAN ORGANIZATION EXISTS BECAUSE people need it, not because of rules and regulations, bosses, reprisals, or material rewards. But in Albany, the state's capital, or in the Administration Building at Willowbrook, this was simply not a consideration. The orders were out, and the subordinates loyally did what they were bid. Everybody employed at Willowbrook fell in line silently—some out of fear, some out of selfishness. Most did out of a deep and abiding disdain for the work and residents who, in fact, were continually and brutally victimized by all the so-called normal people vested with their care.

My persistent clinical concerns over the condition of the 200 residents in my care were disruptive of the modus operandi of the six other physicians in the five-building "baby complex" in which I worked. My clinical expectations and practices exposed the standard neglect and brutality of care that led my new colleagues to complain to the director, Jack Hammond. The sharp difference in my demands for medical resources, record keeping, and diagnostic pursuits to help hone in on the many hidden and evolving diseases and conditions among my building's children. Most annoying to my medical peers was my assumption that we would meet regularly to review cases and medically problem solve as peers. Dr. Hammond, who was still evaluating my skills and energy, reactively responded to the peer complaints that the normally tranquil deficiencies should not be addressed and the prevailing indifferent level of medical practice not be challenged.

Abruptly, after a tumultuous few months at Willowbrook, I was transferred to care for 134 ambulatory children and teens in the prefab Building 76, a federally funded "Hospital Improvement Program" grant program, where I worked for the next full year. Hammond sugarcoated his irritation-factor transfer, asking me to demonstrate my medical standards in a context designated as a model. I felt relieved at the time and trusted the willingness of the director to support my practice. The move was from stone to linoleum. From cavernous two stories with four rigid room spaces to a star-shaped, more intimate space whose children were selected who would show grant monitors the best and ostensible reform orientation of Willowbrook. Five wards each with 30-plus kids with no particular groupings though 20 youngsters were daily escorted to the short off-site "school" as part of the grant deal. Notwithstanding, the health situation was awful with the same spectrum of familiar and rare infectious and congenital conditions that were endemic and epidemic in the closed reality that was Willowbrook.

It was here that I spent the next months, professionally, physically, emotionally woven into the lives of the remarkable 134 children and the workers on our three morning, afternoon, night shifts in Building 76. I was determined to clean the kids up and try to rid the relentless focus on illness to create a developmental habilitation and hoped for exit from what lay ahead of children who reached adulthood and inevitable transfer into the hopeless, suffocating, and separated men's and women's lifetime stone buildings.

Alarmed by Willowbrook's general shocking medical conditions around me that I grew to know through institution wide, monthly twenty-four-hour, coverage duties we all rotated through, I decided to try to befriend and arouse the larger physicians' body. When one has gone through the rigorous medical training I had received, certain reflexes develop. A certain code of performance is fixed in one's mind. Even if one is lazy or incompetent, the call to that built-in system of medical cause and effect, coupled with the veneer of an ethical framework, usually must be honored. I decided that science and top-notch medical practices could not be openly denied nor attacked as controversial. Thus, I began to speak out in each of the weekly medical staff meetings about the need to clean up and standardize our practice across the institution.

Diseases should be monitored, antibiotics should be given in proper doses for proper lengths of time, cultures of infections should be taken to avoid abusing antibiotics, anesthetics must be on hand and used for suturing the constant lacerations. Not one of these things was being done. It was a humble way to begin to push back, the only way I knew at the time.

CHAPTER 6

Adjusting Innocently I

THE PRESSING QUESTION WAS how to release the energy for change stored in the suffering of all the institutionalized residents where possible, their families, and workers alike? What forces could address the systematic abuses that existed? The workers' union? The institution's parents' organization? The professional staff of doctors, teachers, and nurses, each one a person with significant potential power? The family organizations in the community, whose children and relatives with disabilities would all inevitably be driven into the New York State institutional system? How would these natural groups acknowledge each other as the issues crystalized? Who could live with abuse and turn away from responsibility and action?

The workers in the institution were my first hope for stimulating change. Here, whittled down to the post-budget freeze, two thousand strong, was the most terribly dehumanized group of people: those hired to care for those incarcerated in Willowbrook. Mostly people from the poorest areas of New York City and New Jersey, many traveling three and four hours a day to get to and from Willowbrook by subway and bus; mostly black, Puerto Rican, and poor white people; mostly women. These workers were flung into the stench-filled, barren wards without the slightest idea of what to do except hold on and get through each day.

Privately reviled by the administration, harassed daily by job-entrenched supervisors, bereft of basic resources such as soap, washcloths, diapers, and towels, with which to provide even the most minimal hygiene care, the workers were held just a fraction of an inch in status above the residents themselves. Protest led to dismissal or to grinding, subtle reprisals by the caste-conscious supervisors. The wards were for the lowest of the low, the powerless. Once out in the front office, most, though not all, supervisors jealously guarded their status and ingeniously kept the waves of complaints and problems from spilling out of those exitless wards.

The organizations available for the workers to express their interests had long ago been emasculated. The Civil Service Employees Association (CSEA), the sole bargaining agent for the workers, held all employees as members, including supervisors and management staff. In 1970, with an all-white leadership, all-veteran, all-collaborating, all-privileged power circle, the authority of the supervisors over the ward staff was almost absolute. Feelings of fear, hopelessness, and contempt prevented the workers from either joining or turning to their union—the governor's "company union"—for help. These attitudes were tempered out of long and bitter experience.

But this was also a time of militancy and the building of "black solidarity." Yes, a black rank-and-file caucus of workers, the International Union for Advancement (IUA), existed on the grounds. The IUA was led by a small circle of strong people twenty-to thirty somethings, fiercely proud, cool looking, and demanding "black unity" and control. With an office touted to be in Harlem, the IUA sprang into existence in 1968 after a contested elected in which, a real union, the American Federation of State, County, and Municipal Employees Union (a public service trade union) lost out by state decision to the CSEA for representation of all the workers.

The IUA said to the black workers, "Join! Sign a union dues check-off-card." The card was a formal procedure that, suspiciously, went straight to the state attorney general's office. I asked myself, how did the IUA caucus get official dues checkoff, a precious giant step in union organizing, when the CSEA was the sole legal worker representative? Which workers were in the IUA? Nobody would say. Who in my building? Nobody would say. I never knew either the membership of the union nor the source of its apparent power, which it did not exercise. For the workers with integrity and savvy and a feel for self-preservation, there was no choice at either end of the union spectrum. It was the supervisors' rights and the status quo versus what was at best a rhetorically militant-looking group on the attorney general's roster. There was nothing in between. That was that. State labor bureaucrats and sophisticated politicos had covered the ground to stifle any real challenge.

What of the parents? They had everything to gain and nothing to lose, The Willowbrook Benevolent Society, a chapter of the New York State Association for Retarded Children, had carried the burden of the countless families who had turned their relatives over to Willowbrook. Their membership rolls numbered well over 1,200 people. The activists of the Benevolent were essentially confined to the score or so veterans who composed the board of directors and their immediate circle of friends. The organization met monthly with 20 or so parents attending. The bulk of the effort had for years gone "to make life more bearable for the children." Building parties, circus clowns, ice cream, and the like came and went. In addition, money raised from a traditional annual luncheon often went to subsidize the multimillion-dollar Willowbrook budget—for a hearing aid here or there, a few new wheelchairs, TV sets, personal necessities.

The Benevolent leadership, essentially without any effective member participation, relied on one-to-one confrontations with the administration for token concessions. The sons and daughters of the Benevolent leaders were given slightly better consideration, as a way to appear cooperative while still undermining any pressure for changes in the system itself.

Each year at their annual luncheon, the Willowbrook superintendent-director would take the large family-based Benevolent Society to task for not helping enough. It was a profound irony. The Benevolent Society, convinced of their powerlessness, dependent on professional favors all their lives, feeling that being able to even talk to the director was a cosmic privilege, disgusted at the lack of interest on the part of the ranks of poor families who instinctively knew there was no gain to be had in the traditional collaboration. The Benevolent Society posed no threat. Yet all the parents experienced such loneliness, such personal tragedy, such heightened humiliation each time they visited Willowbrook.

Guilt ridden; fearful of reprisals against their sons and daughters if a ruckus was raised; beaten into submission by social workers, doctors, administrators, and ward workers; each family was gripped by a paralysis. If ever conditions existed to weld a reform movement, they existed for these parents. But the key to unlocking the buried fury, the heartache, was still hidden. They were too divided, too brainwashed about the lack of potential for their institutionalized relatives, they had experienced too much personal suffering, and yet were most touchingly gentle and timid. All this kept them powerless and weak.

The families had internalized their second-class citizenship so thoroughly, ears, eyes, noses closed to avoid hurt. It would take time, time to listen and reassure, time to look into the eyes of parents and carefully open them, time to unlock all the locked doors. Someone had to be there when they needed help, stand with them, and interpret the truth of Willowbrook. It would take time to clear the ears and unscramble the jumble of myths, lies, fears—one by one. True, this slow process of growth was agonizing, but momentum would build. There, among the stricken, power would soon flow and collective indignation would arise against their condition.

The community-based organizations of families with labels of "retarded," "brain injured," "cerebral palsied," "hearing or visually handicapped" children and adults existed, but where were they? Willowbrook, in its pastoral and monumental isolation, symbolized the inevitable surrender and defeat of every community family and how their struggle to hold onto their 'special child' was doomed. Despite its size, for community families, Willowbrook was off the scene despite the central role it played in relation to all other human services. For the community, Willowbrook simply didn't exist.

Politically, in the Staten Island community, Willowbrook's top bureaucrats sat on every citizen board and professional structure. The director, as the highest ranking official of the state of New York and the Department of Mental Hygiene, reviewed and approved all grant applications for county community services involving DMH money. Dr. Hammond's wife, as a paid director of volunteers at Willowbrook, sat as a "consumer" on the County Regional Council for Mental Retardation. The head of Willowbrook's Psychology Department was the senior consultant at the only community-based service for children with mental retardation, and virtually handpicked the staff of the community agency and the director of the County Regional Council, and on and on it went.

These administrators used their power to grant a place in the institution for the retarded sons or daughters of supporters, a source of deep relief and gratitude to the parents who understood the writing on the wall. For the disabled in the community, jobs, alternative living arrangements, real comprehensive integrated public school services, transportation, guardianship, and security in the neighborhood existed in token forms or were nowhere to be found.

Any community-based project threatened the established bureaucracy. Hope for the retarded? Forget it. The parents' organizations, so splintered from one another, rallied around this benefactor or that label—brain injury, cerebral palsy, spina bifida. They refused to meet together to take stock of their common needs. Pride and shame together bolstered each tiny parent island. Each was absorbed with scratching for a dollar here or there and influenced to fail by the bureaucracy. Stagnancy prevailed.

The Benevolent Society never understood where natural allies resided in the community. The community groups, through their denial and dependency, were repelled by the institution and the institution-based parents group. Each was isolated from the other. It would take giant convulsions and explosions from within Willowbrook, with the resulting debris falling over the entire state, before a fragile alliance was to be struck and growth of an advocacy-oriented parent and consumer movement ignited. An independent effort geared to the consciousness and specific needs of the community would have to be mounted to build the vital missing unity. This effort would have to be carried on simultaneously with the work of educating parents on the inside. Both were essential if change were to come.

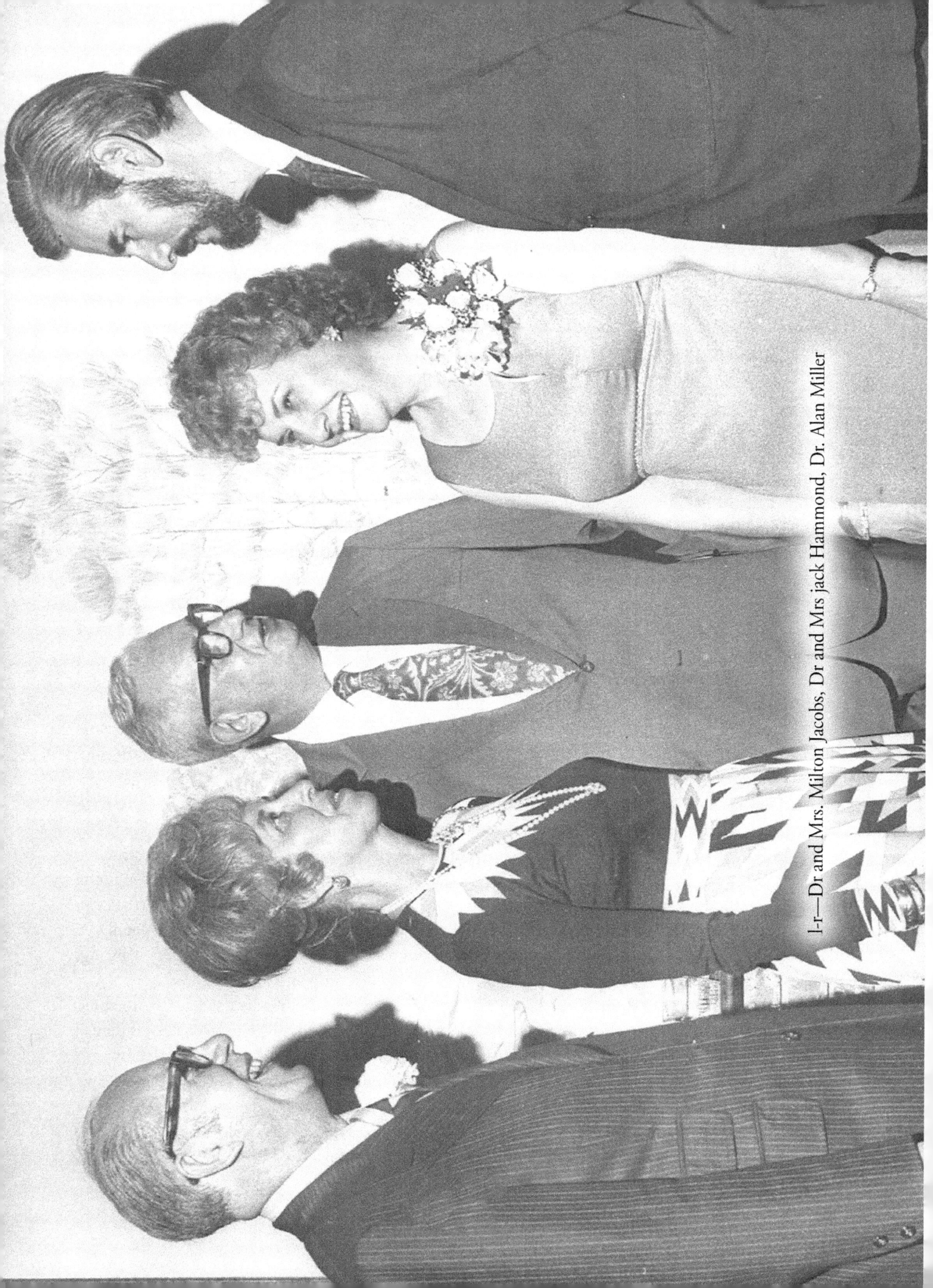

l-r—Dr and Mrs. Milton Jacobs, Dr and Mrs jack Hammond, Dr. Alan Miller

The professionals were the least group in a position to act for change. Here was the white-collar segment of Willowbrook's staff: doctors, nurses, psychologists, teachers, social workers, and occupational and physical therapists. My first two years at Willowbrook, the numbers of social workers and psychologists were pitiably small, altogether not ten to serve the five thousand plus residents. All were housed in a single building, remote from the residential buildings, where they did all their work.

The NYC Department of Education's teachers certified to work with select Willowbrook children were another matter. Young and attractive, most had come to Willowbrook in search of scarce work or in the course of their training and certification in "special education." Shortly before I began work, a serious confrontation had occurred between the more outspoken teachers and the administration. A series of demands related to their status, working conditions, and insisting the ward workers reinforce their lessons when the children returned to their buildings had been presented to the director. A petition they all signed was circulated. A delegation went to Dr. Hammond to seek his action. He issued a blunt rejection and threatened to fire all the teachers if need be. His response apparently was overwhelming to the idealistic group. Lacking any prior alliance with other forces among the ward workers, or any support from parents, the teachers' organization was effectively crushed. Their bluff to quit if their demands were not met was called, and a deep cynicism and bitterness set into the group. The leaders quietly drifted out of Willowbrook, each feeling betrayed and alone, not having understood the long and arduous road that would have to log numerous defeats before the established conditions could be altered.

It was a salient victory for the administration. The teachers had collapsed notwithstanding their valiant moral outrage and threats. The bureaucracy's authority became more firmly entrenched than ever. It was their institution, their island domain, their mandate to maintain the status quo and the control. Two years later, in another struggle, the firing of two teachers who stood for just and concerned service principles would place the administration in a grave situation.

But in 1970, the time had just not come. The work had not been done to challenge Willowbrook. The forces for progress and change had not yet awoken, either inside or outside the institution. Things would get much worse before the turning point.

At the end of 1970, the governor announced a devastating budget freeze throughout the state system, savings that would be rechanneled to build Rockefeller's multi-million-dollar imperial marble and gold Albany Capital Complex. This action crashed into all our lives with inconceivable destructive force. Somewhere in the far reaches of political space, where men manipulated hundreds of millions of dollars and tens of millions of lives through the vicissitudes of their power, avarice, and arrogance, a unilateral decision was made to breach the social contract between government and the people. A decision was made to stop the lifeblood of the New York's public institutions, to block all new hiring, to halt all job advances, to screw down on all costs, to save and scrimp and trim budgets.

Here we were, already strained to the breaking point. Service was already a sham, two to three workers on a ward, no clothes, insufficient food, no furniture. What would a cut do to the residents? Wasn't the public paying even more taxes, producing ever more wealth? Why turn the trickling tap off on the state's most defenseless? As if the answer was not immediately obvious. Who would know? Who would care? The administration clucked, shook their heads, and said it would pass. "These things come and go." The professionals? Well, they'd seen freezes in the past, and it hadn't hurt them. "That's politics." The workers were panic-stricken and used every device to isolate and hide their fears.

The normal worker turnover exceeded 50 percent annually, with first-year workers turning over at better than 80 percent. As attrition hit the ward staff, and the work would double and triple. Despite this, the unions remained silent. The professionals remained silent. The administration carried out the policy from above. The parents were unorganized and had no idea what this would really mean in the toll of lost life, injuries, and further dehumanization forced upon their kin.

It was the system's move to demand more "ransom" for worse services, and the governor held all the strings. I was beside myself with anger. The loss of even one worker had concrete implications of the direst sort. What I could not predict, for I had never seen such a thing happen before, was how the whole fabric of communication and efficiency, fragile as it already was, collapsed as the workers' numbers dwindled. The delicate balance of routines, understandings, familiarity that held Willowbrook together far out of reach of the administration and their supervisors—a balance that takes years to achieve in a job as complex as this one—was decimated. No matter how many workers might be rehired someday, the functional ecology of minimum care giving and safety was irreparably disrupted and, like a forest burned to the ground, would require years of regrowth and stability to again achieve a new balance.

CHAPTER 7

Adjusting Innocently II

DOCTORS: Men who administer medicine of which they know little.

To cure diseases of which they know less.

To human beings of whom they know nothing.

—Voltaire

IN APRIL 1971, I had naively confronted and been utterly rejected by the physicians' organization in a bid to heal Willowbrook's disease. The confrontation began back when I had just written my second enthusiastic report on the medical progress we were making in Building 76 and the adjacent "Hospital Improvement Program" temporary building, 77, with youngest and most capable children. Willowbrook had been what it was for over twenty years. I should have realized that sincerity and motivation on the part of a few individuals could no more alter the nature of the system than swatting a few mosquitoes alters the existence of malaria. I had decided to speak out in the physicians' meetings, hoping by my own demonstration of the efficacy of proper medical care, to raise the consciousness of the doctors and direct it toward cleaning up and standardizing our practice across the institution. The forty doctors in Willowbrook, mostly elderly men and women, 80 percent trained outside of the United States, 40 percent unlicensed in New York, carried the ball on the front line of every aspect of care, or so it seemed to me. Their every word and action was, by definition, incontrovertible law. Each functioned in isolation, practicing his or her own style of institutional medicine. It seemed to me worth the gamble to present my case for proper, ethical care and to search for places where mutual assistance and information sharing would help us all. For me it was a period of inquiry, exploration, and testing, to understand where things stood and what motivated these people. I did not at that time have any idea of the full scope of their power they had allowed to lapse into the charge of the nurses.

At a period of calm, after the 1970 budget-freeze furor had died down somewhat, the incumbent elected chairman of the Willowbrook Association of Physicians and Dentists, Dr. Archie, decided to step down in retirement. He privately invited me to assume leadership of the organization. I insisted that if I were elected, it would have to be on an explicit set of positions that would allow a less self-glorifying posture among the physicians, who were utterly isolated by their immense privileges from the rank-and-file working community.

I asked a friend and fellow physician, Mike Wilkins, who had come to work at Willowbrook on my request a few months after I began to work there, to join with me as a co-chairperson. Mike agreed to develop the platform positions and to run, to share in covering the time-consuming responsibility we both foresaw if elected. Even if we lost, finding allies among the other doctors would stand us in better stead. At the next regular meeting, we submitted our positions we would seek to advance if elected.

PLATFORM POSITION

submitted by William Bronston and Michael Wilkins

The following are a series of positions which we feel are in the interests of patients and professionals alike. We will energetically carry this position to Albany and the New York State Physicians and Dentists Association if we are elected as delegates from Willowbrook State School Chapter. We feel that a consistent and progressive position should be put forth and become the hallmark of the employees of the State's human services sector.

-PATIENT CARE

- Actively oppose the job freeze, budget cuts, layoffs, and all directives from Albany that are budget reduction projects at the expense of patient and employee well-being.

- Press to meet the American Association of Mental Deficiency specifications for accreditation emphasizing highest quality services and relevant to the public.

-HOSPITAL ORGANIZATION

- Support "unitization" of Willowbrook State School* proposed by the administration. A term to describe decentralizing the administration and creating a geographical focus to clusters of buildings to increase accountability and convenience to families in New York.

- Push for mass programs emphasizing productivity of residents and connection with the community versus the present custodial and detention strategy long outmoded.

-EMPLOYEES

- Support all efforts to upgrade all employees' status—wages, working conditions and service skills (emphasis on ongoing in-service education at all levels).

-COMMUNITY

- Develop concrete community relations and coordinate with community programs and services for the neurologically impaired population (consultation, community education, direct services around the clock, etc.)

- Push for coordinated public health preventive machinery in the community concerned with prematurity, neonatal follow-up for high risk births, etc. Support the FAMILY HOSPITAL project to establish a comprehensive Child Development Unit to service neurologically impaired children in the Borough.

-PARENTS

- Build an active and meaningful alliance with the Benevolent Association and all other parent groups concerned with improving resident care through discussions, forums, and creative educational projects to enhance dealing with the problems of their institutionalized family members.

-RESEARCH

- Press for establishment and expansion of clinically related research In all fields of health care, learning, and teaching techniques, communication skills and home care logistics.

-GENERAL

- Call for the immediate withdrawal of all U.S. troops from Southeast Asia, whose support is the single greatest deterrent to realizing the desperately needed health and educational services in our community and our country.

The day we distributed the platform, one of the senior physicians, Dr. Frew, who had been a practitioner in the local community until Medicare and Medicaid were passed, when he promptly retired to Willowbrook, jumped to his feet and literally screamed, "Communists!"—along with every other epithet he could squeeze out. The doctors, to the last one, were petrified. All of a sudden Mike and I were personae non gratae, a status we maintained from then on with our professional "peers."

The day of the election rolled around. The depth of the withdrawal of the otherwise aggressive medical men was only really expressed when Frew, the old "red-baiter," got every single vote in the group. Frew's candidacy opposed ours. It was comical and ominous at the same time. Our hopes for friends and for a modern service philosophy to emerge were dashed. Had we been elected, we might have had a slim chance to influence policy in Albany directly. The vote against us was a rejection of the principles in the platform. The gamble hadn't succeeded, and trying to win over the doctors would have required more time and diplomacy than we could afford. At the risk of being accused of sour grapes, we had to fully free ourselves from continuing attending the organization to develop other forces to confront the squeeze.

I summed up the situation in a letter to Dr. Archie to take advantage of the opportunity to clarify the issues and explain our anticipated conflict with the doctors' organization.

April 15, 1971

Dear Dr. Archie:

After careful consideration, I have decided to notify you of my withdrawal from membership of the State Association of Physicians and Dentists.

I would like to briefly explain my position. As you recall, my interests in the Association followed your strong prompting that I consider myself a candidate for delegate from Willowbrook. At that time, I shared your feeling that the association did not seem to be active nor represent broader interests, which I feel are part and parcel of any health professions' organization. As you recall, I insisted that the only basis upon which I would run was that my candidacy would flow from a principled position placing patient care uppermost. This specifically meant focusing our energies against the forces that were responsible for the savage budget cuts and "job freeze". It was my belief that the colleagues had to take a stand on professional and moral grounds against this situation.

In conjunction with Dr. Wilkins, a comprehensive platform was put forward around which we hoped to rally the other physicians and dentists. We hoped they would see the possibility of a broad alliance of health people occurring, an alliance that will become more and more a necessity as the coming weeks and months will bear out.

At last week's staff meeting, I was shocked by Dr. Frew's slanderous tirade when the platform was distributed, but felt that his blatant reactionary position, a position which I understand has a long history, would encourage the other physicians to exert a more positive thrust. I felt that with the support of you and your wife, plus the friends we have made among the other doctors, that even if we were not successful, at least there would be an opportunity to discuss the issues facing us, the hospital and our patients.

I was quite unprepared for the events of yesterday's meeting. It was clear that our hopes of a small ray of light coming from the physicians and dentists was sheer illusion. Dr. Frew's election without a single voice being raised to even question his position meant that the majority of physicians and dentists either shared his politics or did not have an ounce of courage to oppose him with another, more moderate nomination. Dr. Frew represents the most backward, the most selfish, and the most elitist interests in medicine. The association at Willowbrook, having voted him into office and represented by him, can only been seen by the people as odious to progress in the institution, and solely dedicated to the aggrandizement of a small group in comparison to the thousands working to make patient care something to be proud of.

I cannot allow my name to be associated with such an organization nor can I excuse myself for contributing in any way to its vitality while such objectionable leadership prevails. The Association represented by Frew is medieval! We live in this twentieth century.

Dr. Archie. I trust you will make the necessary arrangements to withdraw my registration prior to Frew's taking your place.

Thank you,
William Bronston, M.D.

This awakening to another rude truth of Willowbrook made it clear that those of us who did care about human services must develop and maintain ties to objective and competent people in the field outside of the institutional system to keep touch with both science and, more importantly, perspective. Working in Willowbrook tended to be numbing, and one could easily lose touch with how out of step the institution was with the standard of care outside its walls. During this early period in Willowbrook, I had seen fine and dedicated people like the young teachers crushed professionally and spiritually in their attempts to bring improvements to the place. The combined phenomena of feeling alone and, in fact, never searching for outside help and confirmation of one's instincts invariably led to surrendering with a "you can't fight city hall" attitude. I was determined that I would not succumb to the overwhelming forces for stagnation in the institution. Six months later, during a grievance hearing, I was readier than ever to actively enter the struggle.

CHAPTER 8

Photos: From People to Things—
Mass Reduction

WE LIVE IN A cultural system where things are more highly valued than people. Vitality is gauged by what we possess: home, auto, clothes, family, friends, TV, knowledge, money. We are conditioned to experience our own value by owning things or having the capacity to acquire things. If we have a life, a dynamic, it has been interpreted as this capacity to consume and surround ourselves with objects. It is an ordeal to refrain from consuming things, let alone to experience ourselves and our relations with other people as basically powerful and productive. It is no wonder that in where "things are king" and people are the go-between, people are easily experienced and interpreted as things, statistics, numbers.

Some things have more apparent social value than others, and so some people have more value. Those people who can retain an image of individuality—a name, a special identity—can temporarily escape being reduced to subhuman, object status. But once the reduction of that identity is begun, an image of being less than human, stereotyped is fashioned, and the rush toward disappearance into a bunch of labeled things gains momentum.

In order for the institution to carry on its operation, it is vital that the individual be submerged and become nameless, without identity. The alchemy of dehumanization from person to thing occurs. Thus, the infliction of violence is no longer experienced as violence, brutality, scorn, regimentation. Such terms are all meaningless, for how can one be brutal to a shoe or a toothbrush? One is compelled to expect stacking, piling, ordering, uniformity, among large numbers of things. Is that not what we have been taught? Keep our things together? Put them away at night? Classify and group things according to similarity?

People are only too ready to make things of other people. People with power do this routinely. The very idea of parity and respect among people—all people—is a contradiction to those whose self-definition is one of superiority. In fact, people with the most power in our society count their power not by money but by the legions of others under their influence and in their control, whose control requires their reduction to the mass—anonymity, namelessness.

EMPLOYEES
MUST
WASH HANDS

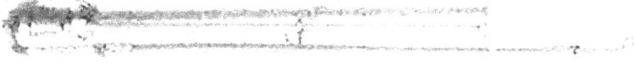

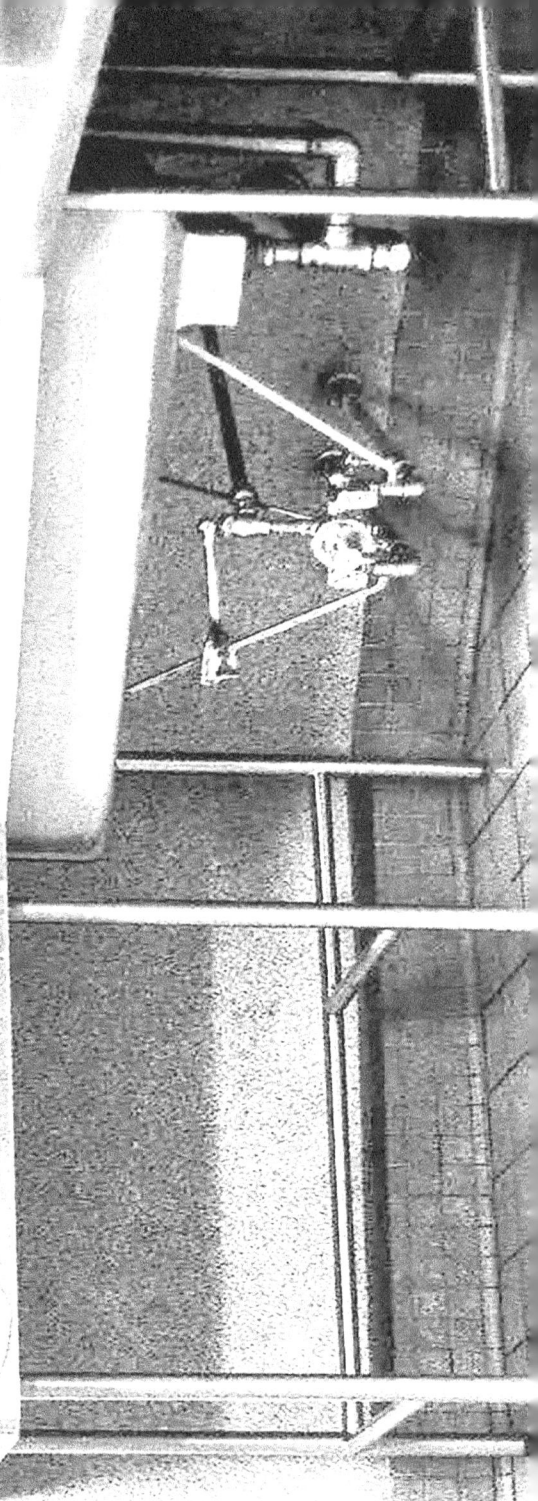

One must actively fight the alchemy whereby the most powerless individuals, those in the institutions of our country, are reduced to things, talked about as things, perceived as things, arranged as things, cast off as things, kept as income property by people—by the few who understand that their own power derives from their ability to practice this alchemy over blocs of fellow citizens. It's stunning how easily we can become things ourselves when, in our own minds, we allow the reduction to occur to others.

Infirmity, powerlessness, and the ability to define oneself as valued are the most real yet fragile facts of life.

Unless. Unless we dare to change ourselves, along with those values and structures that make things more real than people we contribute to the dehumanization. Is that too much to ask—that we save ourselves from certain future destruction from public institutions?

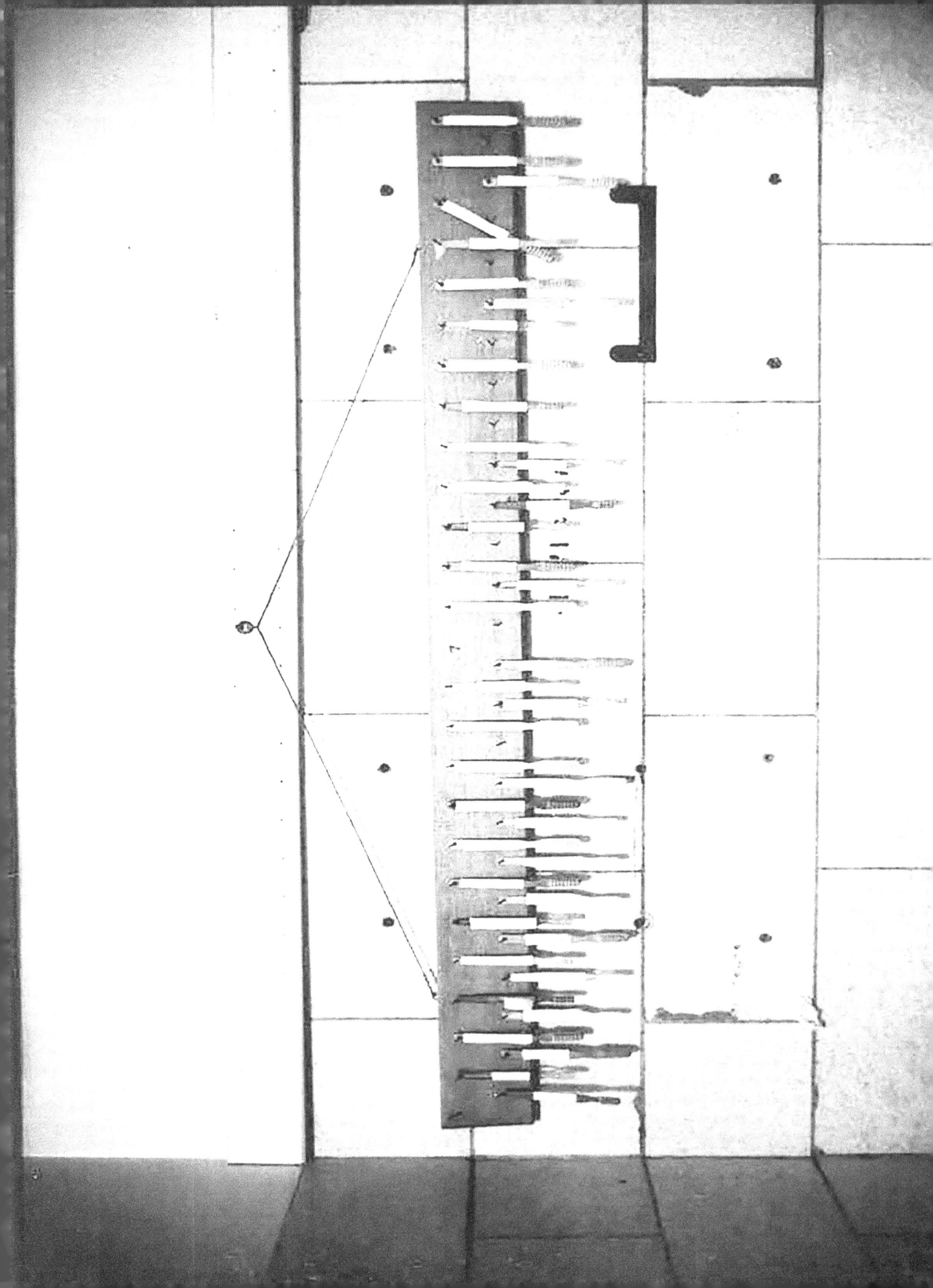

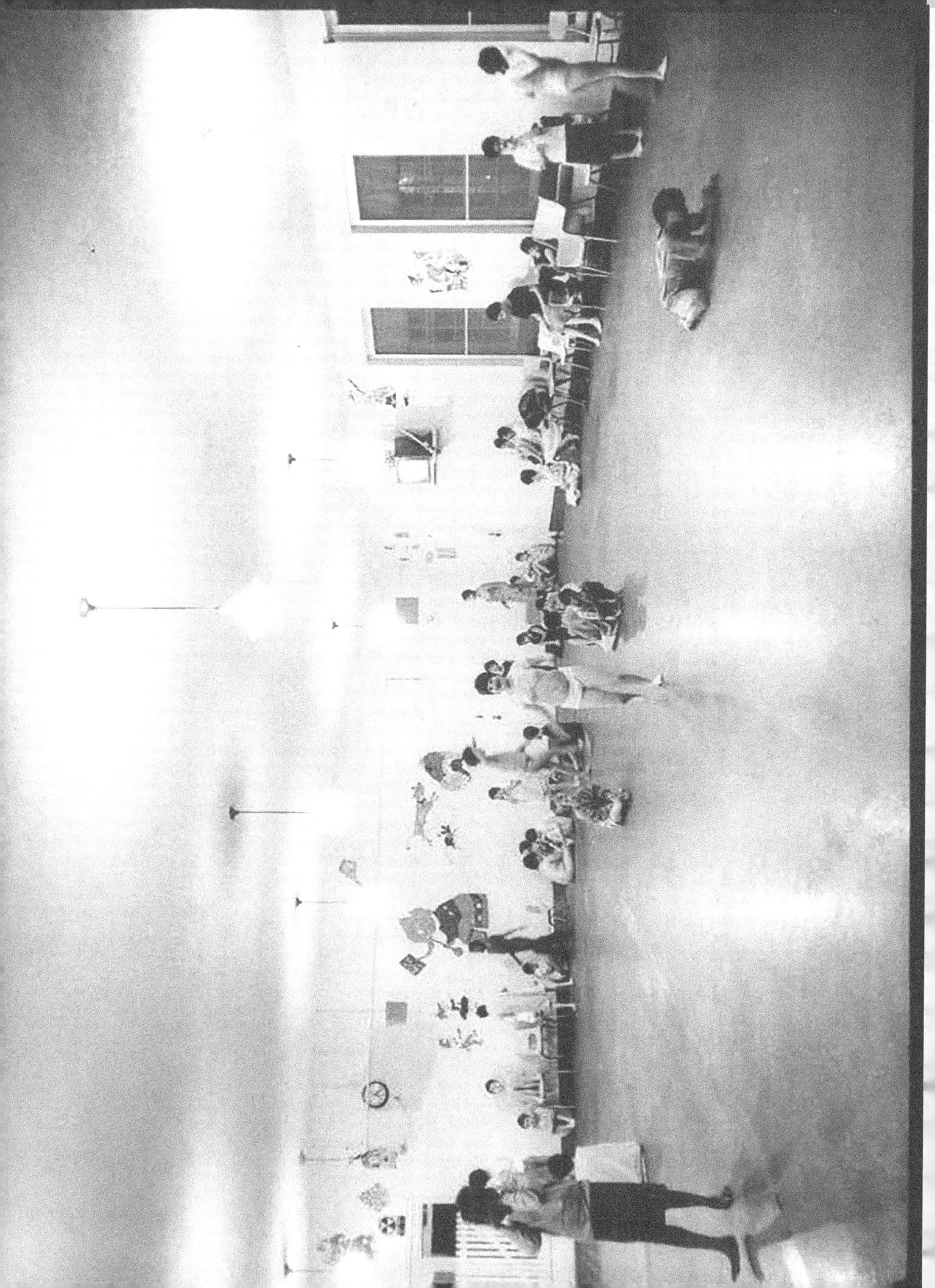

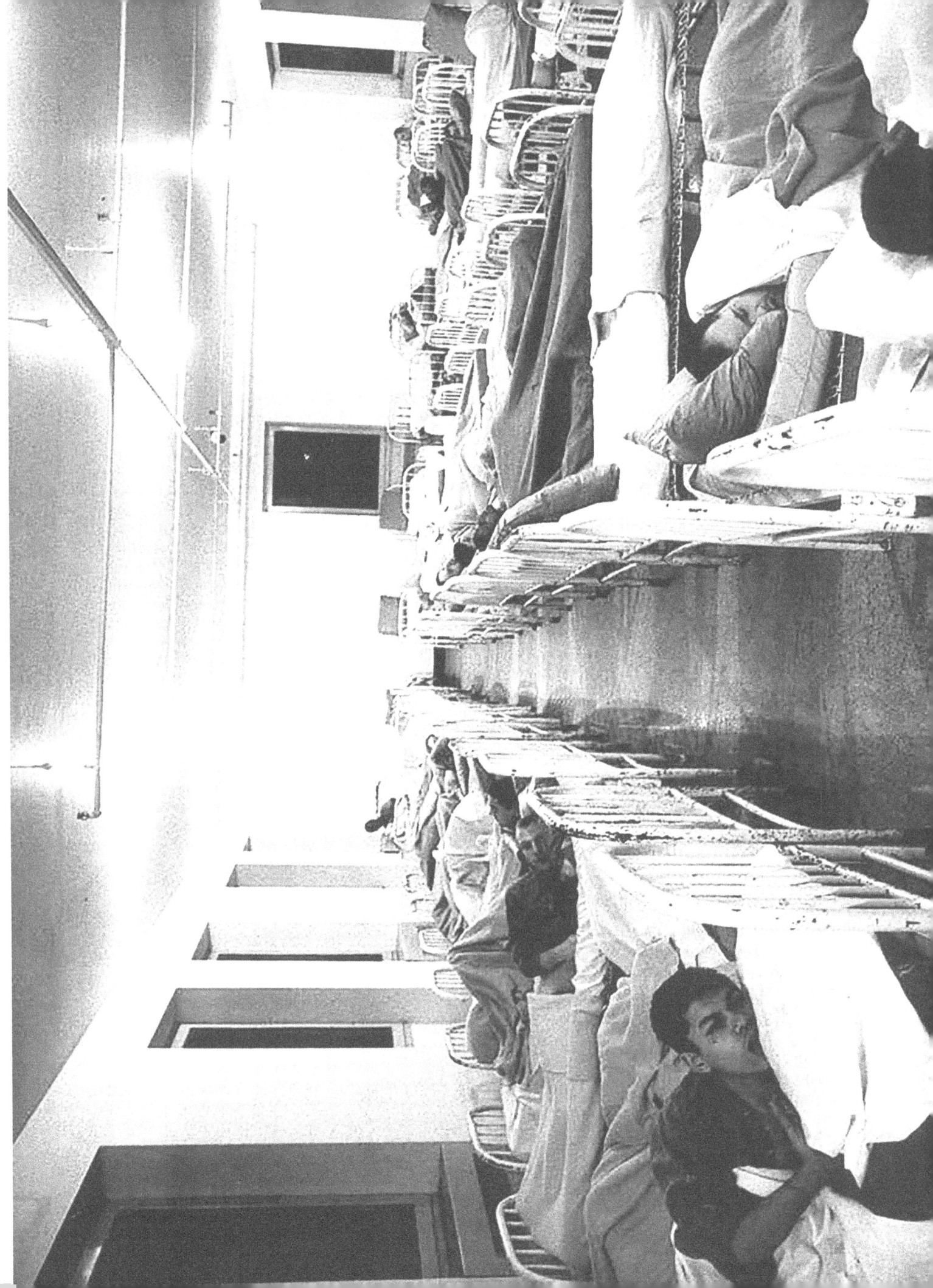

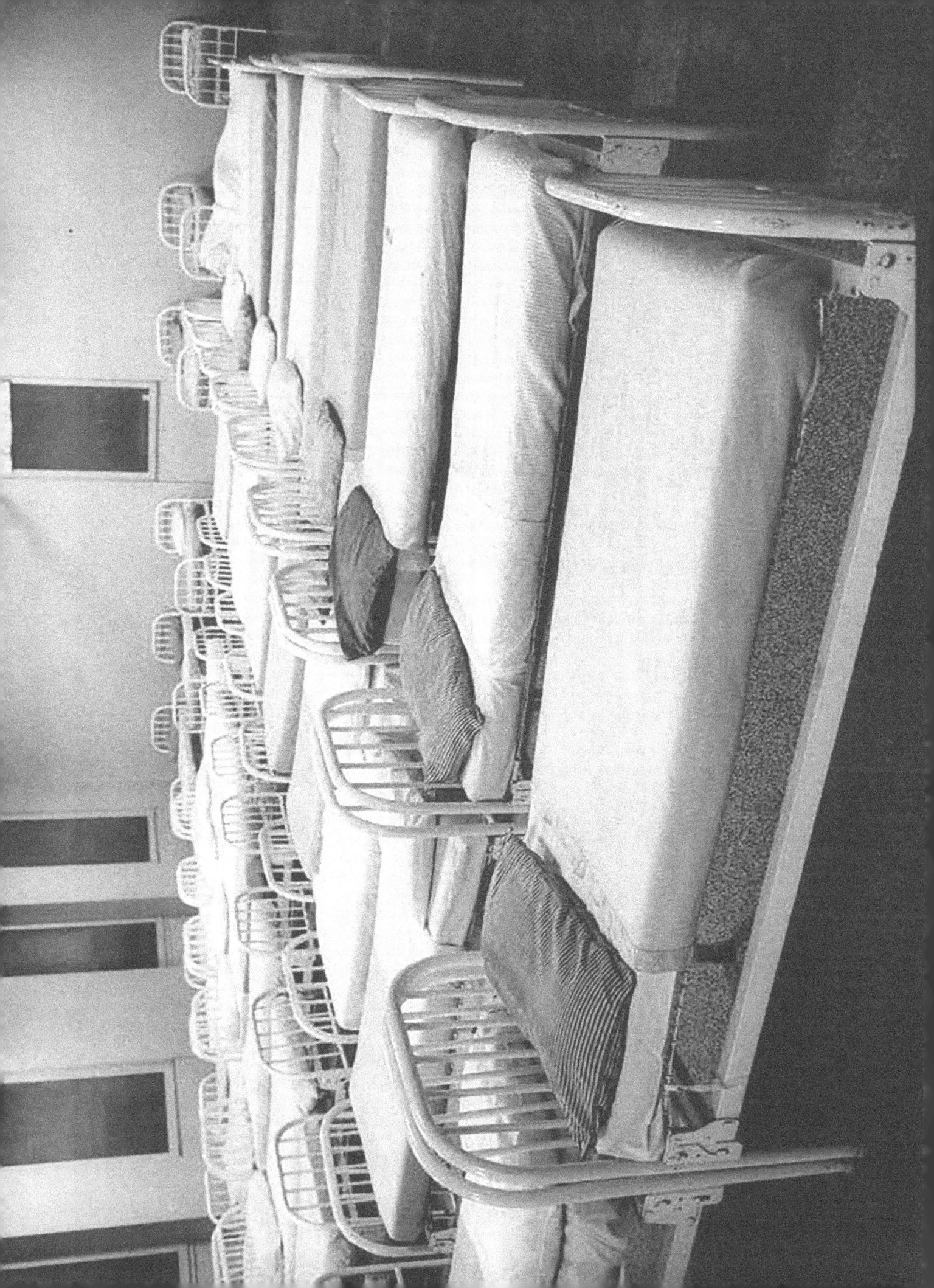

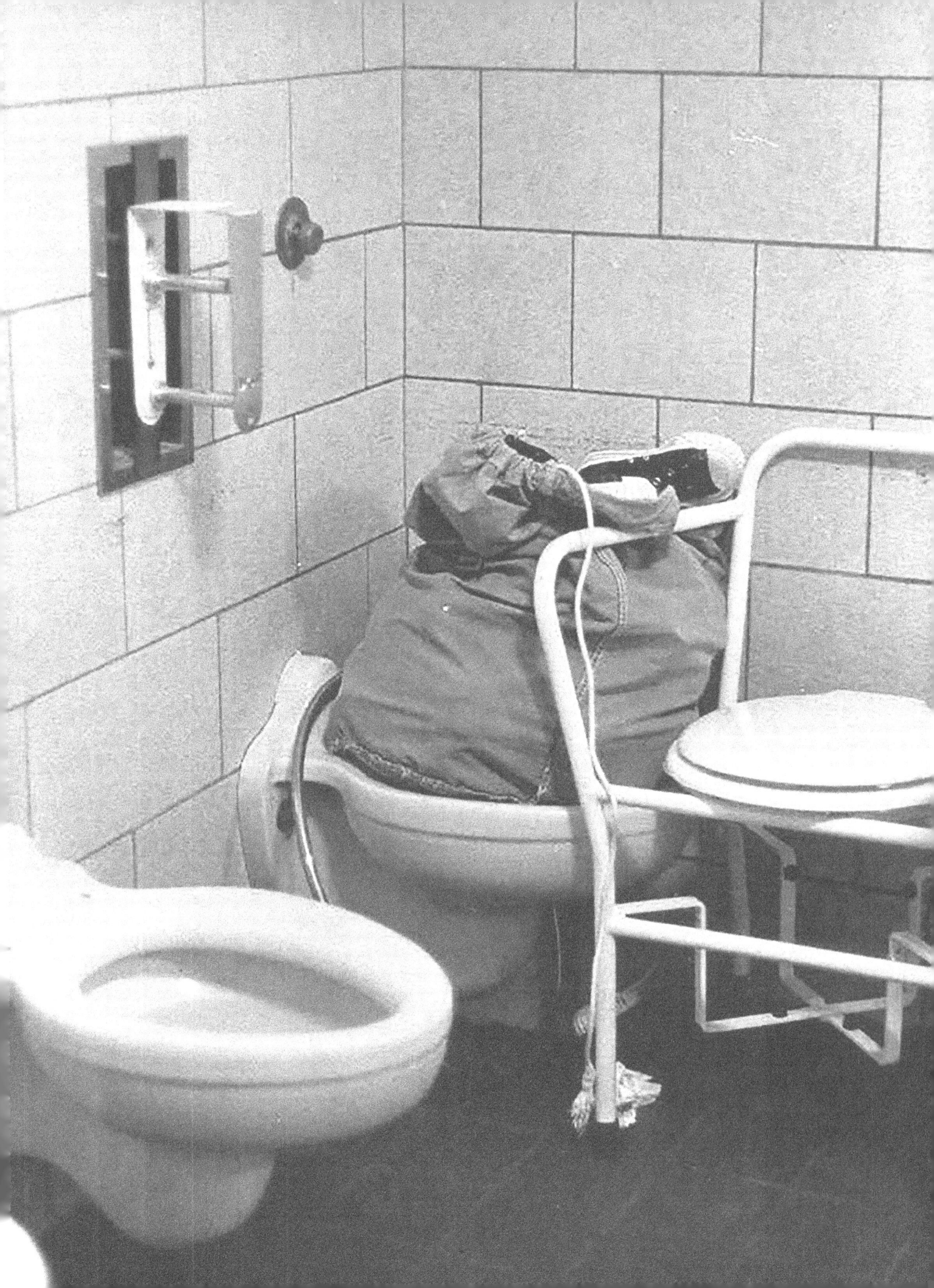

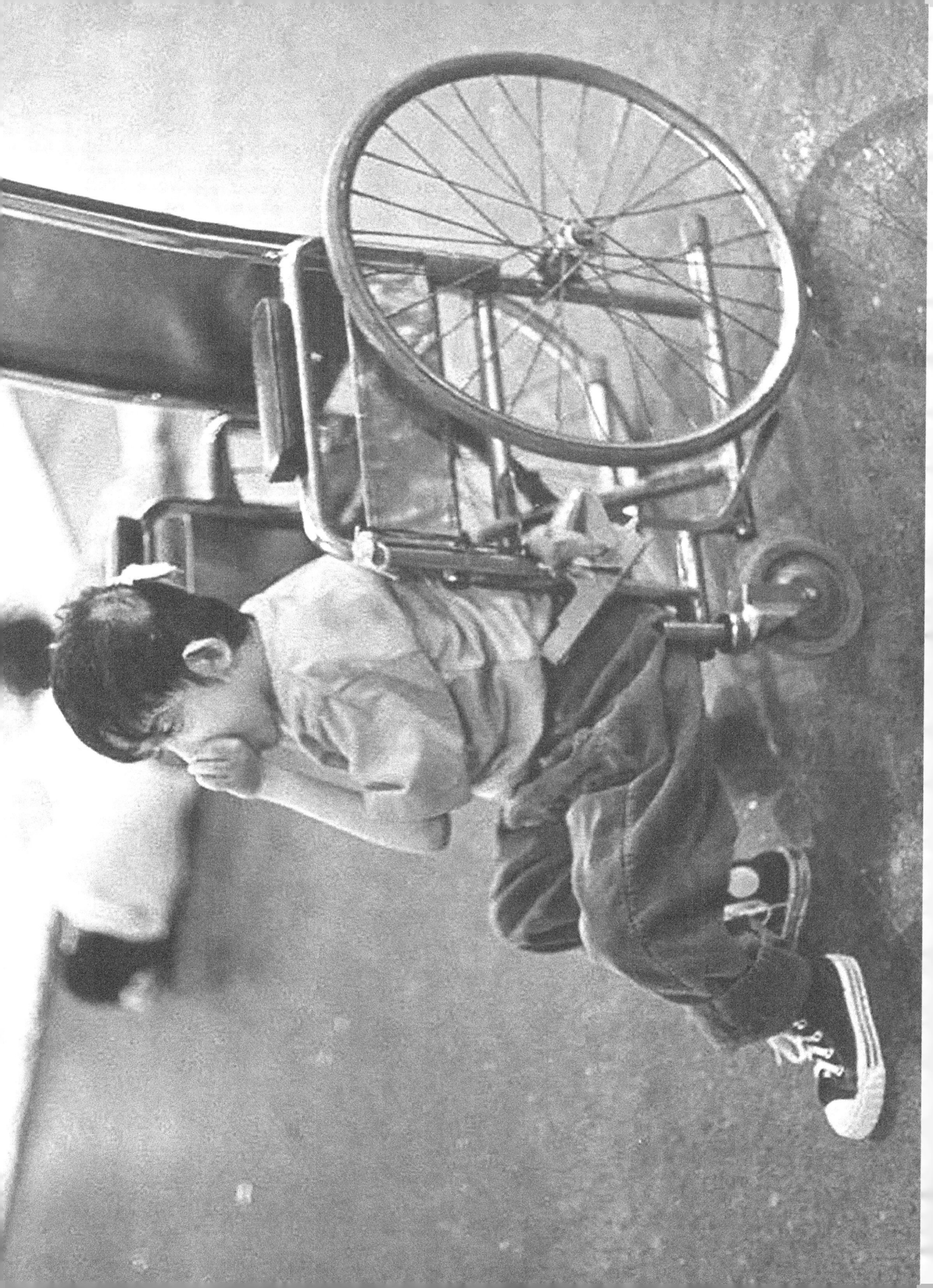

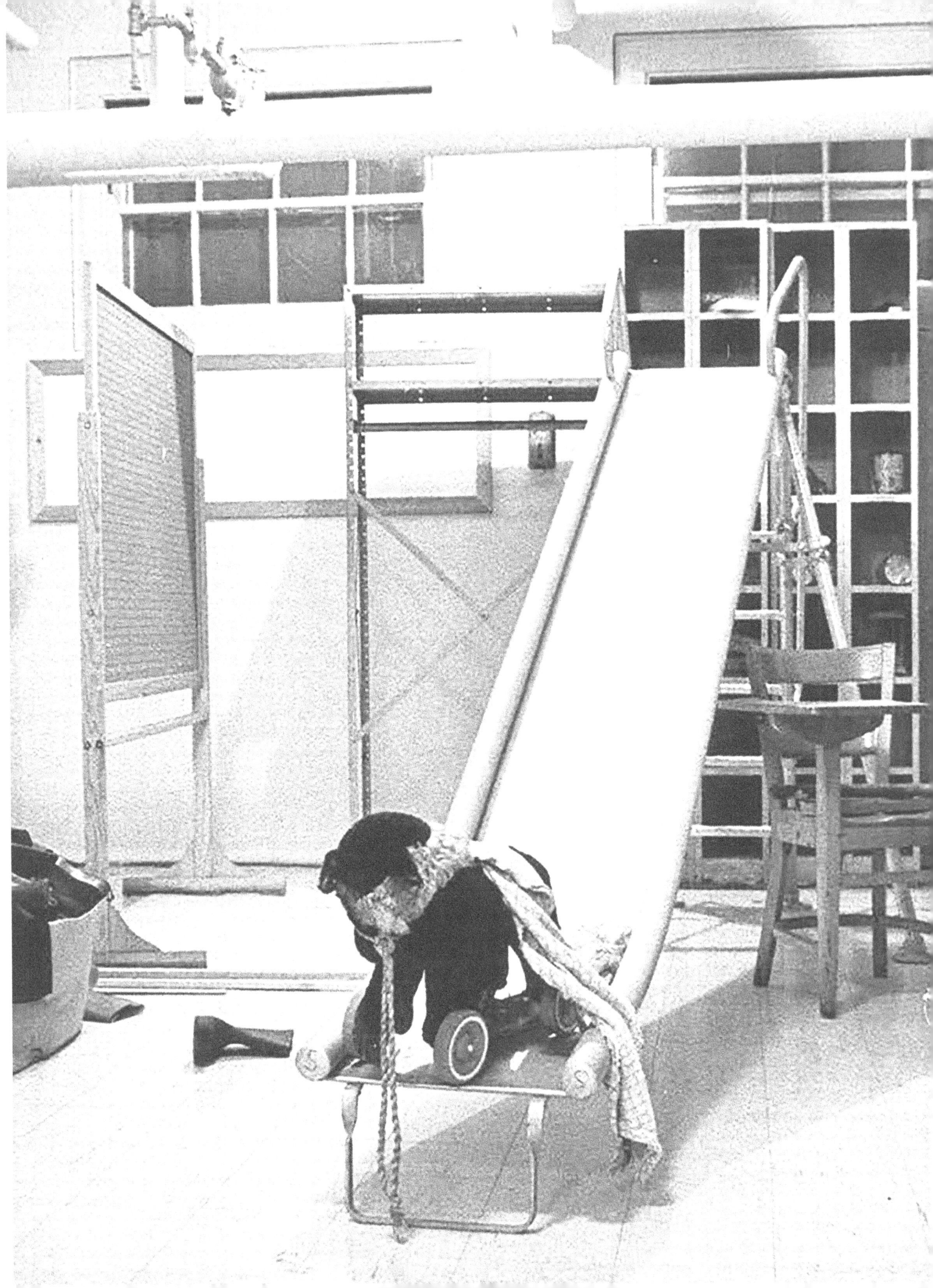

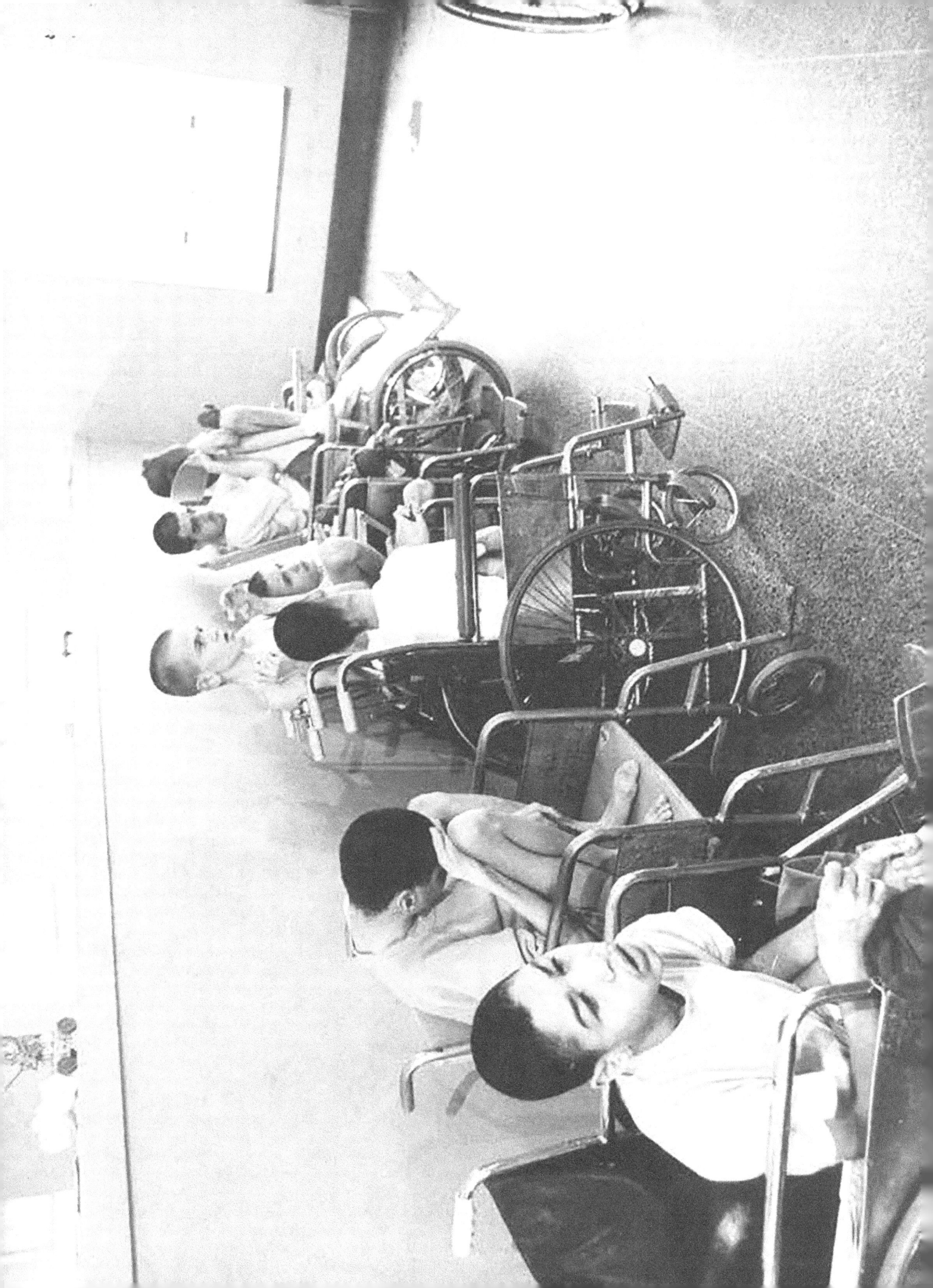

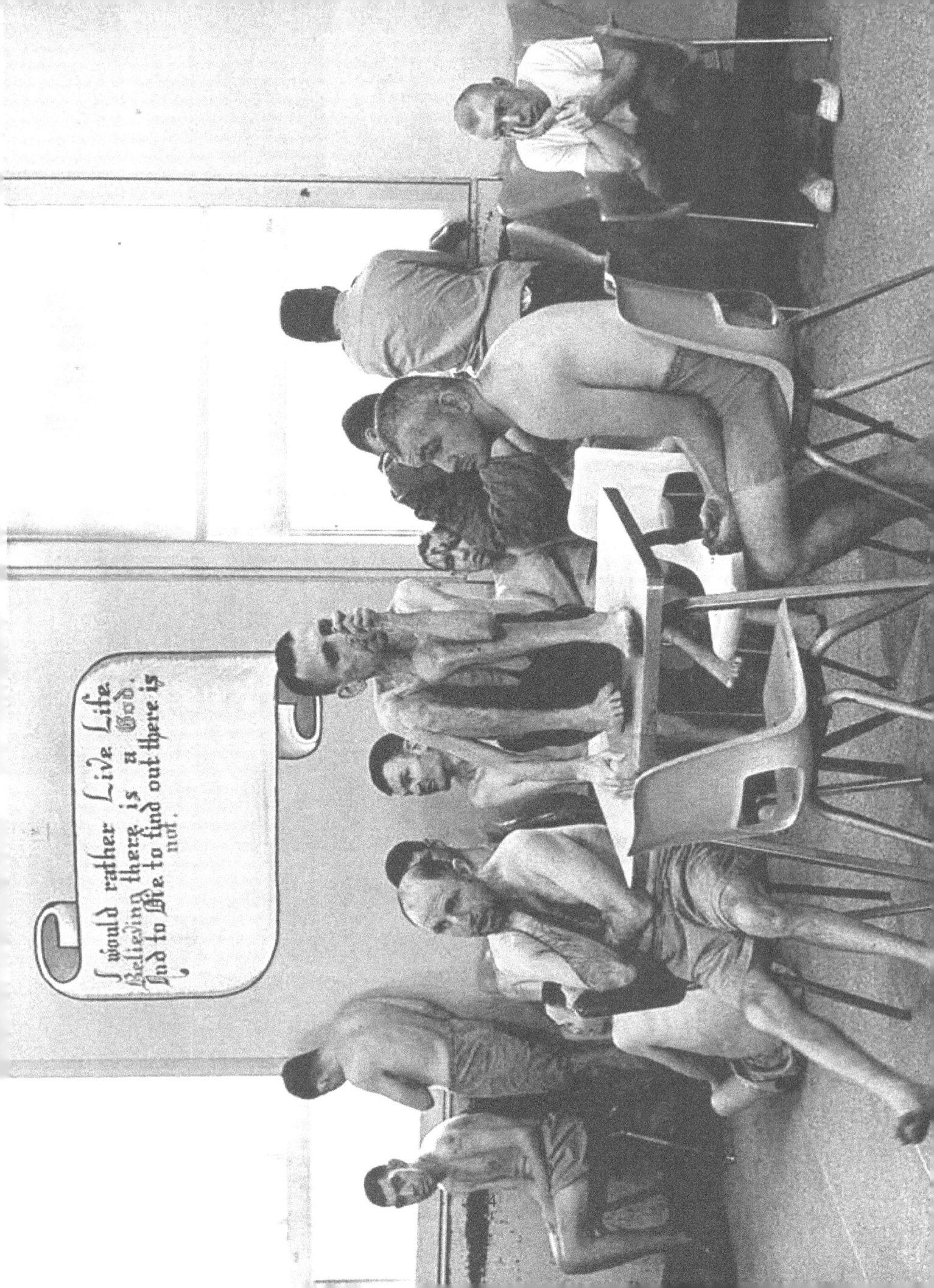

I would rather Live Life
Believing there is a God,
And to Die to find out there is
not.

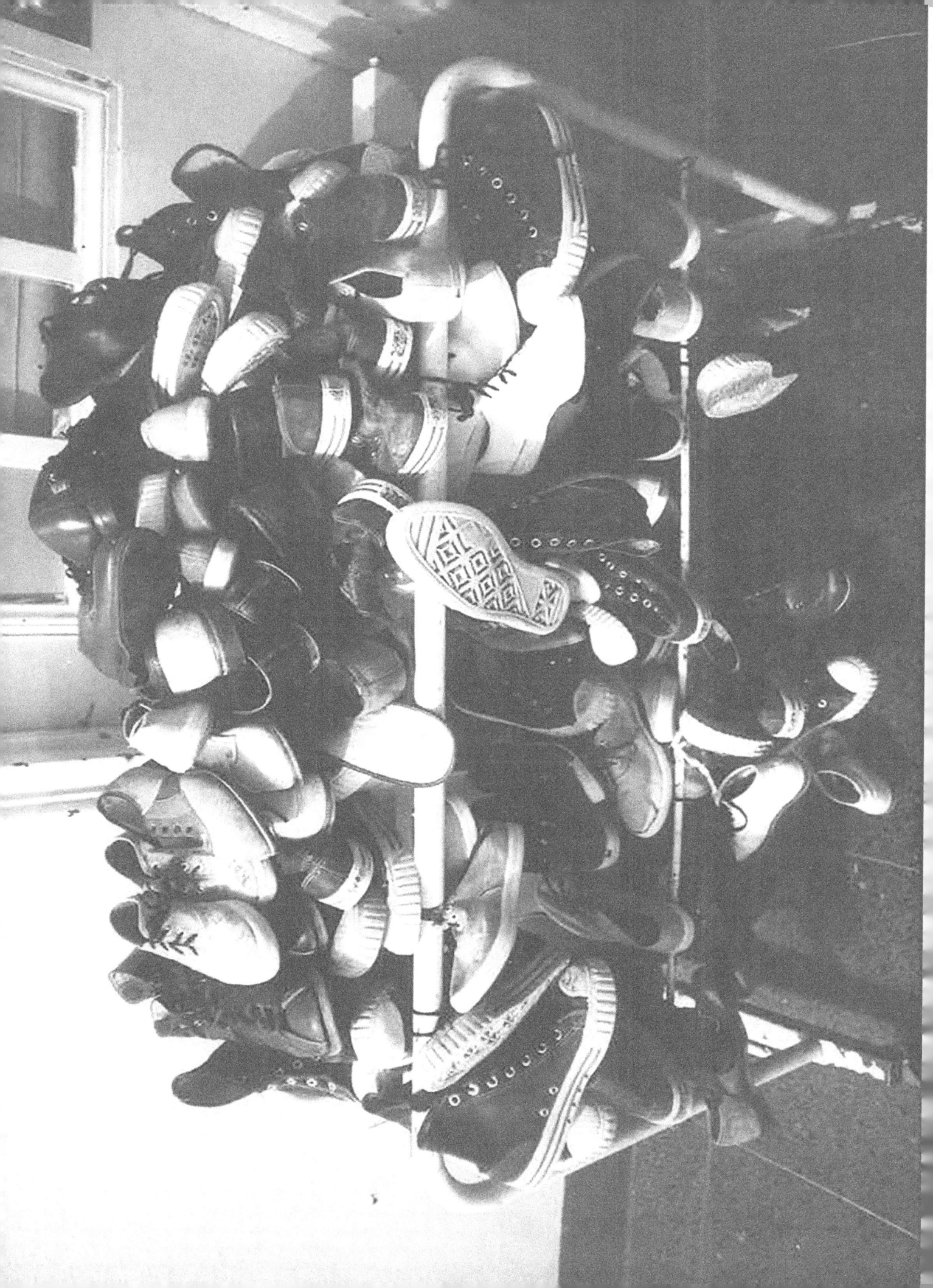

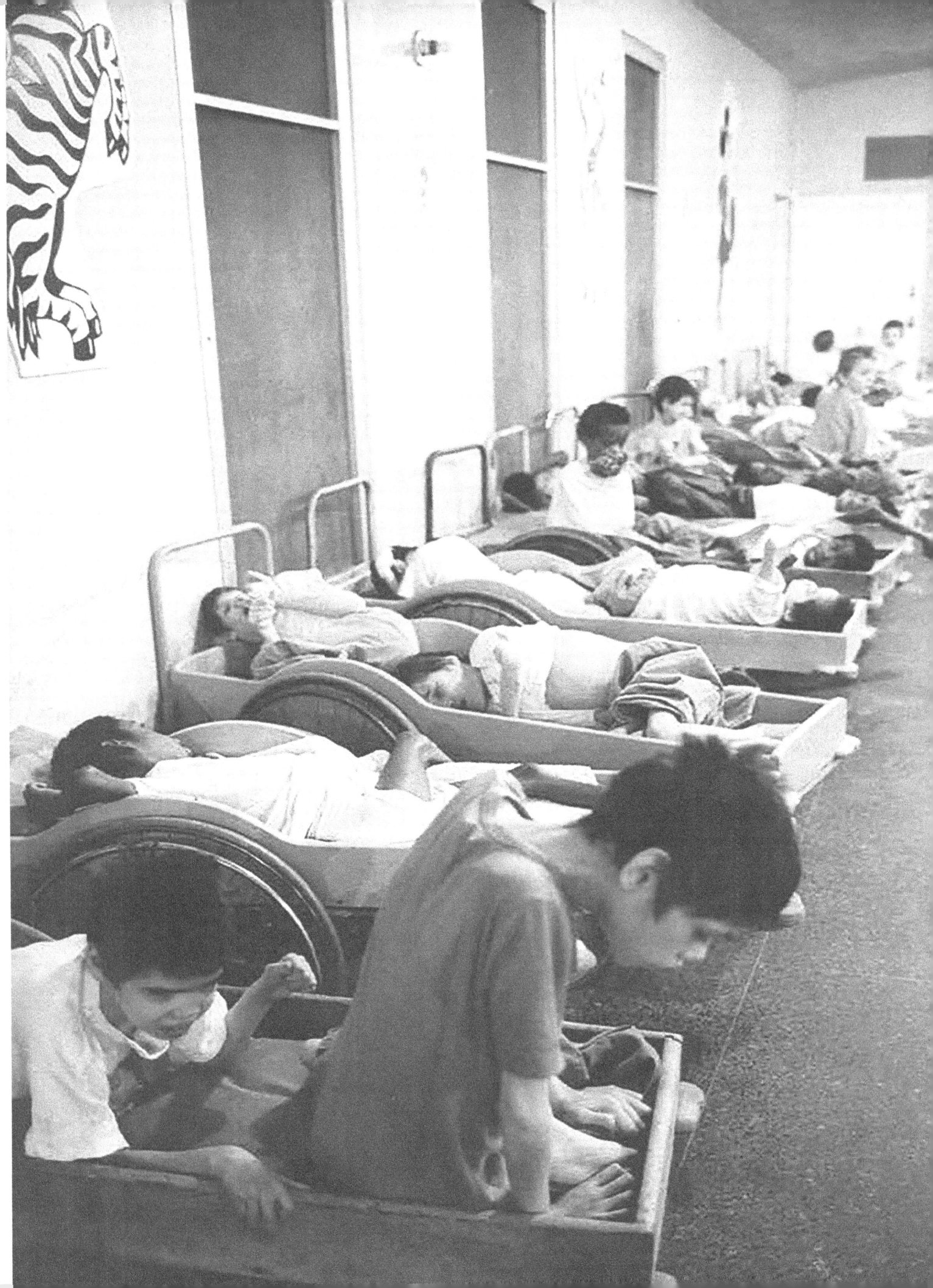

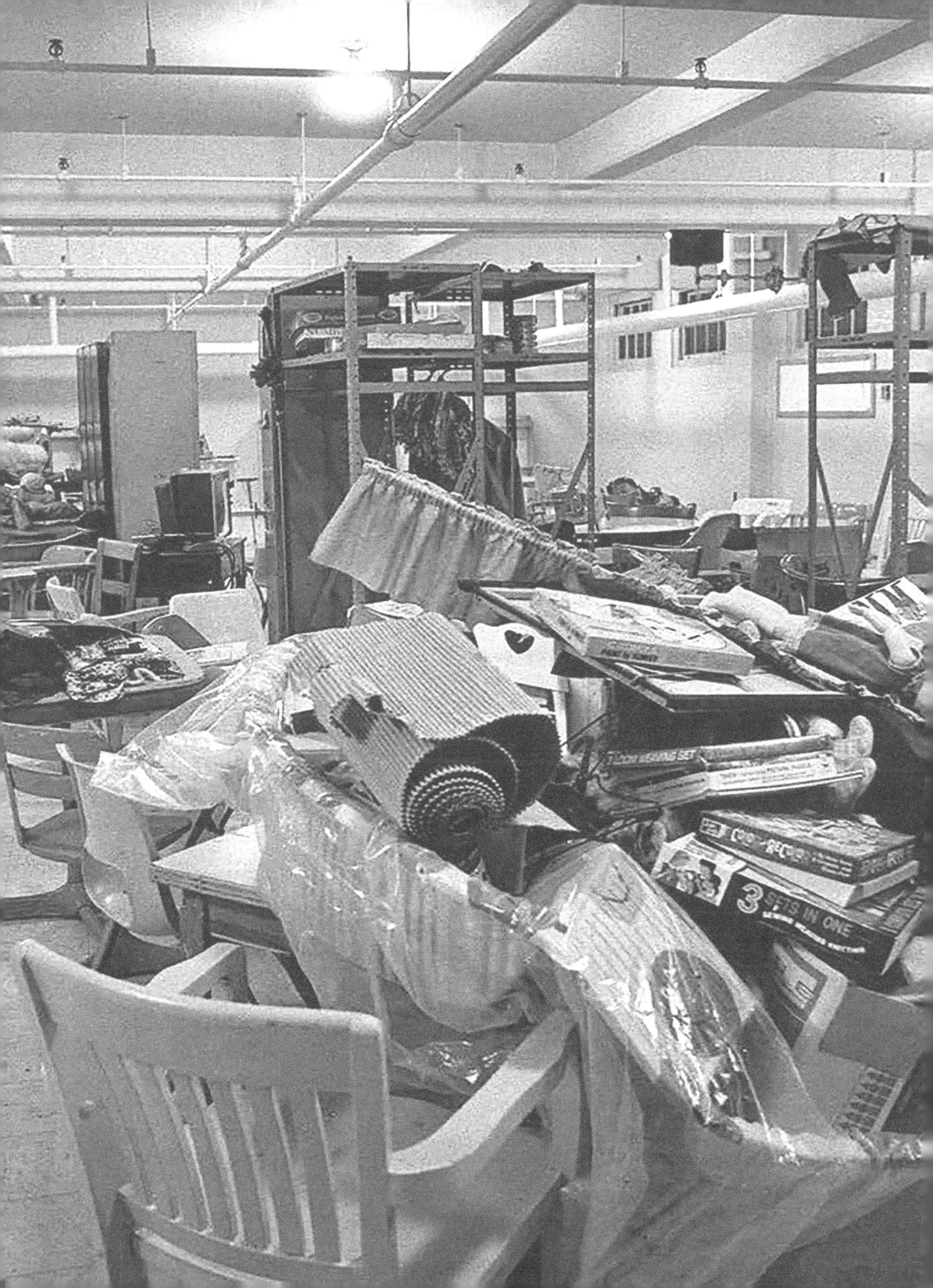

CHAPTER 9

Childcare: The Enemy of Willowbrook

ABOUT THAT TIME, A new state evaluation form called the Utilization Review was introduced in order to systematically get federal Medicaid reimbursement money, at that time $24 per day ($213 for 2020) per eligible resident. The forms had to be filled out by the state every six months for each child. I thought it was a great chance to genuinely review and get a handle on where each Building 76 child was in his or her overall development and to establish a real plan for each one. The administration, however, instructed the physicians not to recommend anything on the form that Willowbrook couldn't deliver. The associate director coordinating my building, Dr. Milton Jacobs, stood firm on the uselessness of the form. "No one will look at them," he said sneeringly, deflecting the true financial intention of the Utilization Review at the medical staff meeting, "but they have to be filled out by order of Albany." If an estimate of a child's performance were needed, we were told to use a heavy hand in assigning severe to profound physical and learning disability wherever we could, and need for continued residential care at Willowbrook. This followed the practice of the institution which had prompted a memo to the physicians instructing them to estimate IQs to be below 65 when filling out Medicaid forms, so that the state would get the maximum federal reimbursements and, in turn, justify their continued operation. I was furious at this fraudulent dishonesty and defeatist attitude. I warned Jacobs that I would only put the truth into the evaluation forms and not limit recommendations because of the absence of services and programs at Willowbrook.

I felt immensely uplifted. I finally saw the situation as a way to justify and deliver the child development program for which I had ostensibly been brought to Building 76. I saw how to break the stalemate and get the routinized building staff back on the road to serving the true developmental needs of the children again. Conditions for a step forward existed in Building 76. I began to meet with each of the five ward worker teams, three daily shifts, teachers, and therapists who were serving each ward scheduled to be reviewed. Over the first month, we completed the forms for the first thirty-five girls. The data and summaries provided compelling criteria for regrouping the children and gave us a perfect mechanism to see how seriously a thorough reorganization was therapeutically needed in my building.

Over the nearly past year of aggressive medical management and duplicate record keeping I maintained, I could track and see the building's public health transformation. I had been able to overcome all the rampant communicable and environmental diseases that were brought under control. I had also ended the prior practice of loading each kid with stultifying tranquilizers. The review order came at a perfect time. After three more intense weeks of completing these for each child, I had had truly inspiring conversations and provided simultaneous in-service training to each of my building coworkers.

The lack of any real individual developmental plan or programming for the children could no longer be denied nor postponed. I had no idea what the submission of the building reorganization plan would unleash from the administration. Nor, I guess, did they foresee the error in opposing progress.

Taking nothing for granted, I itemized all the assumptions and all my observations in the introduction of the plan. A number of basic problems existed. The children had not been regrouped since the building's "model" establishment six years before, despite real changes in the children's natural developmental progress. There was no plan for grouping children in the building based either on their needs or on the best use of individual skills among the workers. All the groups had been clustered willy-nilly for ease of handling. The "brighter" children were forced to deal with and help the "slower" children. The institutional jargon divided the children into two categories: "low grade" and "bright." The degree of disability or achievement among the children was not seen on any kind of a developmental continuum.

The staff members were also grouped for expediency rather than for their skills, interests, experience, or programs. "What will keep the peace" was the governing strategy for staff assignments on each of my five wards. This practice had been nurtured by the Building 76 nursing supervisor, who consistently placed administrative accommodation above clinical service. The need for rational organization and a sensitive communication network in the building was a precondition for change. Ongoing in-service training for the staff and an individualized education program for the children were pivotal.

The inflexible medical model that prevailed in the building, the norm throughout Willowbrook, limited management of the children to "first aid," crisis intervention, and a defensive medical care posture that absorbed the bulk of our everyday attention. Our energy needed to now be turned beyond the daily crisis treatment of illnesses and injuries. The across-the-board educational and developmental needs of the Building 76 children, needs that had gone completely by the board, required immediate and creative attention.

The underpinning of my written plan aimed at clarifying the chain of command in the building that was desperately needed. Frequent program disagreements between the nursing staff and me as to the residents' needs had to be resolved. I proposed that in keeping with the official job descriptions set up by the department, the building MD was the top administrative person and must have ultimate authority for all clinical and child development strategies and operations within the building. The nurses had to carry out these strategies, once agreed upon. I really was unaware that because of the historical slothfulness and unreliability of Willowbrook's physicians, the nursing department had coopted and assumed the daily authority role in practice, while carefully role-playing a diplomatic subordinate position. I insisted that all assignments of staff within the building had to be directed toward meeting the training and care needs of the children. Any changes, orders, or resource allocations in the building had to be evaluated in relation to the programs of childcare and brought to the attention of the building doctor to establish unity of planning and action. Over many months, I had been confronted with unilateral decisions by the Building 76 nursing supervisor that continually disrupted purposeful planning and programming.

The second major area of the proposal was to cluster all the children into our five available ward groupings: (1) slow-learning boys that needed more teaching power, (2) active boys, (3) youngsters who needed an advanced program to be called the "living room" group, (4) youngest and smallest girls, and (5) teens and young adult women. Though a crude division, even this would have radically improved the hodgepodge situation that existed with all manner of children thrown together. I wanted to concentrate the natural training groups together to clarify program relevance and intensity. Even this basic reform, dealing with so many children crammed together, still only addressed the lowest common denominator of care. Up to now, minimizing injuries which resulted from antagonistic groups of children had been the basic grouping rationale. I had inherited the mindless lumping of hyperactive with slower children, those capable with those most dependent, the large with the small, all for ease of ward management, that made every child unnecessarily vulnerable.

Now, it was vital to improve the around-the-clock program and therapy continuity by limiting the overall range of programming needed for each group, a problem of insurmountable magnitude under the preexisting pattern Building 76 had been grouped. The plan called for staff to be thoughtfully reassigned, according to their individual strengths and knowledge, so that true teams could be established in place of casual assignments and program needs of the children, so that the more dependent and less socialized youngsters would receive more supervision and care. All this rested on establishing real contexts and expectations for growth for each child. Up to now, staff attitudes had been deeply pessimistic and expectations ruthlessly low. No worker in the building retained true objectivity about the children, resulting in the complete breakdown of activities and the bankrupt prevailing conviction that the children had "gone as far as they can." Naturally, the children, like all human beings, responded to these expectations and literally played the roles cast for them by their stultifying confinement and lack of staff sophistication.

My proposal explained the rationales for a number of the special settings and programs needed. The living room and a dining program, as well as speech and hearing, recreation, and occupational projects, were outlined. The underlying purpose of the ward to be handled as a living room was to develop each child's capacity for learning—how to live in settings similar to those of a normal home or community dwelling—given the obvious limitations of the institution environment. The ward was to approximate in every detail and expectation a community home, to encourage the children to develop those abilities needed to function creatively and appreciatively at home. Rugs, curtains, individual bedding, room for individual storage of clothes, decorated walls, suitable bathroom facilities, and music listening and visual training systems all had to be included.

The workers to be assigned to the living room ward would be selected to duplicate normal family relations. Here, the workers might either follow their clients into the school settings to assist or be available to work with children who required short-term or smaller group work. Such settings as this were not to be found anywhere in Willowbrook, and so it was not at all surprising that families had real difficulties with their kids when they took them out for visits or home for weekends.

In Building 76, there were at least thirty-five youngsters, a full ward, who desperately needed this socializing input despite their participation in school part of the day, frequent trips outside the institution, and competent eating and self-care skills. Their wards over the years had all been depleted of anything but the most starkly indestructible chairs and tables. Acquiring the needed replacement furniture, gradually from the Staten Island dump, and making projects of repairing and refinishing would cost nothing and involve the children in constructing their own environment. Lamps, radios, TVs, and phonographs were to be added as individual children accepted these items as their responsibility. The decor would be taken entirely from the work of the children themselves in school, and occupational classes and could be changed frequently. Prerequisite to this, the entire ward would have to be repainted and repaired sufficiently to erase every reminder of the unstructured and chaotic present. The entire milieu had to communicate comfort, order, pleasure, and normative living.

The same thing applied to eating and mealtimes. Fully one-half of the building's children still ate in the most vulgar way—stealing food, throwing food, and using their hands instead of utensils. Yet minimal attention was given toward changing these learned behaviors. Food was served on plastic compartment trays with portions run together into a conglomerate mash. Although the majority of our children had received work in self-feeding skills when they were toddlers, most of these abilities were rudimentary. Now in their early adolescence, all the youngsters needed considerable work in preparing them for polished, social eating.

At one time the building had set up a small-scale advanced eating program for a group of boys who went to the institution's school. Workers brought in dishes, stainless ware, and tablecloths. The boys had a rotating table captain, and food was passed around the table to be served. However, this program was spontaneously dropped as staff was lost.

After the program was abandoned, some criticisms surfaced. "Why did only the best children have the opportunity to get this special training when they were able to pick up the skills with little or no training compared with the more significantly dependent children?" "The program took too long in the cafeteria and interfered with the smooth process of feeding the balance of the building's children." "There weren't enough chairs and tables to keep the program going in the dining area." Clearly, all the children in the building did need training in dining.

In addition to inadequate training in more advanced self-help skills, there was a lack of attention to the development of basic sensory and communications skills. Eleven of the children in the building had documented hearing deficits. The majority of these were in special education in the institution school. At least twenty of the most capable children, many of whom were in school or chosen to attend class, had significant speech problems. We needed a full-time person from the Speech Department to take several groups of children in two or three daily sessions and work toward articulation and language skills, not to mention training the ward staff to follow up on the short-term intensive sessions.

All the recreation programs had to be reanalyzed, with new groups set up based on concrete developmental goals for each child. The simplest needs had to be considered: body image improvement and basic coordination, confidence building and integration of physical and social activities, and strength building for skeletal growth and coordination. Specific goals were essential to evaluating progress and integrating the recreation programs with the overall goals of the children. At that time, the crude emphasis was only on getting some of the children off the ward to relieve the custodial burden of the ward workers, which was anything but the setting of rational objectives derived from a scientific assessment of the child's needs. More advanced recreation was needed in the afternoon to focus on structured sports, sportsmanship, cooperation, comprehension of rules, building frustration tolerance, and postponement of gratification for those youngsters at that level of developmental readiness.

Finally, the program proposal that I submitted to the administration spelled out an important role for the occupational therapy (OT) technicians. Their training and skills were geared for breaking down performance tasks into the smallest pieces, exactly suited for people who learned slowly or in different ways than typical children. But as with other developmental approaches, occupational therapy had been used in its grossest and least useful way in the building, as if calling a classroom in an OT setting made it one. The proposal outlined the evaluative or diagnostic role of occupational therapy, as well as its inherent training power. Each child's program should flow from an analysis of that child's unique needs and abilities, and OT groups had to be reformed so that children would be clustered at essentially common levels of achievement for the sake of program unity. Also, OT needed to become involved in the training of basic living skills such as dining and toileting, long since abandoned because the children had ostensibly reached an age beyond these training needs.

I also proposed the establishment of "advanced" occupational therapy. This was a prevocational program that would emphasize mature peer relationships and simple competitive work for the older teens. It would simulate sheltered or real work toward which the young people should and would be directed. This would require modern retraining for the staff, but the benefits would be incalculable to the children, and the staff would gain consciousness of the impact that these programs could have.

The huge design work needed unprecedented conversations with the ward staff that would be thrilling, and I was overwhelmingly optimistic given the unarguable and doable fixes. My most engaged ward staff held their breaths as nothing of this kind had ever even been discussed in their experiences. The institution was changeless, a gargantuan cultural treadmill to them, and their traditional powerlessness and subordination on the job were all they knew.

Time stopped. The profound message was the demand that old attitudes about the hopelessness of the youngsters' progress be abandoned and that the management holding action, fiercely clung to by the nursing hierarchy, be surrendered and replaced. The nurses panicked. They had been the traditional custodians and protectors of whatever routines and services existed. A decision was required by the administration. I had given the proposal to Dr. Jacobs, the administrative assistant for my building, who told me that although he was going on vacation he would review the position and quickly pass it on to Director Hammond.

My usual schedule at this time created considerable periods during the week when I was off duty. Friendly workers in the building began to tell me about unusual comings and goings of the institution's top nursing supervisors and hushed meetings that went on when I was not there. Dr. Jacobs had returned to work. Both he and Dr. Hammond made appearances in the building—but only when I was off duty. For the director, this was truly remarkable, as he had visited my building only twice the entire preceding year. Things had come to an absolute standstill. A small group of senior workers became openly insubordinate to me. The nurses took on a sullen anger, and the bulk of the workers in the building withdrew from the usual warm contacts that were customary between us.

I assumed that Drs. Jacobs and Hammond were investigating the feasibility of the proposal, and I looked forward to the negotiations which I felt certain would follow. But something frightening was in the air. Friends continued to describe how they had become socially frozen out from other workers—the clique who got regular privileges from the nurse. Rumors that I was going to fire a handful of workers and change workers' shifts sprang up from nowhere. I called Dr. Jacobs regularly to pursue the matter of the proposal and was met each time with an annoyed tone and the reply that Dr. Hammond was still reviewing it.

As the days and weeks wore on, the attitude of all the building staff became more fearful and hostile. I could not understand the administration's foot-dragging.

The apprehension and distrust caused by their delay could be cleared in a moment by a strong mandate from the director to act. Instead, the delay continued to fuel the rumors that I was about to invoke some kind of drastic changes.

Finally, I felt the situation had so disintegrated that I demanded a meeting with Dr. Hammond. Two months had elapsed. The meeting in the director's office was my last effort to convince the administration that a disastrous situation had to be corrected. After nearly twenty months at Willowbrook, I had just about exhausted every drop of reason, patience, and persuasion at my command. In this final meeting, I meticulously spelled out how vital the director's positive action would be in establishing a commitment to childcare.

Drs. Hammond and Jacobs were unresponsive to these concerns. Instead, my proposal was pushed aside and the issues were suddenly totally turned backward. "Why did you provoke the Nursing Department and cause all that trouble in the building?" "Why can't you get along with the building nurse who has her job to do?" "Why didn't you produce a program plan when you first entered the building instead of waiting so long?" "Who do you think you are?" "The administration has been battling Albany all along to correct the ills of Willowbrook. Do you think that the director is not doing his job?" "Now is not the time to change anything—there's no money, no staff!" I felt enmeshed in their web of self-serving distortions.

Finally, having worked himself into sufficient moral ire, Hammond jumped to his feet. "Furthermore, Bronston, I am removing you from your building as of today and reassigning you! You have caused too much trouble already. The building will stay the way it is, and you are lucky I'm not preferring charges against you. Now beat it!"

The administration had made a choice. I had to think what this really meant. It was obvious that my days were numbered and that my efforts to work with Willowbrook's administration had to be junked. In civil service, as in the private job sector, employee disfavor results in additional attention by supervisors toward that person, and whether conscious or not, an attempt is made to smooth out the annoyance. The blue-collar workers understood this phenomenon instinctively. But repression was both new and unexpected to me, as a doctor.

This was my second jolting move from a building. I had grown deeply attached to the children in Building 76. In a very special way, we belonged to one another. The work of reducing the fear of the children, the elimination of the carloads of tranquilizers administered to most of them, their improved appearance and performance over the thirteen months all tore at me. I knew that the practices of the older doctor who was taking charge after my removal would undo all that. During my stay at Building 76, many deep friendships had been struck with the parents, as a new hope and expectation for their children had emerged. The parents had come to know that they could demand a better standard of living from the institution. I had urged their participation in planning and defending quality services. Now, the fate of their children would depend, most surely, on what they were willing to do as a body.

CHAPTER 10

The Power to Define

MY PRIOR TRANSFER FROM the children's complex, where I had first started, had been coupled with a request from Dr. Hammond for professional program development in Building 76, an opportunity I took seriously. This second transfer was an act of censure on the part of the administration against the needs of the children and clear repression aimed at me. I had a choice: conform to an intolerable and unethical situation or stand for what was right, regardless of the consequences.

There were some things that were clear and true about what was at the root of the Building 76 affair. If I chose to stand for what was right, two actions lay ahead. First, I had to crystallize a principled position to challenge the administration's repressive and punitive transfer action, separate from my personal pain. This had to be done in the face of the massive vested interest opposing any reform in the institution. Second, I had to implement this stand in a way that would make the issues visible, so that hopefully some relief for the children in the conditions of Building 76 might occur.

I had a feeling that this confrontation would challenge the very core of the institution's mythology. What was to be their priority, bureaucratic and administrative stability (program stagnancy), or the needs of the residents for support of their growth and future lives in the community? In short, was the institution there to control or to serve?

All of my efforts to achieve even the most minor degree of relief for the residents had been totally rejected by the loyal instruments of status quo. Even though my next step would be an internal grievance procedure, I knew I would soon have to reach outside Willowbrook for help.

Dr. Gunnar Dybwad was a friend and teacher from my days at Children's Hospital, in California. Gunnar had been the first executive director of the National Association for Retarded Children, and was currently consultant on mental retardation to the World Health Organization. He since had become professor of human development at Brandeis University. More than a teacher, Gunnar contained within his career the whole modern history of the movement for the rights and dignity of people called mentally retarded and their families. World-renowned and honored, he was the warrior grandfather for thousands. I did not plan to call on Gunnar for active help in the grievance hearing, but I wanted the security of knowing that he was apprised of the situation and ready to come to my aid when needed.

I wrote a letter to Gunnar explaining the situation, from my experience in Building 16 when I first arrived, to the developments in Building 76. I wrote:

Beloved Teacher, I need your help and want to describe the situation I am in. I have been working at Willowbrook State School in NY, in an ostensible "Hospital Improvement" federal grant program here, a prefab building, #76 with 134 mostly pre teen residents. As I began moving more and more toward clarifying what needed doing to improve things in Building 76, the tension mounted in the building and with the administration. An explosion has occurred when I tried to confront the feeling of defeat in the building emanating from the staff, I submitted a draft proposal to reorganize children and workers alike and was forced to charge my building nurse with incompetence and subterfuge in all practices in the building. As a result, the administration quickly made an alliance with the most backward workers, playing on their traditional fears of change and their attitudes about the hopelessness of the children's future. The superintendent, Dr. Jack Hammond, charged that I had undermined morale through harassing the staff with my "political" views (that is to say my views on patient care and the science of child development) and ousted me from Building 76.

I was assigned on eight hours' notice to care for two buildings, 22 and 23, with 200 profoundly institutionalized adult women each, that operates in such disrepair and abandon, not to mention overcrowding, that it is appalling. I feel that the situation absolutely requires a fight. The New York institutions have been under the gloom of the state budget freeze for nearly a year. No one is fighting back and conditions everywhere are deteriorating. I have an excellent lawyer and filed a grievance against the director for acting in an irresponsible way against the best interest of patient care and with intent to punish me for opposing the sub custodial strategy of the place that dehumanizes and degrades both residents and workers alike. The grievance goes directly to the state commissioner, Dr. Alan Miller, since he is the "supervisor" of the director. I will ask to be reinstated to my buildings and be allowed to call a parents' meeting to discuss my program recommendations and reorganization plan with them, without administration interference. My hope, naturally, is to build a parent defense group within Building 76, to stand active and ready to block arbitrary and violent practices on the part of the administration and to join in the treatment program for the children.

I do not know if the first round of this action will meet with success, because I am sure that the administration will use every technicality to deflect the essential nature of my challenge. However, I am prepared to carry the matter into the courts and fight through this thing at any level to expose the conditions that we all suffer under. My lawyers have asked if the program which I submitted to the superintendent would be objectively validated within the professional community, and it is in this vein that I am relating this nightmare to you. I have enclosed a copy of the draft Plan that I gave the superintendent. The draft is very crude and proceeded from the assumption that as the building physician responsible for the health of the children, that included jurisdiction over their primary "disease", developmental disability! I did not refine the proposal because of the rapid progress of events and my ouster from the building. I plan to show how at no level in the building is there anyone who knows what mental retardation means and that that attitude flows from the administration, who puts forth the line that if a child is labeled as severely or profoundly retarded, there is only so much you can do for him or her—a self-fulfilling prophesy. I really think I will need your help somewhere along the line.

Devotedly
Bill Bronston, MD.

According to procedure, my grievance would have to be decided by the commissioner, since my supervisor was the director himself. I had luckily found a pro bono fiery and brilliant labor lawyer, Eugene Eisner. I felt he could help forge the legal framework needed to give time and a forum for the confrontation. It was clear that from this point on, there would be no quarter on the issues. Standing up against the bureaucracy meant risking professional destruction, win or lose. The question was whether the department could be forced to face the larger questions of public responsibility and accountability."

My hearing began on October 14, 1971, and was assigned to Dr. Hammond to adjudicate even though he was the object of the grievance. It lasted five days over a six-week period. I was usually on duty those days and would come to the scheduled hearing after making rounds. A hearing officer presided, appointed to represent the commissioner. Dr. Hammond and his administrative assistant, Dr. Milton Jacobs, essentially my functional supervisor, were always present. My wife, Kathleen, had been so close to the situation that my lawyer and I pressed to have her act as co-counsel to the hearing, to help give us some distance and an independent observer's judgment of the proceedings. Hammond sat at one end of the table, fuming that he had to be answerable in the hearing. Jacobs, with his usual giant cigar, sat next to Hammond. My lawyer, Gene, sat next to Jacobs. Kath and I sat at the other end of the table. The hearing officer, who drove from Albany on the hearing days, completed the circle.

Dr. Jacobs, Willowbrook's personnel disciplinarian, was an outgoing sort. Before the hearing began, he shook his head sadly and said, "Bill, you're making a big mistake by going through with this. This is only going to lead to big trouble and a bad end." I wondered if he somehow sensed that things would never be the same. Maybe so, maybe not. It was just a stirring at this point. The administration had never lost when the issue was who had the power to define right and wrong on the job.

In keeping with the civil service grievance procedure, no official transcript of the hearing was kept. My attorney filed a brief afterward to ensure that the commissioner would have the facts as we understood them. I am including here considerable sections of Gene's memorandum. There is little editing, to allow the reader to get a sense of the closeness of the argument and the stubborn resistance of the administration to surrender its essential definition of their power and prerogatives.

Law Offices   EISNER & LEVY   351 Broadway   New York, New York 10013 / WOrth 6-9620

Eugene G. Eisner   Mary M. Kaufman
Richard A. Levy   Counsel

Eisner & Levy
Attorneys for Grievant
351 Broadway
New York, New York 10013
Eugene G. Eisner,
Of Counsel

MEMORANDUM ON BEHALF OF GRIEVANT

This post-hearing memorandum is submitted in support of WILLIAM BRONSTON, M.D. (trained in Pediatrics and Psychiatry), who filed a grievance with the Department of Mental Hygiene on September 2,1971 protesting his reassignment at Willowbrook from physician in Buildings 76 and 77 where young children are housed to Buildings 22 and 23 where older women are housed. The grievance, as filed, alleges that the transfer was punitive in nature. We submit that the facts, as adduced before the Hearing Officer, more than amply support Dr. Bronston's position; hence, the transfer should be rescinded.

ISSUES

We believe the narrow issue to be: "Did Dr. Hammond have just cause to transfer (punish) Dr. Bronston by removing him from Buildings 76 and 77 to Buildings 22 and 22?"

Another way of stating the issue is, "Should a young, competent, and dedicated doctor, who is specifically brought into several buildings which house mentally retarded children, for the ostensible purpose of developing programs of child development in those buildings, be punished by the director of the institution for having made extensive recommendations for the reorganization of the children and staff of the building, which incurs resentment by outspoken attendants and supervisors who oppose any kind of change, especially change which would require greater effort on their part?"

Of course, we believe that under the circumstances Dr. Hammond was not "justified" in transferring Dr. Bronston as we will describe in this memorandum the facts, as elicited at the hearing, demonstrate beyond peradventure of doubt, that the transfer of Dr. Bronston is only a part of a plan by Dr. Hammond and others to punish Dr. Bronston and others who speak out in favor of change. Unfortunately for Dr. Hammond, the scenario he constructed was designed in such a way as to ultimately boomerang on him and expose his administration for what it really is.

THE HEARING

Dr. Hammond contended that the transfer was not punitive but merely a "corrective" action. A large number of witnesses testified at the hearing which was conducted during five (5) separate days, spanning a period of almost six (6) weeks from start to finish. In addition to the protagonists, Drs. Hammond and Bronston, attendants in Building 76 testified, as well as Dr. Milton Jacobs, the Supervising Nurse, and a Nursing Instructor, In addition, Dr. Bronston introduced twenty (20) exhibits and the Administration, four (4).

In summary fashion, we believe that the evidence shows the following:

That Dr. Bronston is a young, dedicated physician whose background and experience has been in the field of pediatrics and child development. That shortly after Dr. Bronston began his employment with Willowbrook, he was sent into Building 76 to develop "programs" for the youngsters there.

That Dr. Hammond deliberately sabotaged Dr. Bronston's status as the Building Physician because he felt that Dr. Bronston was trying, "from the beginning of his employment, to subvert, undermine and disrupt the institution".

That despite Administration' indifference, Dr. Bronston developed a detailed plan for the reorganization of Building 76, calling for, in part, the reactivation of training programs and the transfer of the Supervising Nurse out of the Building.

That Dr. Hammond and Dr. Jacobs never had any intention of implementing that plan or any plan of Dr. Bronston.

That Dr. Hammond and Dr. Jacobs spread the word throughout the institution that the plan was unworkable because it would completely disrupt the staff in Building 76 and because of a lack of funds.

That despite a shortage of funds, Dr. Bronston's plans for reorganization are consonant with the views of the Board of Directors of the National Association for Retarded Children, to wit: "That there are many improvements which can take place and which can and will have a profound effect on the mentally retarded residents which do not require large expenditures of funds."

That Dr. Hammond and Dr. Jacobs did not support or clarify the responsibilities of the Building Physician (.as they should have done) when there was a conflict with the Supervising Nurse with regard to the methods of patient care.

That Dr. Hammond and Dr. Jacobs used the attendants' confusion and allegiance to the Supervising Nurse as a ruse to get Dr. Bronston out of Building 76.

That conditions in all of Willowbrook, according to a study by Dr. Frederic Grunberg, Deputy Commissioner, have deteriorated to the point where there has been a "lowering of morale, restlessness, irritation, increasing insubordination, and what is potentially and explosive situation among the employees of the institution."

That the Administration has embarked on a program of harassment of Dr. Bronston and others to the point where the Administration has suggested to Dr. Bronston that he resign from his employment from Willowbrook.

That Dr. Bronston has no intention of resigning but rather intends to continue the fight to eliminate dehumanization at Willowbrook.

That the future of decent residential care at Willowbrook State School depends, in large measure, upon the decision of the Commissioner to return Dr. Bronston to Buildings 76 and 77 with a mandate for change.

THE EVIDENCE

We respectfully submit that the aforesaid summary of the evidence adduced at the hearing is, in substantial measure, a capsule view of the "case", we do not intend here to repeat in great detail what was already heard and seen by the Hearing Officer. We would, however, point out to the Hearing Officer (and the Commissioner) the following important facts:

Dr. Bronston was hired as a Clinical Physician I on April 15, 1970. The duties of Clinical Physicians include the following New York State Civil Service Specifications:

Supervision of subordinate persons
Diagnosis and treatment of illness and injuries Assignment of patients to subordinates
Conferring with subordinates on diagnosis and treatment programs
Supervision of nursing care

At the time of his first appraisal by a superior (after four (4) months of service), Dr. Bronston was described as "conscientious; performs his duties with zeal; is aware of the patients' needs." In addition, said appraisal urged Dr. Bronston "to maintain his enthusiasm and be aware of the State Manual Policy".

According to the Department of Mental Hygiene's Policy Manual, as separate from "Civil Service" descriptions, describes the responsibilities and duties of a Ward Physician as follows:

Primarily concerned with the welfare of patients...rehabilitative procedures...and in instituting the therapeutic program.

Ward physicians are responsible for the general supervision of ward employees and shall encourage their proper attitude toward patients.

Consult with supervising nurse...as to their competency and conduct. If the employee's services are unsatisfactory, he should be so informed.

Ward physicians supervise patient employment assignments.

Ward physicians review patient assignments at regular intervals to determine possibility of release from the institution.

At Willowbrook, after an initial period in another Building, Dr. Bronston was asked to take responsibility for Building 76 and develop programs there. Within a very short period of time, Dr. Bronston began to analyze the problems in Building 76 and submitted extensive work reports for change.

Following up on those reports, In the summer of 1971, to be exact, Dr. Bronston submitted his "Recommendations for the Reorganization of Building 76" (Exhibit 9) to Dr. Jacobs. According to both Drs. Jacobs and Bronston, they had several conversations regarding the possibilities of implementing Dr. Bronston's creative program during and after Dr. Jacobs' vacation that summer. Significantly, however, Dr. Hammond did not "discuss" this program with Dr. Bronston until one week prior to Dr. Bronston's removal from Building 76 in late August. Moreover, the attendants in Building 76 were not made aware of the contents of Dr. Bronston's proposal until after his transfer out at the end of August.

The failure of the Administration to discuss Dr. Bronston's "program" with the staffs in the respective departments in which Dr. Bronston was recommending change (e.g., Occupational Therapy, Recreation, Speech and Hearing, etc.) until after his transfer and even then with apparent mockery, is, in our view, a severe indictment of the Administration.

Another mistake in the Administration's scenario, which was designed to bring Dr. Bronston into disrepute with the Building staff, was its public failure to advise the attendants in Building 76 as to the full extent of Dr. Bronston's authority. A cursory reference to the Department's job descriptions alone could have resolved the conflict. The entire "crisis", which was created around the Supervising Nurse, was created and manipulated by the Administration.

Shortly after Dr. Bronston filed his complaints with the Administration against the Building Supervising Nurse on August 19, 1971 (including failure to follow doctor's orders; failure to assume minimal responsibilities with her staff; indifference and inefficiency, etc.), the Building staff was demanding to know "who was boss" in the building and telling Drs. Hammond and Jacobs "either the nurse goes or Bronston goes" because "the tension was too great". In the words of one Administration witness, the meeting with Dr. Hammond (which resulted in a vote of "no confidence" in Dr. Bronston) was demanded by the Building 76 staff because "we wanted to find out whose orders to listen to". Or as the supervising nurse herself testified, "The meeting was called because there was too much confusion and tension—the attendants didn't know who to listen to."

How did Dr. Hammond handle the developing conflict and tension at that meeting? Well, according to the Supervising Building Nurse, Dr. Hammond, in full view of all the attendants, "reassured me that I was running the building". Dr. Hammond also "reassured the attendants that they would not lose their jobs". Who said anything about attendants losing their jobs? Certainly not Dr. Bronston!! Who started the "rumors that were flying around the building that Bronston was going to transfer people out"? Who spread them around, who permitted the attendants to believe the untrue rumors and who advised them that he would not permit that sort of thing? Dr. Hammond, of course!!

The rest of the "story" is now history; Dr. Hammond "reluctantly" succumbed to the "overwhelming demand" of some "clique" workers and transferred Dr. Bronston out of Building 76. The reason why he did it? Well, in addition to responding to an alleged ultimatum given by Dr. Bronston, "Either the Supervising Nurse goes or I go". Compare this answer with Dr. Hammond's testimony in which he said he merely "listened" to the attendants complaints and "would see what

I could do". (compare with Drs. Jacobs' and Bronston's version, "If you don't get the Supervising Nurse out, I'll prefer charges".), Dr. Hammond stated that he wanted to maintain discipline and programming in the building. What discipline and what programming? They are virtually nonexistent in Building 76, as well as elsewhere at Willowbrook! (See testimony of former nursing employee who stated that the Supervising Nurse exercised no leadership in the building because she was so terrorized by a few of the workers). Besides, as all of the Administration witnesses testified, "Dr. Bronston's programs are a waste of time. All of the kids have peaked out; there is nothing further you can do for them."

Can this possibly be true? Dr. Bronston, for one, does not think so. We trust that the Department of Mental Hygiene does not think so either. If there is any hope whatsoever for the future of decent residential care for those at Willowbrook, we urge that Dr. Bronston be returned forthwith to Buildings 76 and 77. We further urge that his return be accompanied by a mandate for change, including the removal of the Supervising Nurse from the building, together with as much implementation of his "recommendations" as is humanly possible.

Finally, we urge that the Administration be directed to cease and desist from its harassment of Dr. Bronston and others who dare to be critical of the Administration. Specifically, we request that the Administration be restrained from imposing an "excessive work load" upon Dr. Bronston; further, that the Administration be directed to lift its ridiculous prohibition against Dr. Bronston and others from meeting with parents on the grounds of Willowbrook. It is high time that the Administration be held accountable to responsible members of the staff who dare to be innovative and to the community at large. We urge that you act before it is too late.

Respectfully submitted,
EISNER & LEVY Attorneys for Grievant
351 Broadway New York, New York
10013 Eugene G. Eisner,
Of Counsel

We waited then. It was my belief despite overwhelming evidence of the collusion by the administration that the commissioner simply could not rule against his superintendent. If they let my grievance stand, based as it was on the interests of the residents, the absolute power doctrine of the superintendent would be breached for any worker to raise similar contests. I knew that the bureaucracy just couldn't let that happen. I knew it before we started. However, we were obligated to adhere to the grievance mechanism to first "exhaust legal remedies" before we could seek public redress in court outside the civil service system.

Gene remained confident. His comfort with legal procedure and experience with protracted battles in the past annoyed me. I was impatient and felt his position was too pat. I understood we would appeal to higher bodies when the commissioner did the logical thing to defend the department. Our trump card would be the leap from the bureaucracy's grievance machine, with its appointed judges, to a public court. There the issues would be properly recorded and dealt with in a more legally sophisticated and due process way.

Even though I discounted the likely ruling in the hearing, Gene's confidence that we could succeed there made me experience a sense of suspense. Maybe, just maybe, they would concede, fearful of our next steps. I desperately wanted to get back to the children in Building 76 who I was fighting to serve and had come to miss terribly. I had many friends in the building who kept calling me about the children replaced on massive tranquilizer doses after I had stopped that abuse. Two of our boys died of illnesses that went undetected until it was too late.

I had played our cards and was powerless to do anything to help directly in my old buildings. All that was left was to bury myself in my new assignment and hurt. I was hardening. My anger was changing me. Something inside me was turning to steel. I calculated more carefully, watched everything more scrupulously. I was ever so much more vulnerable, as the workload in adult women's Buildings 22 and 23, my new assignment, was impossible. This struggle might last a long time, much longer than I cared to think. I had to settle in and intensify the education of my new ward coworkers and a whole new group of parents and family members.

Gene was but a phone call away. Just knowing that, that there was real support very close, helped more than I could say. We didn't count how many times daily he had to listen to me rant and rave on the phone so that I could keep my cool at work and lighten the burden I placed on Kathleen when I got home.

On February 16, four months after the hearing had begun, the commissioner made his decision. A letter came to my home. I read it without feeling. I understood the department so well. Their pulse, their brain, and their instincts had become as familiar to me as the simplest disease I had learned in medical school.

Form 26-D.M.H.

ALAN D. MILLER, M.D.
COMMISSIONER

WILLIAM VOORHEES, M.D.
FIRST DEPUTY COMMISSIONER

ROBERT PATTON
SECOND DEPUTY COMMISSIONER

STATE OF NEW YORK
DEPARTMENT OF MENTAL HYGIENE
DIVISION OF MENTAL RETARDATION
AND CHILDREN'S SERVICES
NEW YORK CITY METROPOLITAN REGIONAL OFFICE
2 WORLD TRADE CENTER, 56TH FLOOR
NEW YORK, N. Y. 10048

ROBERT W. HAYES, M.P.
DEPUTY COMMISSIONER
FOR MENTAL RETARDATION
AND CHILDREN'S SERVICES

SIDNEY LECKER, M.D.
ASSISTANT COMMISSIONER
FOR CHILDREN'S SERVICES

February 16, 1972

Dr. William Bronston
168 Cebra Avenue
Staten Island, New York 10314

Dear Dr. Bronston:

In accordance with the provisions of the grievance procedure for employees of the Department of Mental Hygiene, a third step review of your grievance was conducted on five separate days during the period October 14, 1971 to December 7, 1971 on the premises of Willowbrook State School. You were represented in these proceedings by Mr. Eugene C. Eisner, an attorney.

You are aggrieved because the Director of Willowbrook State School relieved you of responsibility as Clinical Physician for Buildings 76 and 77 and assigned you to serve as Clinical Physician in Buildings 22 and 23. You allege that your relief and reassignment was unjustified and punitive in nature, and you have demanded that you be returned to the performance of your former duties in Buildings 76 and 77.

You and your attorney sought to demonstrate by submission of documents as evidence and by testimony of yourself and others that you were and are a highly competent physician with a deep understanding of the nature of mental retardation, that you were capable of devising plans and programs, which, if implemented, would materially aid and improve the condition of the retarded children in your care, and that your efforts to bring about much needed program improvements were thwarted by uncooperative employees over whom you had little control and ultimately by the Director who changed your assignment.

The Director and others who spoke on behalf of the management of Willowbrook State School raised no question about your professional competence but indicated that your potential for making an important contribution to the care and treatment of mentally retarded persons had been seriously impaired by your inability or unwillingness to develop cooperative and constructive relationships with your colleagues and fellow employees, that you have, in fact, by your remarks, attitude and behavior, caused tension, confusion, and division among the employees in Buildings 76 and 77 and that you have caused or permitted an atmosphere to be created in those buildings that is not conducive to effective treatment and care.

I have made a careful review of the material submitted on your behalf and on behalf of the institution and have analyzed the reviewing officers' reports of the testimony offered during the review by representatives of both, sides of the issue. It is my conclusion that Dr. Hammond believed he was faced with the prospect of a complete breakdown in the processes of providing minimal care to the children in Buildings 76 and 77 as the result of open conflict between yourself and key members of the staff, that you had failed to demonstrate awareness that you, yourself, might be part of the overall problem, and that no other acceptable course was open to him but to remove you from further contact with Buildings 76 and 77. It is my determination therefore that, Dr. Hammond's action in removing you from a position of responsibility in Buildings 76 and 77 was reasonable and prudent and was taken to protect the interests and welfare of the residents of these buildings. I am not convinced that the Director's action in reassigning you was punitive, as you have alleged, for the reason that procedures prescribed by law for the application of disciplinary penalties were and are available to him for that purpose.

In the event you wish to appeal my determination, you may do so by contacting the Grievance Appeals Board, Office of Employee Relations, the State Capitol, Albany, New York.

Sincerely yours,
Alan D. Miller, M.D.Commissioner
cc:
Mr. Eisner
Dr. Hammond

CHAPTER 11

The Parent Ultimatum

I HAD BEEN EXILED to a darkest adult women's building chamber, ripped from Building 76, where the struggle went on unabated. In Building 76, I had invested diligent work and care into nurturing the parent community as the key possible stakeholders for change. Willowbrook's in-house parent body the Benevolent Society's approach had always been "get whatever you can." The new approach must be built on a sense that people had rights. All the residents had been continually and unnecessarily injured by their institutional stay. Families all described to me the inexorable decline of ability in their sons and daughters after their institutionalization. "She used to talk when she came." "She was toilet-trained and could eat with silverware." "Now I can't take her to a restaurant." "He just was blind one day." "They just told me he couldn't see and didn't explain why." "I'm afraid to come." "I don't know what I'll find next." "It terrifies me." Without exception, the mountainous data pointed to the fact that the institution caused mental retardation.

The parents had simply never been told that it didn't have to be this way. It was not their fault if New York State refused to provide them with modern and progressive services. No, they were not bad parents, ignorant, or inherently powerless. The parents' questions naturally became "What can we do?" "Doctor, you're the only one that ever told me these things. What about the other parents?" "We've gone to the director each time Martha had a cut or bruise on her, and he said he would look into it." "If we didn't like the situation, we could always take her home." "We wrote and wrote and never got an answer."

My reply was always "Get together with other families. Talk with each other. See what is common between you. Go onto the wards each time you come, instead of waiting in the hallway. Check the bathrooms, linen, and clothes areas. Look at the food, not in relief and gratitude, or numbly, but as change agents. You are paying taxes. Some of you are paying fees. Don't feel the state is doing you a favor—you're paying them. They have a sacred obligation to serve you in the best way. That's the agreement between the public and the government. It doesn't have to be the way it is!"

The parents wanted me to do something. They would say, "What happens if you leave? Won't the administration get rid of you for telling us these things? Then things will be back to the old way." There was a great temptation to play God, to join with them in the worry of what would happen if

I weren't there. All would be lost unless the parents truly organized, developed their own political understanding, and found new outspoken militant leaders.

Months and months of such counseling, discussion, and struggle went by. There was something keeping the new ideas and the parents' new sense of themselves from being converted into action. It had its roots in their timidity and lack of confidence. Some held back, feeling that their tragedies were a private experience, unique. Many feared failure at such a huge undertaking that might renew their already encrusted sense of inadequacy. But most of all, I think deepest of all, the families experienced the sense that their sons and daughters were really too damaged—and what alternatives were there? "What should we ask for?" "What is right?" "Joseph could never come home. We could never care for him." "Patricia couldn't ever work. She's too retarded." "Doctor, can you really expect Samuel to change? He's thirty-two and has been here twenty years!"

At the heart of the parents' inaction and doubt was the profound schism between the gut experience of being a parent of a devalued person and their head sense of what was right to do. The abiding instinct to hold, protect, and preserve that special person is deeply buried and very powerful. These parents were a ball of pain, sadness, tenderness, hatred, and frustration all wrapped together, yearning for normalcy, to do what is right, to feel parenthood, when that is brutally denied by society and the professional community's perverse advice. The families, more often than not, pursued a driven course. They relied on feeling, hoping against hope they had done the best thing over the years. The parents' primitive instincts of love and protection obscured their consciousness of their new dignity of taking risks and making decisions about what was civilly and socially rightful.

I do not mean to cast the blame on the victims. The choices available to the families of institutionalized people are disastrous, ruinous, and dehumanizing. Yet, they are masqueraded as absolutes and as reasonable and appropriate. I'm trying to touch something that puzzled me—the conflict that I saw the parents' experience as their awareness grew of alternatives to custodial institutionalization. It forced me to continually reexamine my role as a clinician and also as a parent with children of my own. Even though I knew why the residents were deteriorating before my eyes—that high-level political, economic, and social factors were at the root—I wanted something done! Now! I couldn't stand by, witnessing the daily deprivation, barrenness, and violence. Often, I invested energy that might have been used for systemic changes in trade for risks that could achieve some immediate relief for a person.

I understood why the parents hesitated, shrank from the investment in a different kind of future for their sons and daughters. They were wracked with the issue of survival today for their loved ones. They were parents, and they cared more than can ever be set forth in words. Their sacrifice, what they each endured watching their child changing into an animal state but fearing it could be worse if they spoke up, can never be fully documented. The psychological cost to every family led to tension, illness, breakup, drinking, withdrawal, and all those things that traditional researchers seem to link with some internal weakness in families with "handicapped" members. Their self-awareness are the consequences of second-class citizenship and the acceptance of the institution as responsible and right.

I tried to somehow transmit my insights to the parents, to fuse with their deepest instincts and basic energy. I discovered how to do this day by day, through trial and error, searching for the unique connection, in each family, between their fierce protectiveness, their drive for privacy for their son or daughter, and their capacity to share and join with other families to organize for protection as a matter of right and principle.

What should be made clear is that the experiences of the parents and families of kids and adults with disabilities are not necessarily unique to them. There are universal parallels between these parents and all parents. At any time an altercation might arise in any schoolroom, wherein a child might be punished or unfairly excluded, should the principal or teacher who may have committed such an offense be contacted? What are the risks of doing nothing or of intervening on behalf of a child? What if a relative is in an institution for the elderly who is abused in some way by a welfare department? These dilemmas about whether to act or to remain silent grip us all when special problems or special needs arise in our lives. The family-or friendship-based challenge to become entangled in an adversarial situation with the system is greatly magnified in the case of the institution families. The hesitations, the doubt, and the fear that action can only bring more trouble are the bindings that all people experience but rarely share. There is a social basis for sane and moral human service practice, accountability, and relevance to the people. This is the struggle for every human service worker to be open to identifying with the people he or she serves, sense the depth and pace of growth in the family's awareness, and grow alongside.

The job at Willowbrook was to help the parents avert entrapment. This had to be done by raising their consciousness and understanding so that they would no longer mistakenly embrace the institution as a symbol of security and relief, so that they would no longer accept the label of "mental retardation" as an irrevocable sentence upon liberty for their sons or daughters. They were wholly innocent of how such concessions and surrenders of their citizen powers resulted in massive institutional abuses. Connecting the instinct for protection with a knowledge of—and equal instinct for— rights and growth is a learned phenomenon.

Finally, in late 1971 and on into 1972, a basic change began to come about in the Benevolent Society membership. The parents were gradually igniting to protest.

These parents were not usually old members, and it was predictable that a confrontation between the old and the new ways would arise. The monthly meetings of the Benevolent began to overflow with two hundred, three hundred people. Resolutions came from the floor and were voted in by the new parent activists. The old board was voiceless. The realization of an impending fight that meant something, one that defined enemies who were real enemies, drew out parents whom the old guard had painted as apathetic and non-caring.

Parents organized in three buildings in which Mike Wilkins and I had provided support and encouragement. They demanded the administration account for itself first-hand. The dam was broken, never to be sealed tight again by intimidation, false promises, and contempt. The entrenched circle of administrative leaders at Willowbrook couldn't cover their priorities of social control and tradition in the face of the parent demands for accountability and human service.

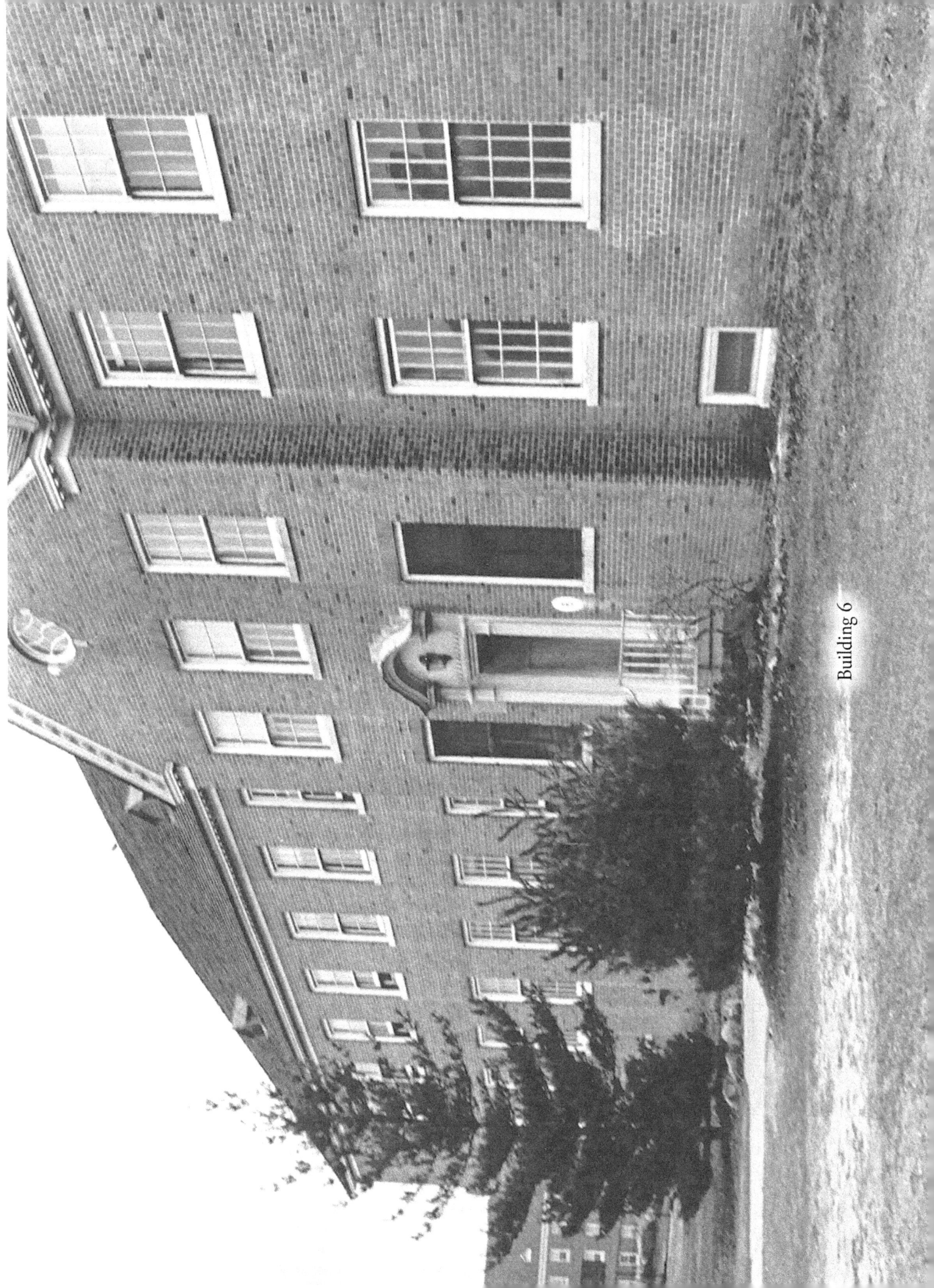

Building 6

Mike, an outstanding physician, took great pride in his clinical skills, which he loved and studied to improve. Mike made friends with just everybody. More importantly, he had time for everyone, no matter how small the need. He delighted in helping people in every way. He loved being a fine doctor and took extraordinary care of the people in his all men and boys buildings, 6 and 8. Like me, Mike was an organizer at heart and an astute political theorist who had long been active in supporting progressive causes. He was from Missouri and spoke plainly in a country way. All this was enough to get him on the bad side of the Willowbrook administration. Mike hated filth, the abuse of medical care, the violence, and the racism at Willowbrook. He turned to his ward workers and the parents, as I did, for support and helped them understand what was wrong and why.

Liz Lee was the social worker assigned to his buildings. Energetic and equally offended by the conditions, she spent her time with the families, counting on Mike to provide the needed information to help her counsel the parents about how to contribute to the program needs of their children. It was only natural, though calculated, that they began to encourage meetings of the families in their buildings and to support the just anger and demands of the parents. Both Mike and Liz had lived in Staten Island for a number of years and had been heavily involved in civic affairs. They were both well-known and trusted for their judgment and integrity. As the parent meetings progressed and conditions in the institution deteriorated, the situation could not help but spill out into the community.

Jane Kurtin, a diligent and skilled journalist for the *Staten Island Advance*, who knew us all, sensed the magnitude of the drama and began to probe the Willowbrook situation. We had been working with Jane as we organized parent groups in the community by sponsoring educational forums with well-known speakers to improve services for children labeled mentally retarded. Our strategy was to create settings where the various competitive and irascible little parent groups in the county would concede to gather together with the Willowbrook parents, and put their major anti-institutional and minor differences aside, to mobilize in solidarity.

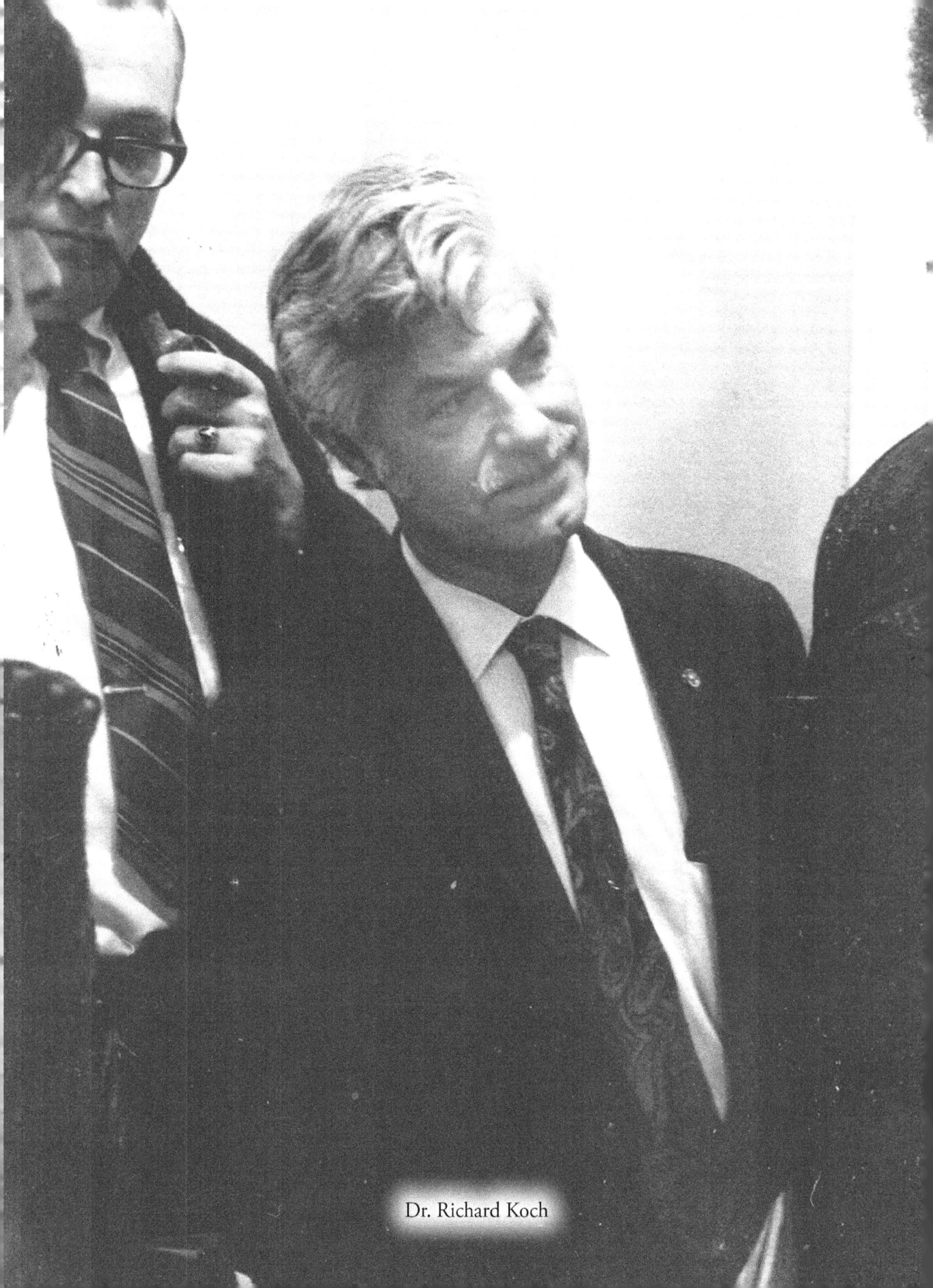

Dr. Richard Koch

An enormous assembly was held at the local community college when I invited Dr. Richard Koch to come from California to speak. His topic, chosen by the parent organizations, was "Institutions: Yes or No." Mike and I toured Dick through Willowbrook before his talk, and Jane came along. It was her first in-person look, as the administration was constantly on guard against a recurrence of earlier media exposés, even though nothing drastic had ever developed from them. Dick's visit to Willowbrook was Jane's first chance to see for herself how things really were. What she saw opened the door wide, and in November of 1971, Jane mounted a series of articles that were printed on the *Advance*'s front page about what she had learned and seen. The combination of the parent mobilization in the institution and the community, the newspaper stories, the confrontation around Building 76, and the hearings—all had humbled Dr. Hammond. The loss of control and the humiliation that Hammond experienced in being locked in place by Albany clearly pushed the man beyond his capacity to rationally cope.

Mike was still not a permanent employee, as the job freeze had halted his final tenured appointment. On January 5, 1972, Dr. Hammond took advantage of this vulnerability and issued a memo terminating both Mike and Liz, refusing to give any reason. He undoubtedly hoped to relieve his misery. The drive to get the pair rehired became a rallying focus to which all other issues were attached. Never had parents spoken up so strongly, so convinced that this was the last straw! It was significant that the drive was not on behalf of their sons and daughters directly. It still made more sense to them to respond emotionally and politically to the fact that two good people had been taken away from them. It was not a sustained conviction that a battle had to be waged each and every day to open more opportunities, insist on more accountability, and create the social conditions that would transform their children into respected citizens. This level of consciousness still remained on the agenda for the future. The parents' movement was naturally aimed at reforming Willowbrook, to make it a better place. The idea, the paradigm shift that the whole system of institutionalization and dehumanization was the brute to be swept aside, rather than individual bureaucrats and politicians, had not yet been internalized.

Maybe the most important observation that could be made was that even the most militant parents still somehow felt that the solution rested with some responsive individual in the department, or with the governor. If the governor would just come to Willowbrook to see the inhumanity. But the governor sat somewhere, remote and imperial as the city of Albany, never setting foot on the grounds of Willowbrook to see what his state policy had done to the people. This governor who was responsible for the deaths of his own guards and prisoners at Attica State Prison earlier in the year.

The parents could not yet see that change would come from their power, independent of the bureaucracy's tiny yields. This deep and traditional trust of the state and its "respectable" leaders still persists and persists, denying the virtue of the multitudes. And yet, the parent organization, the Benevolent Society for Retarded Children, Willowbrook Chapter, after two decades of humiliation and manipulation by the state, rose out of its timidity, depression, and agony. It was the end for the unchallenged old way. Events followed one on another, and the house of cards built by the department's arrogance, pseudoscience, and secrecy began to collapse.

Reprinted from the **Staten Island Advance**

Willowbrook: Inside the cages

By JANE KURTIN

The boys in building 5 pick at the sores on their naked bodies during the endless days they spend on wooden benches, curled on the floor or leaning against the alls of their ward.

They don't understand the indignity of being perpetually naked or the repulsiveness of their drooling. They don't understand that people are afraid to tough them.

Showers are given communally in open stalls. Beds are jammed into massive rooms and stand not more than 12 inches apart. If these severely retarded boys have any are not visible — only row upon row of institutional white iron beds.

Called for lunch, the 60 or so young men responded at one. In a single, chaotic wave, they used for the door which would open and eventually lead to food.

Some, crying and screaming for reasons not easily understood, tried to push their way past one of the three attendants who watched over them. Some who slipped to the floor, began to crawl out.

The attendant, a pleasant woman, stamped her feet at the doorway and shouted to the boys on the floor to get back.

Whatever the boy in Building 6 might learn, employees explained, has to come to them from normal persons. But the normal persons aren't rushing into Willowbrook State School to help and the employees can't.

One case of a young man we'll call Alan, who created problems for already overtaxed employees was told by a member of the professional staff this way: "Alan's record shows that for quite a while before he was put in seclusion he was having problems in school. The significant thing about this is that he was in school and of an IQ which deemed him educable.

"Eventually, Alan bit one of the female attendants who couldn't handle him, and in May of 1969 he was put in seclusion.

"In January of this year a letter was sent to James J. Murphy, deputy director here at Willowbrook, from another ranking official in the institution.

"The letter informed Murphy that Alan had been i seclusion for over a year and his condition had deteriorated drastically because of his isolation.

"Murphy was apprised of the fact that Alan ate, slept, urinated and defecated in one room and that he should have been transferred to another building where attendants would be able to deal with him.

"Eventually, after a long struggle, Alan was out for about a month. He's back in seclusion, however, because he scratched and attendant. He's 21 and no longer considered educable.

"The terrible thing is that he was not destructive in school and if he'd gotten help with the problems he had then, all of this could have been prevented."

Say retarded children being neglected

November 15, 1971

Parents protest cutbacks at state school

By JANE KURTIN

While about 100 of their parents marched outside and protested crippling budge cuts, severely retarded patients in Willowbrook state school spent yesterday in darkened, barren rooms, wailing at the concrete walls that mark the boundary of their world.

Some, half-naked, huddled in corners or behind a very few open doors. Others wandered aimlessly, flailing their arms, or sat rocking quietly in plastic chairs.

For parents who have been visiting their retarded children at Willowbrook for dozens of years, it is not the sight of distorted faces or pathetic deafening cries that shock the senses.

For those people — who long ago faced the tragedy of their children's retardation — it

is the apparent level of neglect at the school which encouraged a march.

Asking that their names be withheld, parents described scenes where children were marched into a dining hall, naked, and marched out again minutes later with only the food that they could grab from the tables clenched in their hands.

Those adults who regularly bring their children home on weekends explained that they are always extremely hungry and thirsty when they arrive and that the first hours together are devoted almost entirely to eating.

One woman, whose son was transferred to Willow brook three months ago, said that he has lost 20 pounds since his arrival at the institution.

In one ward, a visitor was greeted by women patients who rushed frantically to be able to

say hello, make conversation and be hugged.

"These people," and employee at the school said, "are in desperate need of contact. Many of them don't belong here and could, if they received intensive training, go back into society.

"Because of the staff shortage," the employee continued, "they are lumped together and receive no programming. They regress terribly."

Diseases, a member of the medical staff claimed, ran rampant throughout the institution and cannot be effectively controlled because of the severe overcrowding.

"This place is like the Congo," a doctor claimed. "We have sickness here that you just don't find anymore in the civilized world."

A visitor yesterday saw a bleak, empty room which, ac-

cording to employee, was until recently occupied by a woman kept there in solitary confinement "for three years."

Because of the already insurmountable problems of dealing with residents, and employee commented, "rebellious or individualistic patients are punished by isolation."

With no staff to handle them, problem cases are sometimes confined in these empty rooms for years with nothing more than a mattress, the employee claimed.

Dr. Hammond gave the current hospital patient census as 5,200. The institution's capacity, according to state standards, is 4,500.

The anger and frustration of the parent who carried placards yesterday at Willowbrook is not directed at the attendants in the school, they said.

"They do what they can" a father commented, "but it's like a drop in the bucket.

One man observed, "The animals at the Staten Island Zoo have more space and get better care than the children at Willowbrook."

"We have to decided," and employee said, "if the people here are going to be treated like nothing more than protein garbage or human beings."

Two women were arrested yesterday and accused of blocking traffic at the parent's demonstration. The received summonses after police say they refused and order to move from the middle of Victory Blvd. in front of the institution.

At their next regular meeting, January 24, 1972, a list of grievances was set forth from the Benevolent families. It was circulated to all the members as an official document and was formally presented as well to the department officialdom. Following the drafting of the list, the members of the Benevolent recorded a vote of no confidence in the Willowbrook administration. The governor and his appointed commissioner of Mental Hygiene for the Empire State were clearly identified as the source of the problem—and thus, the potential source of the solution. This put them both at the apex of the situation.

CHAPTER 12

The Conspiracy

THE FIRING OF WILKINS and Lee instantly became a cause célèbre for parents and concerned citizens in New York. The administration must now make a move to protect itself and to retake the initiative. Both Mike and Liz had been exemplary workers. They had brought about significant improvements in Building 6, a building packed with young, adult men whose lot was wretched beyond belief. Under fire from parents, the local press, and the public, Dr. Hammond had reacted by lashing out against Mike and Liz, whom he perceived as the cause of his torment. Mike called Geraldo Rivera at WABC-TV to discuss the situation with him. Geraldo had been a lawyer and a friend of ours before turning to his Channel 7 *Eyewitness News* role on TV. As a television reporter, he began to focus the glaring light of publicity into the murky corners of Willowbrook, visiting unannounced, repeatedly, with his camera crew.

The month that followed could only be described as a melee. Even the old guard of the Benevolent Society could not condone Hammond's action in the firings. The parent outrage grew as the full weight of the ABC TV penetration continued. The night of January 27, after considerable back-and-forth communication, two meetings were held. The first involved Dr. Miller, Dr. Grunberg (the deputy commissioner over all mental retardation and children's services in New York), Harold Wolfe (the public relations officer for the department), and Edward Jennings (a liaison person for the department). The Benevolent leadership had made a firm demand to "rehire Mike and Liz, or else…" The president of the Benevolent, Tony Pinto, and four other officers attended the meeting, held at the department's commissioner's offices in Lower Manhattan. It seemed endless. The parents relentlessly pushed their demand, while the department chiefs searched for a way out without losing face.

BENEVOLENT SOCIETY FOR RETARDED CHILDREN

Non-Profit   Non-Sectarian   Voluntary   Tax Exempt

Willowbrook Chapter of the New York State A.R.C., Inc.
1150 Forest Hill Road
Bldg., "L"
Staten Island, N.Y. 10314
Telephone (718)-983-5204

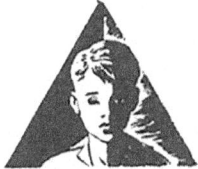

A Non-Profit Tax Exempt
Organization of parents
and advocates to help all
individuals who are men-
tally retarded, wherever
they are, regardless of
color, creed or age.

January 11, ~~1974~~ 1972,

Dear Dr. Hammond

     I am submitting in writing the non-negotiable demands presented to you orally by the Executive Committee of the Benevolent Society for Retarded Children...Their implementation must be expedited without delay to bring some measure of relief to Willowbrook State School.

     Conditions at Willowbrook State School continue to deteriorate with no committed relief in sight. Recent TV and news coverage has focused on these appalling conditions affecting the residents and the staff. Despite the critical understaffing, employees have been removed without charges, ie. the removal of Dr. Michael Wilkins and Mrs. Elizabeth Lee of the Social Service Department.

     1. Demand the immediate reinstatement of Dr. Wilkins and Mrs. Lee to full working status at Willowbrook State School.

     2. Demand written charges, if any.

     3. In the absence of formal written charges, the status of Dr. Wilkins and Mrs. Lee become that of permanent employees with tenure.

     4. In the event there are formal written charges, an open hearing before an independent panel, eg. The American Arbitration Assn., with parent participation.

     5. No further suspensions or firings of Social Services Dept. or of Physicians without written charges to the employees and B.S.R.C., with charges made public to all parents, and the opportunity for open hearings by an independent panel, including parents.

     6. Recognize the right of active parent participation in developing administrative policy and implementing the care of residents at Willowbrook State School.

     7. We demand the immediate revocation of all directives to any and all personnel restraining contacts of any kind with parents, both individually as well as in groups.

     8. We demand a formal policy statement supporting full contacts among ~~between~~ parents, staff, administration, and residents.

     9. We demand a declaration of Willowbrook State School as a "Disaster Area" and request Federal and State emergency funds and assistance by the Dept. of Mental Hygiene.

     10. We demand the lift of the budget freeze together with the replacement of all lost personnel to the December 1970 levels.

     11. Stop all admissions to Willowbrook State Schook, which is already over its maximum census.

     Copies of this document ~~were~~ have been sent to Dr. Alan Miller and Governor Rockefeller. A motion from the floor of the Benevolent has demanded that the Benevolent Executive Committee inform Dr. Hammond that if these basic demands have not been met, ~~that~~ a vote will be taken at the January 24th meeting to declare Dr. Hammond no longer the recognized Director of Willowbrook State School.

The Statewide Federation of Parents of Patients in New York State Institutions, another important parent organization, has called for a thorough Federal investigation of Willowbrook and the other New York State Schools, the removal of the State School System from the Department of Mental Hygiene, an immediate creation of a State Commission excluding Department of Mental Hygiene to study the entire problem of services for the Handicapped with recommendations patterned after the California plan within 6 months. Locally, the Federation has staked itself on the reinstatement of Dr. Wilkins and Mrs. Lee declaring that no Director or the State Department of Mental Hygiene can again usurp sole power to make unilateral decisions related to the vital interests of parents, relatives, and residents of the institutions in New York State.

Rehiring Mike and Liz meant admitting a mistake and conceding accountability to the parent community. But, over the table that night, there was no way out. The parents had demanded that Dr. Hammond and others in his top administration be removed. The compromise that was finally struck was that the commissioner would call Hammond and gracefully rehire the fired pair. In exchange, the parents would suspend the demand to clean house, on the department's word that the situation would be rectified at a later date. At 3:00 a.m., the session ended. A statement was jointly drafted by Miller and Pinto, to be released to the press. Once printed, it became a legal public agreement.

Unknown to the parents, a second meeting was being held in the home of Jack Hammond. Equally tense and late, there gathered a circle of people including the key administrators; the leaders of the two employee unions (CSEA and IUA); several Willowbrook churchmen who had, throughout, stayed staunchly loyal to the administration; and some major politicians from Staten Island. Most astounding of all, a fact linked to at least one Island politician, the FBI had become heavily involved in a collaborative attempt to discredit Mike and me rather than allow the issues to be centered on the quality of care provided by the state. Early that morning, Jennings (the department's liaison man) traveled from the Benevolent meeting to Dr. Hammond's home to inform Hammond of the commissioner's agreement. It was grave news, news that the people in that living room could not tolerate. The fact that the parents would demand the rehiring of the fired workers from Dr. Miller had been well-known. Whether he would concede had not been known. What transpired then became evident later that morning

At about 9:00 a.m. that morning, Pinto and Wilkins arrived at Willowbrook to meet with Dr. Hammond, as they understood was the implementation of the agreement for the previous night. Unbeknownst to any of us, the FBI had made periodic visits to the administration followed by their provision of assistance in planning how to handle press coverage and the provocations that had since received widespread exposure in protest struggles.

When the two men entered the Administration Building, they were met by pandemonium. Employees were swarming throughout the building in a state of hysteria. Each building had received a call from the secretaries of the administrators to say that Dr. Hammond was being held "captive" in Administration Building 1 by Mike and me. The parents allegedly had taken over, and Hammond was to be fired; supervisors would be next. The workers were instructed to come and defend Hammond!

Coming as it did from the Administration Building, the message was crystal clear, and the old-timers responded in force. Dr. Hammond was nowhere to be seen. The two unions, through their leaders with outside help, were circulating hundreds of a mimeographed three-page anonymous denunciation of Mike and me as "sinister subversives" who were plotting to seize the institution and purge all loyal employees. The stapled unsigned hate sheets were everywhere. The supervisors were in frenzy, and their mood was being orchestrated by their trusted leaders and second-echelon administrators who feared that if Hammond went, they would surely not survive.

The situation was dangerous. Pinto and Wilkins were physically wedged in and menaced by the throng. Despite their efforts to explain what had in fact happened, they were shouted down and forced to leave. The local press had been alerted and given the story that despite the agreement to rehire Wilkins and Lee, the workers of Willowbrook were solidly against it and would continue their protest until assurances had been secured that Dr. Hammond was firmly in control. From nowhere, a line of Willowbrook buses drove up, and the demonstration leaders announced that all were to drive to Albany and demonstrate against the commissioner's decision to "fire Hammond." Virtually every supervisor on duty, fearing for his or her job, with visions of waves of irate parents descending on their sanctuary demanding redress, got into the buses and left. No provision was made for ward coverage. Hammond, clearly part of the staged revolt, was cloistered in his home.

Who had obtained the buses? Who had organized this "spontaneous" walkout? Who had authorized that the hate sheets be printed in the Administration Building and collated by telephone operators under the eye of the chief secretarial supervisor? Who had given the top administrators' own secretaries the order to call workers off the job to "save the situation"? None of these questions were asked. In fact, the whole affair went like clockwork. It is almost inconceivable that such an event could have occurred if it had been the ward workers walking off the job, demanding an end to their desperate job conditions, and mobilizing their forces. Had the sanction come from their midst, scores would have been disciplined or worse. The event would have been one of extended administrative reprisals, with the supervisors standing against the challenge. Here the situation was reversed. All the supervisors and loyal employees left their stations without question from the administration about what was happening back on the wards. The administration's reaction had just begun. A climate of chaos was to be fueled to the bursting point.

The following day, hundreds of the contrived three-page, stapled hate sheets were reprinted, again anonymously, under the chief secretary's management, and again the telephone operators collated the piles. This time the piles were picked up by the three Willowbrook churchmen and top administrators and carried into the community to try to arouse the sentiments of Staten Island against the threat to plunge the county into "revolution"!

On February 1, the administration made their next move. This time with practiced confidence, the Building 1 executives informed each building supervisor that a mandatory meeting would be held for all employees in the Willowbrook auditorium. The workers were ordered to attend. The head of the education department, in an absolutely unprecedented move, canceled all classes and ordered all teachers to attend. At the meeting, onstage was the recently elected head of the Physicians Association, Dr. William Frew. With him were the institution's rabbi, the Protestant chaplain, a Catholic priest, and three workers from Building 76 who had been used by the director to help in my ouster. Coincidentally, I was off duty and unaware of the meeting. As the hundreds of workers filed in, completely in the dark as to why they had been mustered, they were surrounded by scores of supervisors who lined the auditorium walls with placards which read, bronston and wilkins out, fire em both, better dead than red, wilkins—no!

The program began. Passionately, Dr. Frew called on the workers to line up with the administration and demand an affirmation of "the Willowbrook way" with Dr. Hammond at the wheel—Hammond, the best director they ever had. Each of the spokespersons followed suit, amid the support of the standard-bearers in the auditorium. The workers were baffled and cowed by the forcefulness and by the show of authority before them.

As precisely as it had begun, the event ended, and the workers were sent back to their wards without an opportunity to raise a question. The administration had exercised its maximum political strength. If they couldn't win the disgusted workers over, at least they would make it clear that to dissent was an immensely risky business. Who would refute Frew or the churchmen or the women workers who screamed racism against the two white doctors? So went the administration's thinking and their plan.

However, the afternoon shift meeting did not go smoothly. Even the most dedicated Willowbrook professionals went home at four o'clock. Why should it be any different this day? They held power. The morning shift meeting went without a hitch. Thus, the scenario was shifted, with Frew and the other chiefs leaving the job to their subordinates to recreate the morning's success.

Again, the PM shift workers were summoned to attend the assembly in the auditorium. The placards were still about the walls. This time, the three women from Building 76 led off, accusing Mike and me of everything that came to mind. Suddenly a worker rose and blasted the group on stage. "Wilkins and Bronston are the best doctors here, and you know it. They're the only ones who come when we call. They care about the residents!" So fierce and unexpected was the challenge that the onstage speakers were stunned into silence. The rumble grew from the captive audience. Somehow, the people on the stage sensed that they had lost the initiative. A worker had spoken back! Immediately the assembly was dismissed like a second-round-knockout fight. Never again would the administration chance such an assembly. The press release the next day described the assemblies as a massive worker protest against Mike's rehiring. "Twelve-hundred workers turned out to support Hammond." The charade had accomplished its objectives. To any outsider, the workers were on the rampage.

The parents' fear and distrust of the workers was intensified. The workers were defending Dr. Hammond, who had fired Mike and Liz. The workers were defending the Willowbrook that Hammond perpetuated, that they had seen exposed on TV. The administration had already been sowing the seeds of the parent-worker conflict to insulate themselves from family complaints about conditions. The parents, rarely able to see their relatives' doctors and held at bay by the building nurse or supervisor, had been taught that if abuse occurred and it happened on the ward, there was only one person to blame—the ward worker. So deep went that resentment against the workers that it was simple for the administration to play on the division between worker and parent.

Isolated and on the defensive, the bureaucracy of Willowbrook desperately needed a shield, an ally—willing or not—to sustain itself. It was the workers' job security that suddenly was at risk if parents succeeded in asserting their wishes—so the administration said. Always at the margin of unemployment, the ward workers fearfully and reflexively clung to their niche. They were trapped, and the administration knew it. No one would refute the press statement of what had happened.

Now the scene was set for the finale. In a pang of conscience, carefully weighing the conditions created for him, Commissioner Alan Miller had to opt for the welfare of the Willowbrook residents and, in due respect to his employees' wishes, renege on the published agreement to rehire Wilkins and Lee. Mustering the expression and language to convey the ethical dilemma, Dr. Miller grappled with his conscience for the people of New York to see, and on February 3 notified Mike and Liz that they would not be reinstated.

For a brief moment, everything stopped while we, transfixed by all that had happened, digested the subsiding of the storm and understood the logic of what had happened. Although unable to cope with the needs of the residents, the administration had creatively and energetically responded when the threat itself came near.

It took a little time for the magnitude of the plot to be pieced together. Information about the calls from Building 1 filtered through. People who had been privy to the meeting that night in Dr. Hammond's home told us about what had happened there. The printing of the hate sheets, the production of the placards for the phony assembly—news of all this reached us from the myriad of friends who, though unable to openly risk their jobs, privately described the staging. In a fit of anger, Dr. Hammond accidentally told me about the FBI's involvement. Finally, the local state assemblyman and head of the New York Assembly Banking Committee, Lucio Russo, in his typical self-effacing manner, took credit in a newspaper article for helping block Mike and Liz's rehiring.

The Benevolent Society, on behalf of the residents and families of Building 6, and Mike and Liz, filed suit in federal court against the principal conspirators. They charged that the firing had been a violation of free speech, right to assembly, and due process. In addition, as a second legal cause, the parents charged that the department had breached a public contract to rehire Mike and Liz, a contract sealed by the joint press release from the January 27 meeting.

The state was in real trouble, caught red-handed in a massive public fraud that included a sizable chunk of respectable men. At nearly the same time, in mid-March, the Legal Aid Society of New York, the National Legal Aid and Defenders Association, and the New York Civil Liberties Union filed the monumental "right to treatment" class action lawsuit on behalf of all the residents and families of Willowbrook that I had been working on with them behind the scenes.

The strategic importance of the class action suit required that it receive full attention, ahead of the controversial conspiracy suit that was strategically never pressed further in the face of the atomic thrust of the Willowbrook class action. Characteristic of the pace of litigation, even the class action suit was to sit for nine months before a hearing was held in federal court on an emergency order. And the wave of events rushed on.

During this sequence of events, every major TV network in the greater New York area was in and out of Willowbrook every week. Never had such diligent and intelligent reporting attended a public issue. Mental retardation—its causes, its status, its problems—could be seen every night on some channel. Ratings on the TV viewing of the Willowbrook footage, outstandingly filmed by Channels 7 and 11, skyrocketed off the charts. Willowbrook became a symbol of abuse and degradation to every New Yorker.

The body blow to the department was staggering. What might have been a small game, a small embarrassment, began to take on huge proportions. Commissioners, legislators, and even the governor could be badly discredited from this exposé. The movement was still very fragile. The gravest weakness was that the parents knew what was wrong, but they did not know what alternatives to demand. In the end, the department would weather endless attacks on their incompetence and immorality. Unless a real, positive alternative was put forward, they would prevail, because they held the mandate, the power, and the permanence.

There were two ideas that needed general public understanding. The first was that people, all people, regardless of how injured or different they are, grow and change continuously. They develop. All human services had to respect that fact and remain committed to a real future for every child and adult with a disability. The institution denied this. The second imperative fact was that the department was always, and would always be, opposed to broad social needs in favor of narrow political and economic gains for the benefit of those at the top. Only a small group of us understood these two facts. We had learned them the hard way. Only a small group of us had the knowledge and the credibility to say these things openly and honestly. It stood to reason that every effort would be bent to isolate us, limit the audience and the spread of organization among the many like-minded people about New York.

CHAPTER 13

For the People, a Choice

A GREAT BREAK CAME—DICK CAVETT had become interested in Willowbrook, partly as a result of a call from a parent celebrity, Malachy McCourt, and wanted to do a full February, 1972 show with both sides present on national TV. We were terrifically scared about the red-baiting "hate" sheets that had just been broadly disseminated around Staten Island and could provoke any kind of crazy physical attack on our multifamily wood-frame home from our ultraconservative neighbors. There was a real risk that the department, with its great prestige, would glibly extract itself with a facade of confidence, but it was worth the risk. Miraculously, a show was set for a week away!

Geraldo Rivera, who had done the ABC Channel 7 breakthrough, would start off with his film clips and personal story. Mike Wilkins would follow to talk about what services could be like if they took a place in the community based on citizen rights. Bernard Carabello, an ex-resident who had been at Willowbrook for eighteen years, and Bernard's mother would talk about how a person with cerebral palsy from a Spanish-speaking family could get thrown into a warehouse. Diana McCourt, Malachy's wife and mother, who had been blackmailed into submitting her daughter to the experimental hepatitis inoculation research program to gain admission to Willowbrook, would talk about that and what parents had to know to free themselves of these terrible decisions. My job was to talk about the California service system as compared with New York's, and doing the "cleanup" and assuming the guardian role.

We didn't know whom the department would send down. The night of the show, we were all terribly nervous. Would we be able to say what we felt and believed? Would people, millions around the nation, sense the drama and importance to their lives that our struggle in Willowbrook symbolized? Were we the right handful to tell the story? At the same time, we were all elated. This show would make or break the effort to deal with the department's suppression of information in its effort to keep Willowbrook an isolated issue, rather than as indicative of all the scores of New York State institutions. Two weeks hence, legislative hearings would open in Albany to look at New York State policy for people with special needs. The department would have to stand before citizen groups from all around the state. The budget freeze, the closing of community services, the expansion of institutions, the unaccountability of the system would all become points of departure for every citizen spokesperson.

The Cavett show would be the first "testimony" in the overall public policy debate on institutions, yes or no? The show went on. Cavett—glamorous, inquiring, quick—came on and began his probe. The department had sent its public relations head, Harold Wolfe, a man with carefully combed hair and a meticulous black suit and vest, who was the top public information—apologist—officer in Albany. The second person was a curiosity, a new face in New York, having recently arrived from California. Quiet and gentle, almost to an embarrassing point, balding and also meticulously dressed in black, Robert Hayes had been an administrator in the largest Southern California institution for persons with mental retardation, Pacific State Hospital—the Willowbrook of California. We did not know at the time, but Mr. Hayes would replace Dr. Grunberg, then commissioner of Mental Retardation Services for New York State.

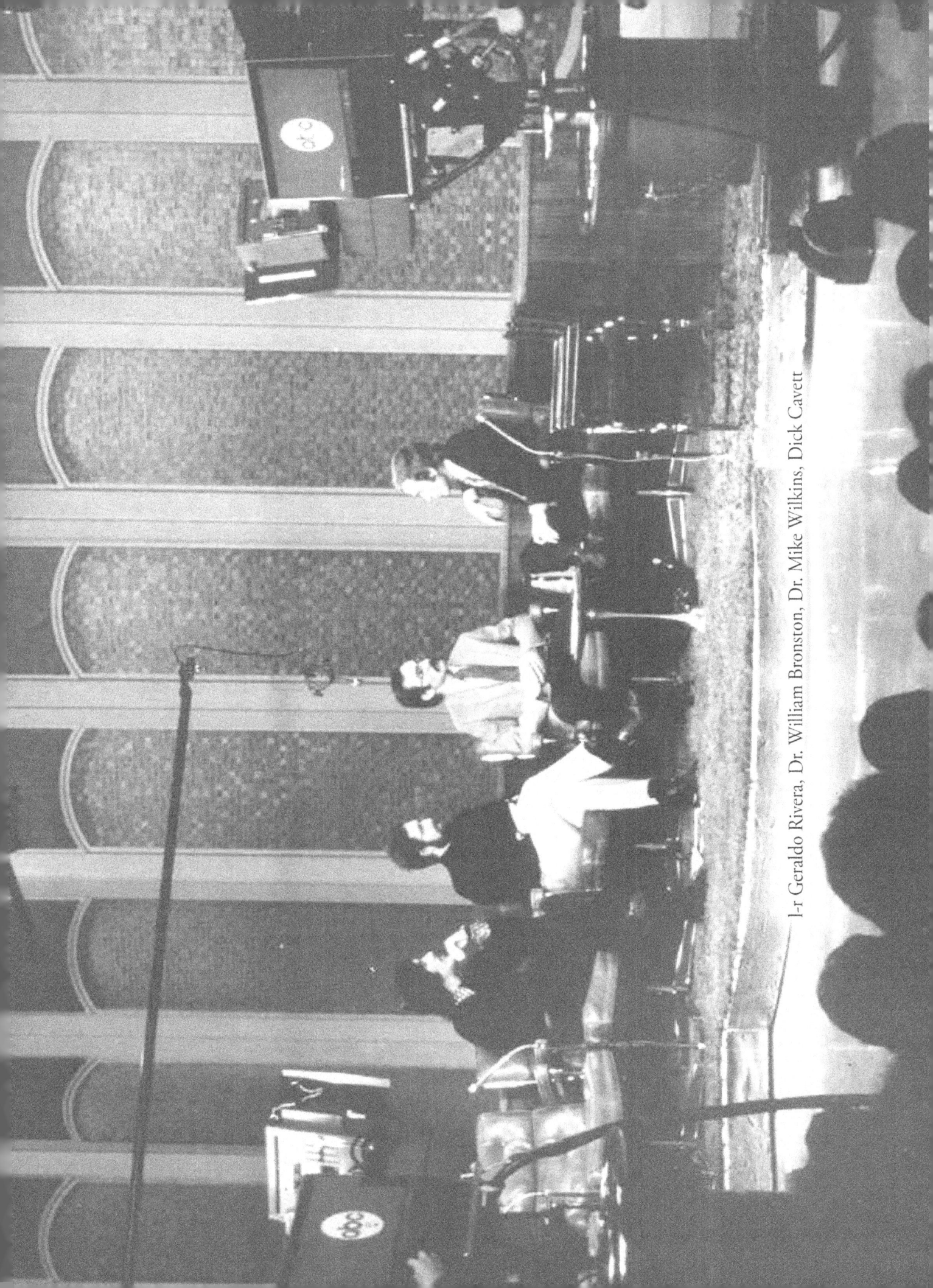

l-r Geraldo Rivera, Dr. William Bronston, Dr. Mike Wilkins, Dick Cavett

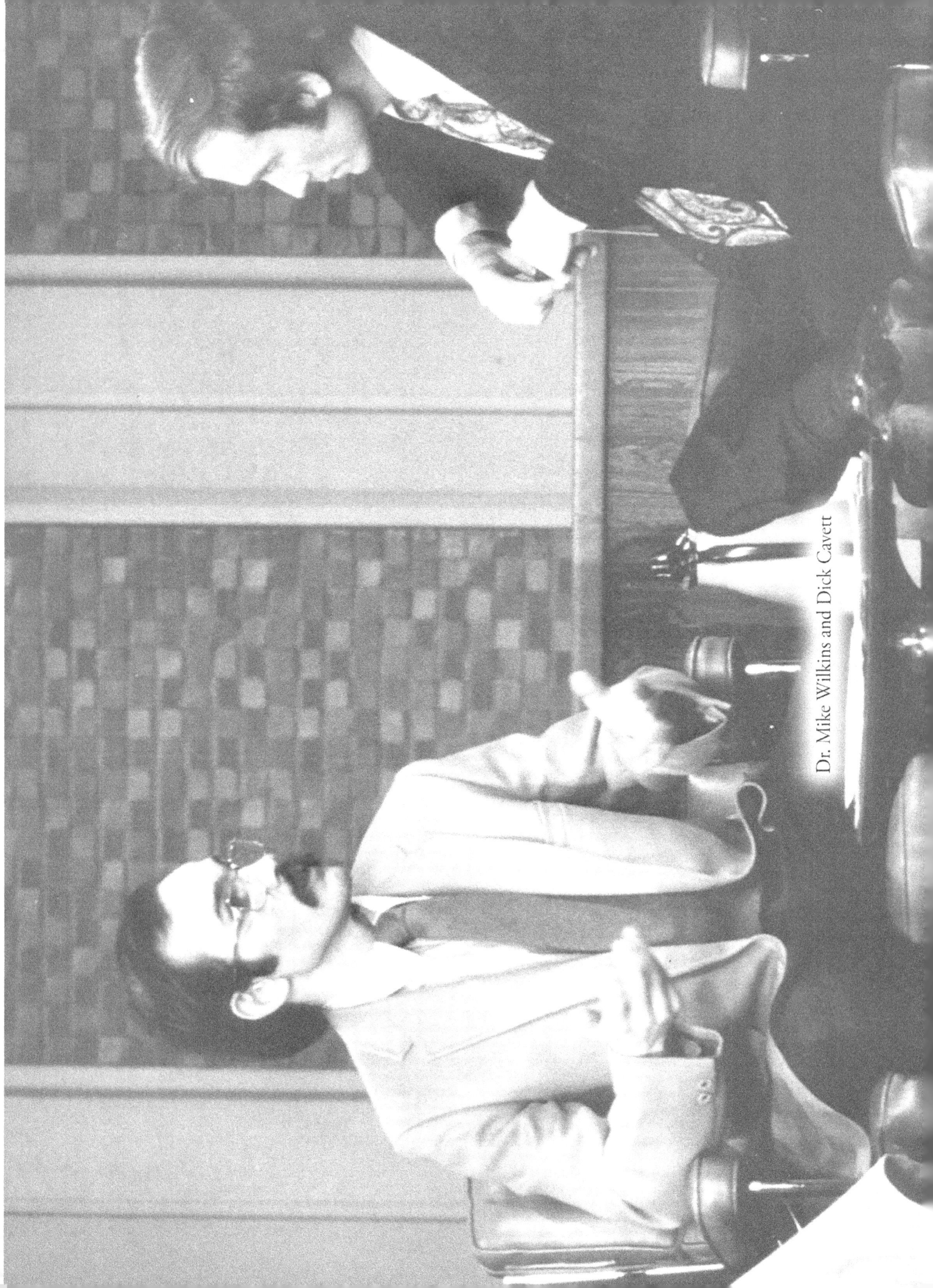

Dr. Mike Wilkins and Dick Cavett

We did our part in about fifteen minutes. ABC TV clips from Geraldo's exposé with his powerful verification were shown. Cavett asked about the anonymous hate sheets that I was able to read aloud, almost in full, over national TV that immediately showed the desperation of the state's effort to distract attention and discredit Mike and me from documenting the horrors from the inside. Then Cavett called on the department representatives to do theirs. It was all Mike and I could do to keep in control during the filibuster that followed. We knew we had to shut up and let the bureaucrats have their say, but it was hell.

Making a deft leap away from all the carnage, Wolfe took off on the department's virtue and intentions. "We plan to...We've always stood for...But the legislature... We've always been the leaders...good people...caring...committed...dedicated to the public...Look at our 1965 Master Plan...it didn't happen just because...Now how can you believe all you've seen is true...We are reality...We are righteous...We, we, we...Just...Upright...Honest...Look...Look!"

For twenty minutes, we sat quietly; then I couldn't take it anymore. Courtesy or not, the disease and death, the brutality, the suffering, the tears of parents, the smell, and the contempt were the fabric of the impeccable suits and shined shoes of respectability droning on before the country. Wolfe and Hayes were like two super funeral home operators selling their wares, trading death for money and power. They were undertakers, apologists for massive crimes. I, finally, fiercely interrupted, and I professionally said so! Once the ice was broken, it was a rout. The two mothers took over and with their extraordinary integrity and genuine compassionateness and buried the bureaucrats in their own self-serving misrepresentations and cynicism.

It was over, all of a sudden. The hour was up. Something had gone out into countless homes. All of us were exhausted, drained from the test. There had been so little time. Such precious little time.

I have traveled all over the country since that show. I am still amazed at how many people remember. People said they were glued to their sets. They understood. They, too, saw the salesmen for death and felt rage when they saw the pictures of the degradation.

The sides opposing each other were etched sharply. That was our greatest hope. What the people would do with the experience and knowledge in their own communities was theirs to decide. We had done our best and had a war in our yard to pursue.

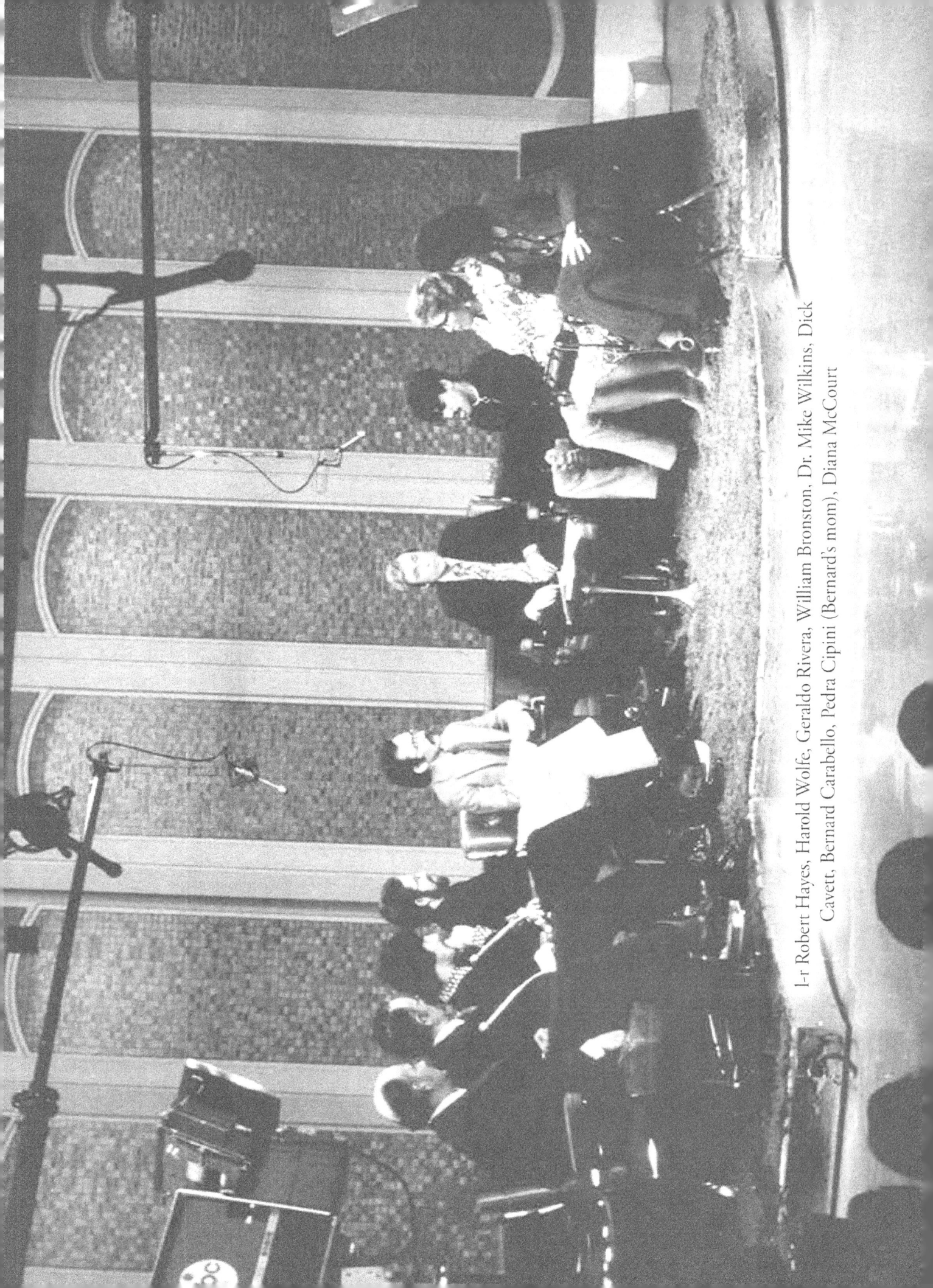

l-r Robert Hayes, Harold Wolfe, Geraldo Rivera, William Bronston, Dr. Mike Wilkins, Dick Cavett, Bernard Carabello, Pedra Cipini (Bernard's mom), Diana McCourt

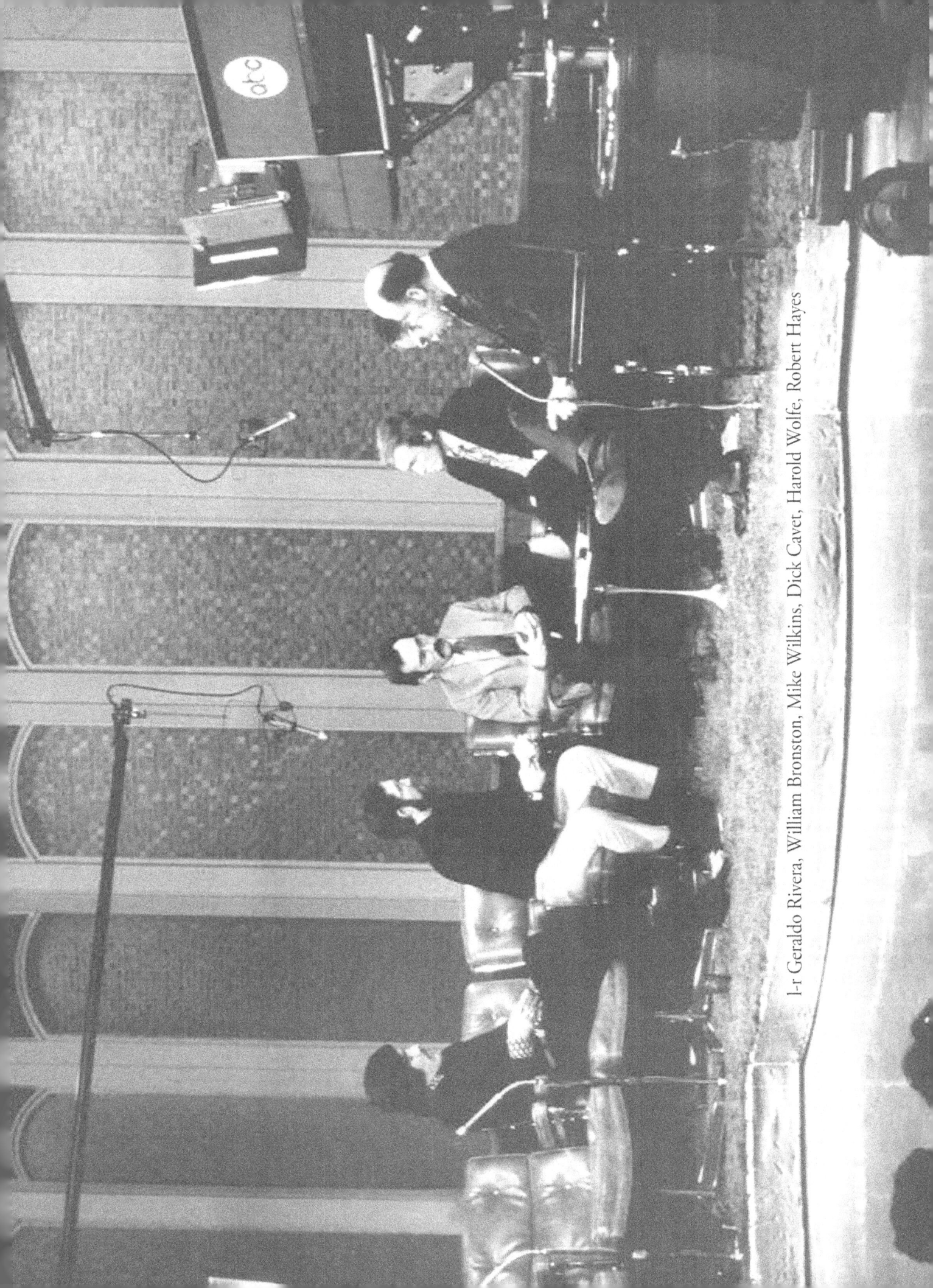

l-r Geraldo Rivera, William Bronston, Mike Wilkins, Dick Cavet, Harold Wolfe, Robert Hayes

CHAPTER 14

Willowbrook: A Testimony before the Legislature

In February, shortly after the Cavett show, it was time for the annual hearings of the state's Joint Legislative Committee on Physical and Mental Handicaps. Historically, those hearings had been a pro forma exercise dominated by what the Department of Mental Hygiene and the Governor dictated should happen. This year, the two-day hearing was packed. Thousands filled the great auditorium in Albany. I think more than to place their age-old grievances before the remote legislature, people came sensing the importance of the occasion, the importance of the times.

Traditionally isolated, feeling alone, angry, guilt ridden, and powerless against the great bureaucracy, people came to find one another regardless of the legislature's predictable inaction. In recent years, Joseph Weingold, the executive director of the New York Association for Retarded Children (ARC), had been installed as the executive consultant to the committee. That conflictual sweetheart relation with the department to gain prestige and token attention had stultified any real truth telling and blocked any important or systemic challenges to arise from families in these critical hearings. The ARC had to be seen as a legitimate advocate, and Weingold's chair alongside the New York Legislature was a symbol of the status the state parent organization held in the eyes of the establishment. This was the magnet for attracting membership that carried with it the belief that protection was at hand. Yet for years, as budgets and survival conditions fell to intolerable, The ARC played ball, shared in the whitewashing, kept the facade of official concern intact, allowing the craven political depredations to annually go unchallenged.

The air in the hearing was electric. Standing ovations, cheers, camaraderie bubbled among the citizens, parents, and concerned field workers that filled the huge auditorium, as speaker after speaker broke free from subordinate timorousness and told their awful personal stories for the first time. It was for them a strategic breakthrough, to see their potential might, to peer into a different future. For the first time, they came searching for friendship and first-class citizenship.

Mrs. Rosalie Amorosa, a mother of a boy in Willowbrook, spoke during the first day, expressing the feeling of parents around the state:

"I suppose I should come up here today and say something nice and polite, but I don't feel very charitable lately. I find it so hard to understand why it takes mountains of publicity about the conditions of our state schools before most politicians become embarrassed and start to jump on the bandwagon; and then we have all sorts of investigations and hearings. Personally, I think the parents should run the hearings at their respective state schools and we should summon the politicians to come and testify. After all, we know what our kids need, but who listens to us—we're only parents you know.

When I passed by the Albany mall today, I got very sick. One billion dollars and it's not finished yet. I don't deny that the legislators needed new office space, but why didn't the state economize and build plain, ordinary office buildings? Instead, the state decided to economize on our kids. I look at that mall and then I think of the building my son lives in at Willowbrook. The roof leaks, the Celotex blocks on the ceiling are falling down, and it desperately needs a paint job. You build super highways, grand malls, world trade centers, and then you "cut the fat out of the budget" of the Department of Mental Hygiene. Well, you didn't cut the fat out of the budget, you cut the fat out of the hides of our kids.

When we tried, over the past year, to tell you how badly our kids were hurting as a result of the freeze, we were continually ignored. The Board of Visitors at Willowbrook sent Governor Rockefeller a telegram in which they vividly described the bad conditions they found there. Their telegram was also ignored. It was only after two young professionals brought the press and television into Willowbrook, and all hell broke loose, that the politicians started to sit up and take notice. And do you know what? As a reward these two young people were fired. Now that's what I call real justice. I couldn't be polite or charitable today if I tried.

The state keeps putting money into the state schools, but they will never improve. For the parents, state schools are the court of last resort. People are forced to place their children into state schools because there are no state-run community services for our kids. My own son was put out of public school because his teacher couldn't handle him. I had no other worthwhile program to put him in; and I'm sure he could have used a wide variety of programs, such as behavior training, good recreation programs, and possibly a sheltered workshop setting. Many children are placed in institutions because of the lack of these essential services in the community.

It is only when the mother is on the verge of a nervous breakdown, or the whole family structure starts to go, that parents are forced by circumstances to institutionalize their children. The state then becomes the keeper of the living dead. Having a handicapped child isn't always the easiest thing to accept, but if we had the right kind of help in the community for our children from the time they are born and as they grow up, the burden would be easier to bear. It is only when we know our children aren't getting a fair shake, and when we have to come up here to Albany like beggars looking for a handout that we become bitter and resentful; and today I stand here bitter, resentful, and very uncharitable."

The second day, I had the honor to testify about Willowbrook.

"The Pandora's Box of our state school system for the retarded has been open, and our citizens have had a true glimpse of the misery, loneliness, and stench that have existed within for so many years. We must completely correct this legacy of suffering that has been heaped upon tens of thousands of families in our state and upon the helpless who still continue to decay under the present system employed to meet the needs of the handicapped here.

The essence of that system has been to separate people with special needs from normal interaction with society and to relegate them to non-productivity. The concept that the state school is the final common pathway for all afflicted children and the primary strategy for the state of New York has made the general public come to accept institutionalization such children and adults, disregarding the deep instinctual protest against such a surrender on the part of every mother and father. In short, the practice of institutionalization, historically, has led to an ideology which has gripped the nation and the state of New York to the present day. In turn, this ideology, that retardation and developmental disabilities are fixed stigma, untreatable, and worsening, has reinforce the inhuman anti-scientific practices current in the Department of Mental Hygiene and the state school system."

Removing these children from society, concentrating the "handicapped", offering no hope of return to society, are the strategies of those who have no strategy. Willowbrook, Letchworth, and Rockland Institutions are examples that represent the end points of ignorance, irresponsibility, educational and scientific bankruptcy. It must be clear to the people who are in a position to correct the situation of the Willowbrooks of our state, how unthinkable a task it will be to remold the state schools into serviceable resources. Of all places, the state schools have become imbued with the legacy of dehumanization. It grips every policy, every administrator, the overwhelming majority of professionals, and by default, every ward service person charged with carrying out the job defined from above."

First and most important, when a child with a developmental disability is identified in the community at large, it is ultimately the family's decision whether to institutionalize the child or not. For the moderately through profoundly handicapped, where mass public sector services do not exist, the decision is made by society because society supplies no alternatives. Often this decision is made just by the virtue of the label assigned to a child. As the Willowbrook State School administrator was quoted in Medical World News, January 28 issue, "…our population—grossly retarded, Down Syndrome, cerebral palsy patients, spastics, epileptics, hydrocephalics". This sort of labeling clinches the sentence to institutionalize. Most parents have never been told that a diagnosis is not a sentence but signals the need for preventive and supportive services in the community instead of shame, hopelessness, and surrender.

Second, when the parent admits their child to a state school, the instructions are to allow the child to "adjust" and not to visit for up to three months, deterring the presence of parent advocacy. The family is dealt with much in the way a funeral contracts for the body of the deceased. This is usually the last time the family sees the doctor in charge and has a real sense of how their child is doing. From this point, every inquiring phone call is met with the stock reply that the child is "doing fine and there is nothing to worry about" as defined from the institution's perspective of what it expects from the child…a perspective illustrated by the mass media over the recent weeks. From this point in the history of the child, "doing well" means become a member of a herd of compliant animals. From this point, communication with the family, if they do not persist in visiting regularly and become a "nuisance" to the institution, is confined to terse requests for consents to perform surgical manipulations, notification of serious and critical illness and, finally, death. No progress report to the family, with set goals, is ever required because under the institution's ideology, there can be no progress. In short, any real role that the family may still wish to play is systematically crushed, leaving feelings of devastation, frustration, and defeat.

Third, the definition of the "retarded" as sick and, therefore, requiring medical-psychiatric management—becomes another strategic blow against habilitation. Willowbrook is run on the medical model, where physicians dominate all key decision making from administration down to the ward's doctors, who are hired in pseudo-psychiatric terms and emphasize the medical aspects of the child in lieu of developmental and vocational definitions. Checklist terms such as "cooperative", "destructive", "assaultive", "self-abusive", and "disturbed" capsulize each child and determine the expectation of the staff. The doctors' judgment is supreme and unchallenged, despite its narrow focus and the fact that the child is always defined by his or her liabilities.

There is no public health control at Willowbrook. There is no medical correlation or summary of illnesses, except those conditions defined as communicable diseases by law. At any given time, no one knows the extent of illness in the institution, not only because there is no two-way recordkeeping system, but because the expectation of the doctors coincides with the "laudable pus theory", where, because the children are "retarded" and because conditions of filth, epidemic, and endemic disease, lack of scientific and planned treatment exist, a state of chronic illness, debility, malnutrition, acquired insanity, deprivation, and deformity is accepted as normal. It is only the dramatic incidence of violent injuries—gashes, soaring fevers with wrenching incapacity, and overt and often preventable illness that attract attention. In short, crisis care is the order of the day. The minimally trained ward attendants are relied on to do case finding which they then present each morning to the building doctor, who rarely leaves the sanctuary of the treatment room to see for himself what afflicts the vast population under his care on the wards. Treatment orders are quickly scratched down on the order sheets with seldom a note of the physical findings. If the child is not followed daily because of fulminating illness or the specific request of the physician, the patient is again submerged in the mass, not to be seen again until the next crisis. Crisis care recognizes no past and admits no future. Thus, the highest level of common denominator of service exists in the area where it is theoretically best equipped. Compliant doctors among all the NY state institutions are interchangeable from building to building; where thoroughgoing knowledge of the residents in our charge is practically deterred, and continuity of care is totally undermined."

I went on to describe how in each of my various transfers from one building to another that I had not received any off-service and clinical briefing from my predecessor nor, in most cases, even met him, and that this total lack of orientation was the custom, rather than a matter of oversight. I described the administration's negligent delay and unconcern about remedying specific conditions that endangered the safety of the patients and compromised the effectiveness of the medical staff. I told the hearing in some detail about the preventability of many of the rampant physical scourges and the economic savings to the state in following such a program, aside from the advantages to the patients. I described the elementary, straightforward practices with which we had eradicated a major portion the medical problems in Buildings 76 and 77. I told the hearing how Willowbrook creates the behavior it describes and about the farcical "progress notes" routinely transcribed on the individual charts, all pointing clearly to the institution's assumption that each resident was "here to die."

I discussed how this attitude resulted in a total lack of planning for any developmental goals and education or training simply did not exist for most of the children. I told how the children were labeled and lumped into crude management categories. I described the routine massive misadministration of drugs and the everyday physical injury and degradation; I described the gradual descent of the disabled child into pandemonium. I told of the heartrending state of the parents who, hopelessly, must watch their children in their inevitable descent. I placed the blame for every sin of omission or commission for every condition of Willowbrook squarely on the people who, by virtue of their leadership mistraining, perpetuate the culture of the institution.

"There is no end to this description. There is virtually no nook or cranny in Willowbrook, no relationship, which does not have the stamp of sadness and pain, hopelessness, or cruelty. The ward workers, like the patients, are the innocents, both victims of forces and notions forced upon them. They toil together in an insane and savage alliance, while the privileged professionals and supervisory staff and their lieges, the administrators, who know better, have, like Dr. Strangeloves, learned to live with Willowbrook and defend it against change

Willowbrook is not, and can never be, a medical care facility. What it spawns in the way of disease and misery makes it a medical disaster zone. Willowbrook is not, and can never be, a school. What it teaches by virtue of its architecture and the expectation that prevails is the exact opposite of human growth and development. Willowbrook is not, and can never be, a decent residential center.

You may feel that Willowbrook and the other state schools can be reconstructed, but this will take hundreds of millions of dollars, and in the end you will still have a monstrosity that is a bottomless well for tax dollars without a product. If you decide to provide funds to Willowbrook in the face of the incalculable suffering that now exists there, it must be accompanied by a plan that will guarantee an eventual and complete replacement of the state school system, through growing accountability in the hands of parents and consumers. Only under these conditions can the legacy of hopelessness and violence flowing from the concept that the handicapped are worthless, be relegated to the past."

CHAPTER 15

Editorials

WHEN YOU ARE TRYING to decide who your friends are, it is useful to balance two things: what are they doing for you, and what are they not doing that they could be doing? The whole area of what is omitted in a relationship is very swampy, but it is often the most important criterion in making a judgment about the integrity of allies. Judging the integrity of the department solely by its token reforms and promises, and ignoring its omissions and deceptions, would ignore the truth. One had only to refer back to the institution wards to know that the department had no intention whatsoever of responding to the outcry against the inhumane conditions. Change might be coming, but with no urgency nor any sense of priorities related to people's lives. What was missing told the story of the department's integrity.

There was another agency, the omissions of which should be noted and taken very seriously. The information cataclysm and the TV and press exposure of Willowbrook that was unleashed are not to be underestimated. The *Staten Island Advance*, by editorial policy, had the story on the front page for nearly two months. The TV networks were in and out of Willowbrook weekly. But standing monumental and silent was the nation's number one newspaper, the newspaper of record, the *New York Times*. It was as if Willowbrook was a provincial episode, irrelevant to the *Times*, The fact that the chain of responsibility ran around the governor's office, the state's Executive Budget Bureau, and the unimpeachable prestige of the psychiatrist who ran New York State Department Mental Hygiene did not seem to pique the curiosity or newsworthiness of the scandal by the *New York Times*. It was almost as if very high in their editorial circles, a decision was pending on what to do. What would the line be? Most importantly, to maintain its positive image, how often and how hard would the *Times* press its position, when a position was finally decided upon? The *Times* must have known, and certainly knew then, the magnitude of the connections that we were stumbling upon and groping to understand. We interpreted this silence as a sign of how really explosive the situation was.

Finally, almost after everything was said and done, a *Times* editorial appeared on February 26, 1972.

The New York Times

Published every day by The New York Times Company

ADOLPH S. OCHS, Publisher 1896-1935
ARTHUR HAYS SULZBERGER, Publisher 1935-1961
ORVIL E. DRYFOOS, Publisher 1961-1963

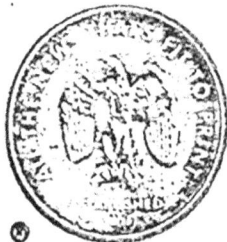

The Willowbrooks With Us

It is part of the tragedy and the disgrace that inhuman conditions at Willowbrook, a state facility for the mentally retarded on Staten Island, have persisted through repeated "exposés" and full-dress inquiries. The current storm over the degradation of the human beings institutionalized there must not be allowed to fade away in still more inaction.

New York State's current fiscal stringency has had an especially severe impact on Willowbrook, on other state facilities for the retarded and on the entire mental hygiene system. The budgetary freeze has caused an attrition of personnel at institutions already understaffed. A single attendant at Willowbrook may now be required to care for as many as fifty or more brain-damaged youngsters crowded into a single small room.

Governor Rockefeller's response to this most recent exposure of conditions at Willowbrook is utterly inadequate. He has merely restored some money previously cut from this year's budget and has promised modest increases in the year ahead. There is little question, however, that this additional state funding will still leave every institution in desperate straits.

Beyond staffing requirements, real and immediate as they are, lies the need to make fundamental policy decisions. Are huge institutions that offer only custodial care the most effective answer to the needs of the mentally retarded? Governor Rockefeller seems to think that building huge buildings solves every problem when often it only makes them worse. California has pioneered with a decentralized system of small institutions and day-care facilities. Its experience indicates beneficial results in terms of helping many of the less severely retarded as well as holding down costs. Permanent institutionalization may cost as much as $8,500 annually while day care, more appropriate in many cases, may cost $2,000 or less.

Legislation announced by Democratic leaders yesterday is to be introduced in Albany on Monday to reform New York's backward system for dealing with the mentally retarded and developmentally disabled along the lines of the California model. In the meantime, more funds must be found even in this period of budgetary austerity. The state dishonors itself by its dehumanization of these helpless children.

Then, silence again. The *Times* had done its thing for the public. Their pursuing the issue, as a matter of moral obligation, as the valiant little the *Staten Island Advance* had done, simply was not genuine. One wonders if the discovery of a Buchenwald in Queens or Brooklyn would have been treated as conservatively. Maybe "news" means something else to the papers of the wealthy and the powerful.

Then, silence once more. No risk had been taken even though the position was hard-hitting. In fact, all the editorial did was to summarize what had been said by the previous three months of press coverage of Willowbrook.

Nearly three months later, after the federal class action suit had been filed delineating the massive crimes against humanity, the across-the-board accusation of the department's violation of almost every constitutional guarantee of the incarcerated citizens in Willowbrook, the *Times* printed an enormous guest editorial. It was written by—of all people—Dr. Jack Hammond. Hammond had repeatedly and publicly sworn his absolute loyalty to the department. He never acted without permission from above. The matter had gone too far. Almost like a voice from the grave, the department had used the flaccid *New York Times* to salvage its credibility on the policy of institutionalizing human beings. With no apparent concern for seeking a voice from the parents or advocates of change, the *Times* had provided a forum for the department (through Dr. Hammond) to lay out the age-old and twisted version of how residents and their families in Willowbrook should be grateful and how the public should understand how devoted and shining were the sacrifices made by the institution to cope with those that nobody wanted.

New York Times Guest Editorial

Another View of Willowbrook By JACK HAMMOND

It has never been the policy of this administration to forewarn the employees of impending visits by the press or by official visits and whether they arrived announced or unannounced such visitor have always been promptly escorted to all parts of the institution with no special preparation made for their visits.

The comparisons which have been made between the retarded in the various community centers in New York State and elsewhere and the profoundly retarded multiply handicapped whom we have at Willowbrook State School have also been distorted. Almost all of the Willowbrook population in this category would be found "non suitable" for enrollment in those community programs.

With rare exception little or nothing has been shown on television or described in the newspapers concerning the many programs for the training and education of our somewhat more capable patients and the better living conditions that naturally follow for those patients who have self help skill and who can feed, bathe and dress themselves.

Nothing was shown of our fine school department or infant therapy complex, or work of the physical therapy, occupational therapy or recreation departments. No mention was made of our several unique programs for the habilitation of younger patents and the preparation of our young adult patients for community living. Our volunteer program the largest in any of our institutions, involving several thousand volunteers, understaffed and overlooked has been maligned.

We at Willowbrook have for years been in the forefront of to fight to improve the living conditions, the staffing and the programming for our most helpless residents the unpleasant conditions, serious overcrowding, shortage of help and absence of visible programs in so many areas of Willowbrook State school have repeatedly been reported to the proper officials and to the parents organization. To the extent that more money was made available during the past few years there has been improvement in these areas, but not enough.

A great disservice has been done to the many sincere dedicated, hardworking employees of this institution who labor under the most trying circumstances. No recognition has been given to their herculean efforts. Instead they have been criticized shamed and even abused. Their morale has been devastated.

The anxieties of many parents who had placed their profoundly retarded, often multiply handicapped offspring in a residential setting as the only alternative to disruption and decompensation of the rest of the family, have been aroused. They are now beset with doubt and feeling of guilt.

Somehow the public seems to have gained the impression that New York State provides no services for the mentally retarded other than that which is available in our residential facilities. Somehow the fact that only approximately 2 percent of the mentally retarded reside in our institutions and that 98% of them reside in the community, mostly with their own families seems to have been overlooked. Over 50,000 mentally retarded youngsters between the ages of 7 and 21 years are enrolled in special classes in the public schools throughout the state. More than 26,000 mentally retarded youngsters and adults who are either too young too old or otherwise ineligible for public school classes are being helped to remain in the community by 200 community based programs, representing a total state and local expenditure of $14,000,000.

Let us beware of false prophets. While absolutely agreeing that our community based programs are essential, we must bear in mind that there will always be some for whom there will be no alternative but a residential placement unless society chooses to return to the ancient practice of abandoning it's helpless members on the mountainside.

In their effort to stir the conscience of society and to call attention to the need to improve the care of the institutionalized retarded and to expand community-based programs, the media have rendered a great public service.

However, one must bear in mind that Willowbrook State School, which has been the focus of the recent publicity concerning the mentally retarded serves a very severely and profoundly handicapped population. Seventy-seven per cent of our patients are severely or profoundly mentally retarded. 39.1 per cent are non-ambulatory with severe spasticity due to cerebral palsy or other neurological condition; 30 per cent have histories of convulsive seizures; 52.8 per cent have no speech; 60 per cent are incapable of adequately attending to their own personal hygiene; many are hyperactive or disturbed.

The sight of one individual with a combination of such afflictions would cause great distress and anguish to anyone with any compassion at all. The sight of large numbers of such individuals gathered in one location such as Willowbrook is even more distressing.

The reader or viewer should realize that with 5,000 patients at Willowbrook, of who about 4,000 are as described above, there are numerous buildings housing these individuals which replicate themselves.

Some of the media repeatedly zeroed in on this target population, frequently at the most inopportune times such as when the residents were being showered and were therefore naked as they entered and left the bathing areas; or immediately after mealtime when unavoidable food spillage had not yet been cleaned up and patients were being toileted, presenting a distorted picture.

The media have never been barred from Willow State School. When media representatives did visit they were always shown a balanced picture that induced a number of our problem areas. In turn, the media always previously presented a balanced picture to the public. However, during the recent publicity many of the media representatives absolutely refused to see anything but the most unpleasant situations.

It was not necessary for media representatives, accompanied by scores of irate parents and indignant officials, to barge in through the back doors of buildings, climb over residents and disrupt employees in the performance of their duties in order to obtain factual information about conditions in the institution.

> Members on the mountainside
> Jack Hammond, Director of the Willowbrook
> State School on Staten Island

I was incensed! The ground was prepared for the last ideological collision with the old-line leadership. A circle of parents, who had led the demand for public accountability, with the participation of a few leaders of family organizations in the community, asked for a reply from the inside. I called the *Times* on their behalf. There was not much they could do but edit down our collectively agreed-upon and exhaustive rebuttal as much as possible, using an "equal space" agreement, and immediately submitted. A rejoinder showed up two weeks later.

THE NEW YORK TIMES, SATURDAY, MAY 27, 1972

Willowbrook, Continued

By WILLIAM
BRONSTON MD

The public has been grossly misled by the self-serving and self-justifying guest editorial, "Another View of Willowbrook," which appeared on the Op-Ed page May 6, 1972. The parochialism of its author, Dr. Jack Hammond, Willowbrook director, and the Department of Mental Hygiene in trying to convince anyone that Willowbrook alone is under attack, or that this issue has arisen from mass media exposure and parent outrage, denies historical reality.

•

In the United States there has been a steady drive from the community of families of the "handicapped" and progressive professionals to foreclose on the legacy of charity for the "handicapped" and the second-class, hat-in-hand citizenship that befalls those families.

•

At issue are, two fundamentally antagonistic outlooks. On the one hand, a philosophy which accepts the brutalization and reduction of human beings to a subhuman condition, as has been amply documented in the state institutions.

Opposing this, our position was that people with special needs, labelled developmentally disabled, the physically disabled and others, must be accorded the full spectrum of human—and constitutional rights with regard to care, treatment and education. The former view, held generally, by the chiefs of the Department of Mental Hygiene, leads to policies and practices that justify human losses and the systematic exclusion of a block of people from the mainstream of society. The latter view is based on respect for all people and must lead to a complete overhaul of the contemporary practices of seeing and serving people with disabilities. We would expand services in public schools to meet special needs, establish preventive and cooperative health services, develop major planning for normal homes for all handicapped people in every neighborhood and program massive occupational training.

•

As a physician and permanent employee in Willowbrook, I have been in charge of five buildings since beginning work there. I have had access to every building and responsibility for the care of all the residents at one time or another. It is from this firsthand knowledge that "Another View of Willowbrook" is so odious and mendacious What underlies Dr. Hammond's repeated depiction of the residents in Willowbrook as "77 per cent who are severely and profoundly handicapped" is immediately at odds with the one-third figure given by the Commissioner as being people who belong in the community.

•

Furthermore, In order to collect maximum-Federal (Medicaid) repayment, the physicians are officially instructed to estimate low I.Q.'s. Finally, then are five psychologists at Willowbrook for 5,300 residents, I.Q, testing is performed in the most perfunctory way with reports rarely exceeding a short paragraph. The numerical I.Q. values assigned are designed to legitimize excluding people from the token school and rehabilitation programs available, and are on average, five to ten years out of date. How can anyone who understands human growth and development seriously talk about 4,000 people in one sentence as if describing an amorphous mass or herd of beasts, without communicating precisely this image to the public?

•

The allegation that the media "zeroed in on this urgent population at the most inopportune times," revealing nakedness, filth and misery, is an outright falsification.

I have made rounds at every hour of the day and night (unlike the director of Willowbrook who relies on administrative subordinates, who occasionally visit the wards, for his information). I can attest (and will do so in Federal court) that the conditions shown over TV are daily fare for over 75 per cent of the residents and, in fact, the media did not show the worst of the situation. Only first-hand can the unspeakable wretchedness and sadness be appreciated.

•

The boast that the media have never been barred from Willowbrook is preposterous.

As for never forewarning employees or buildings of visits from outsiders, I have personally overheard more time than I can count, phone calls from the administration's secretaries and the nursing office to building supervisors telling them to clean up because this or that politician or visitor was on the way. So universal is this practice that if an unexpected person enters a ward, the attendants will carry serious grudges against their coworkers for not informing them. Granted, this may not be a policy, but it is a practice.

The claim that the comparison between children in the community and

those in Willowbrook is unfair is particularly interesting. First, it must be said, that I personally visited a number of the facilities shown on TV and, in fact, was trained in one of them.

The children were identical at all levels of functioning. What was incomparable was the overwhelmingly low expectations of the staffs and the night and day different environment that, at Willowbrook, led to a child being labeled "unsuitable" according to Hammond, vs. making "wonderful progress" in the personal community centers.

The "great disservice" done to the employees by the true exposure of the conditions at Willowbrook may have aroused some anxious moments for my co-workers, but it certainly does not take any vision to see the connection between the exposure and the smashing of the job freeze that has hung like death over the state, the forcing of service reorganization and exploration of programs to begin to meet the needs of resident and workers alike. What the Civil Service Employees Association union had been unable or unwilling to do, fight for better patient care and working conditions, the lawsuits and parents'

organizations have begun to do.

•

When the parents rose up, Dr. Hammond talked about "agitators and communists" among the parents. When the C.S.E.A. strike was called, he pleaded for these same parents to bail the institution out, denouncing the workers for their irresponsible indifference to the welfare of the children. With the employee crisis over, back he goes to attacking the parents for being filled with doubts and guilts.

The contention that "Another View" makes that 98 per cent of the people with disabilities who are in the community receive services is a flagrant lie. In February, organization after organization testified before the Joint Legislative Committee on Physical and Mental Handicaps in Albany, building a mosaic protest against fragmented and token services, exclusion, mismanagement and a profound lack of any less drastic alternatives than the institutions offered by the state. The question before the people is simple: Do we accept failure and inhumanity or do we take a giant step forward for people with special needs?

Dr. William G. Bronston is clinical physician at Willowbrook State School.

CHAPTER 16

Dogfight: The Collision of Concern

How EMBROILED THE DAYS were, those late months of 1971 and continuing right through the next year. Starting with Jane Kurtin's visit to Willowbrook and her articles in the *Advance*, the struggle went on day after day, both in and out of public view. Inside Willowbrook, in keeping with its deeply established reflex to survive, the bureaucracy continued its relentless campaign to rid itself of what it perceived as offenders, defilers of the faith, and betrayers of the conspiracy of privilege and power held so dearly for over 150 years in the state of New York.

Conditions worsened inside Willowbrook. The exposé was outside. The bureaucracy had control inside. My premonition of a no-quarter survival situation unfolding with the administration was being borne out. As in, Buildings 22 and 23, where I had daily clinical responsibility for between 450 and 1,000 adult women. It was impossible to provide even the most basic surveillance of such a large group of people. It was imperative to keep a record of the situation, as well as making clear that this administrative assignment was irresponsible and again flowed from traditional policies.

My status as a permanent employee was the only reason for my not having been fired. As a permanent employee, charges would first have to be proven and aired in a public setting. It was inevitable that such a serious and legitimate-looking move would be made by the bureaucracy to quash the challenge I represented. Essentially, the administration need not participate in any further confrontation. The situation itself would provide the ammunition needed to discredit any worker in the place if the administration was so inclined. By that, I mean that no worker could complete either work that what was expected or what the regulations called for, where shortages of staff and lack of meaningful organization existed! At any point, a careful inquiry would easily provide evidence of work uncompleted, care gone unprovided, and what could be construed as negligence. The more responsibility possessed by a staff person, the more work that had to go by the board. The more people one is responsible for (a building ward worker for thirty to fifty residents; a nurse for two hundred people; a building supervisor for two hundred, plus all her workers; and the doctor for two buildings, meaning at least twice all the people that a building supervisor might be responsible for), the more impossible the situation becomes. I professionally opted for resident care and refused to do all administrative paperwork until a safe caseload was assigned. This didn't mean stopping work; it was only a formal way of defining that the administration, despite its facade of legality and concern, was utterly indifferent to the fate of everyone in the wards. Having more work than was possible to do, I had to choose between bureaucratic paperwork or taking care of the daily flood of medical and traumatic injuries of the adult women in my care, plus maintaining accountability and communication with their families. I decided my situation required the filing of a drastic grievance for an unsafe workload in order to prevent having charges brought against me. The implications were enormous as any worker in the institution could and should use that mechanism to force the administration's hand.

My attorney, Gene Eisner, advised me to keep meticulous account of everything that went on, to put my observations and protests in writing. In the meantime, he and I filed a set of three new grievances.

Law Offices   **EISNER & LEVY**   351 Broadway   New York, New York 10013 / WOrth 6-9620

Eugene G. Eisner   Mary M. Kaufman
Richard A. Levy   Counsel

December 8, 1971

Commissioner Alan D, Miller, M,D,
State of New York Department of Mental Hygiene 44
Holland Avenue Albany, New York 12208
Re: William Bronston, M.D.
Willowbrook State School

Dear Sir:

Please be advised that Dr. William Bronston has requestedthat I file the following grievances on his behalf:

- relief from an excessive work load
- relief from administrative harassment so as to permit the Doctor to meet the needs of the persons under his care,
- relief from the Director's decision denying Dr. Bronston the right to meet with concerned parents on the grounds of the Willowbrook State School at anytime.

I would appreciate your office informing me as soon as possible the date of the grievance hearing.

Very truly yours,
Eugene G. Eisner EGE: js
cc: Dr. Jack Hammond Director Willowbrook
State School 2760 Victory Boulevard
Staten Island, New York 10314
cc: Dr. William Bronston

Despite the filing of this protective grievance, the administration's first step toward my removal was not long in coming. I received an "unsatisfactory" job rating for the year. Even when you know the score, it's hard to believe it when your worst suspicions about a situation come true. Gene immediately appealed the rating with the state Civil Service Board.

MEMO TO: Jack Hammond, M.D., Director
FROM: Dr. W. Bronston
RE: Performance Rating

I am in receipt of the report of unsatisfactory performance that I received by registered mail. The report is clearly an expression of an irrational and punitive attitude which you and your immediate subordinates have pursued since July, 1971. The charges are all covered by either the active grievance being pursued in relation to my transfer from Building 76 or in the pending grievances lodged in December.

It is crystal clear that this performance rating does not reflect unsatisfactory behavior on my part but monumental irresponsibility on your part as is reflected by the enormous record of institutional mismanagement over the past years. I plan to appeal this document directly to the Civil Service Board and it shall be added to evidence of the continual harassment leveled at me by the administration at Willowbrook State School in its attempt to stifle my protest against the inhuman conditions within the institution and active effort to modify these conditions wherever possible,

cc: Dr. Murphy, Deputy Director
Dr. Alan D. Miller, Commissioner
Dr. Gunnar Dybwad Dr. Burton Blatt
Mr. Eisner

In early 1972, the New York Civil Liberties Union, the National Legal Aid and Defenders Association, and the Legal Aid Society had filed the *New York State Association for Retarded Children, Inc. et al, and Patricia Parisi et al v. Hugh L Carey as Governor of the State of New York et al*, New York class actions suits against the governor, the Department of Mental Hygiene, and the Willowbrook administration for violating constitutional rights of all the residents of Willowbrook. The complaint demanded the right to education, right to treatment, right to protection against cruel and unusual punishment, right to due process and equal access to the benefits of the law and society, and right to real opportunity to live decently. I had been asked to be an expert witness for the parents against the state. My job rating was a move to discredit my testimony and challenge my "good standing" at work.

Both Gene and I were concerned that I could not win my appeal against the unsatisfactory rating, after our earlier experience in appealing my transfer from Buildings 76 and 77. And much more was at stake for the state this time. My credibility would be a strong asset in the federal trial, in which the governor was at the top of the list of defendants charged with abuse in the Willowbrook class action suit. So, what possibly could be expected from the Civil Service department in my hearing? The commissioner would have to line up on the side of "law and order," department-style, against childcare. Nevertheless, it was important not to miss the opportunity to build a written record of explanation and interpretation that would ultimately strengthen the parents' hand. In my job appeals, we had always had the courts as a strong card, regardless of the decision of the bureaucracy. All these complex maneuvers exhausted me, and I longed to relax. But that was impossible. Each day, a new situation would come up. Each day the collision of values presented themselves and required clarification.

To detail the dogfight would tax the reader beyond reason. A few of the documents highlight the kind of thing that was going on and might be instructive to those who find themselves torn in similar situations, now and in the future.

September 29, 1971

MEMO TO: Dr. Murphy, Deputy Director, Bldg. #1
FROM: Dr. W. Bronston, Bldg. #23

I am in receipt of your memorandum regarding Utilization Reviews. There is in excess of 160 Utilization Review forms to be completed in Buildings #22 and 23. In reviewing the schedule for October, I find that I am on 11 duty days, 3 of which are staff meeting days. In order to complete the Utilization Reviews by the institution deadline I would have to perform 15 reviews per day—given the opportunity to sit down with the workers for half day periods twice weekly performing a maximum of 5 Utilization Reviews per week. This would require 33 working days or nearly 4 months' time working at maximum efficiency.

At present in the building we are at minimum coverage. There are barely two or three workers on each ward on the best of days, making it impossible to remove a worker from a ward for fear of hazards to the residents from insufficient supervision. In addition, as you know, orders* must be written monthly. This again requires careful discussion, the effects of the medication on each of the patients, the review of their seizure records and listening to many complaints, misunderstandings, and problems associated with each of the patient's care. At this point, despite having been in the building since the beginning of August, I have only been able to complete 150 of the medication rewrites between the two buildings. Again, this is due to more than half the days I am on duty having to cover four adjacent buildings and meeting myriad problems that spontaneously arise to smash any planned or scheduled work.

I am deeply concerned about the Utilization Review process. I sincerely believe it is vital to patients' care, and yet because of the material conditions in the buildings, which I do not believe the administration is fully aware of, it is physically and clinically impossible to meet the deadline. I hope that you will investigate this matter and if necessary encourage and open discussion among the building physicians and nurses. I am firmly convinced without any doubt that the inclining staff shortage and requiring the spreading thin of our efforts and time is resulting in accumulated hazard to residents and to us as employees who must oversee their well-being.

WB: vf:23

Each person receiving tranquilizing or anticonvulsant drugs had to have their orders renewed and signed off based on a detailed report of their condition each month, or the medication would theoretically automatically lapse. The usual way that this was handled for many building physicians was to have a worker copy the previous month's order and the physician would run through and sign the pile of sheets, month after month.

April 20, 1972

Jack Hammond, M,D,
Director
Willowbrook State School Staten Island,
New York 10314

Dear Dr. Hammond:

I received your memorandum of April 18th. As has become your custom in your vicious attempt to harass and discredit me, the memorandum is filled with distortions.

In my April 14th memorandum to the deputy director, I stated that I would not be an accomplice to your administration's long-term practice of defrauding the federal government by falsifying Medicaid forms. I stated that we must be allowed to fill the forms out truthfully, despite official instructions to the contrary. To the extent that my direct service work is discharged and time permits office work, I shall discharge my responsibilities in the best interests of patient care. I would appreciate, in these immensely trying times, if you stop issuing threatening memorandums which interfere with my work and which tie up precious time and energy to answer. It is perfectly clear that your inability to constructively rise to the challenge of letting the truth about Willowbrook be known and participating constructively in the transformation of this immensely tragic and brutal setting leads you to acts of cynicism and vengeance. What you do to discredit yourself in the eyes of the public is your business, but if you continue your personal vendetta against me, I will certainly be forced to contemplate appropriate court action against you and any subordinates in your administration who are urged to carry out your policy of suppression. Despite numerous efforts to bring patient care and patient rights to your attention through memorandums that I have sent to you and to your deputies, I have yet to receive a single adequate reply. I believe I have the right, on behalf of the patients, to demand some recognition of their needs. What are you doing about Barbara A. and Carol K. interfering and disrupting my meeting with ward staff, the 111 women that I recommended for privileges on the grounds from Building 22 and Building 23, lockers for personal belongings for residents in Building 22 and Building 23 among the most prominent matters that I have brought to the attention of the administration?

Your concern for paperwork to the exclusion of people is a mark of your true commitment and characteristic of your administration's flagrant failure to serve the people.

William Bronston, M.D.
Clinical Physician I
WB: kb
cc: Eugene Eisner
Alan D. Miller, M.D.

By May, the situation was out of control. The grievances I had filed in December, which I had hoped would settle the situation, were completely up in the air. Relations with the administration, since Dr. Hammond was still being defended by the department, were simply blown out. Nothing but stalling was happening.

Time after time, Gene had written to push for legal relief. The department used every technicality it could to avoid the grievance hearing, as the issues were not pure and would set a precedent the administration couldn't afford. The concept of "a reasonable and safe workload" was to be avoided at all costs. If the ward workers could define what constituted a safe client number to serve, the speedup, where fewer and fewer people were required to do more and more work, would be powerfully stopped. The CSEA leadership in Albany would be shown for their statewide sellout. In all their contract negotiations, they had never demanded the setting of safe working limits, nor did they advocate for the meaningful definition of the workers' roles in human services. The other physicians, as degenerate as their role was, were beginning to grumble about the demands being made on them as I kept explaining how dangerous the situation was and how liable they were if a death occurred through negligence.

Gene was laying the groundwork for a due process challenge that we would raise if the department continued to refuse to hear our grievances. Civil service regulations required a hearing be held within a finite period, long since passed in my case.

We set forth the ultimatum:

Law Offices **EISNER & LEVY** 351 Broadway New York, New York 10013 / WOrth 6-9620

Eugene G. Eisner Mary M. Kaufman
Richard A. Levy Counsel

Mr. John J. Lagatt
Director of Mental Hygiene Employee Relations New York State
Department of Mental Hygiene 44 Holland Street
Albany, New York 12208
Re: Dr. William Bronston

Dear Mr. Lagatt:

We are somewhat at a loss as to the procedure being followed by the Department of Mental Hygiene in this case. Moreover, your letter of March 1972, in our opinion, only darkens what have already been murky waters.

Dr. Bronston filed three grievances with your Department on December 8, 1971. Although the Commissioner's Office made numerous attempts to have Dr. Hammond respond to the grievances, apparently his efforts were unavailing. In the meantime, while your office has been "concerned" as to whether the grievances should be heard at the second or third step of the grievance procedure, the oppressive nature of Dr. Hammond and his subordinates' behavior towards Dr. Bronston continues. Specifically, Dr. Bronston has had no relief from the excessive work load; Dr. Bronston has had no relief from the mountain of correspondence he receives daily from Dr. Hammond and his subordinates (all of which of course require "immediate" responses). In addition, of course, Dr. Hammond still refuses to permit Dr. Bronston to meet with any parents on Willowbrook grounds.

Why Dr. Bronston cannot have an immediate hearing at the third step of the grievance procedure is a complete mystery to us. The language of the Order grants such a right. As we indicated in our earlier letter, Dr. Hammond flatly denied Dr. Bronston's request for relief from an excessive work load as far back as October 22, 1971. Dr. Hammond also denied Dr. Bronston's request to meet with parents on Willowbrook grounds on November 5, 1971. The day-to-day harassment of Dr. Bronston has not ceased; as a matter of fact since the filing of this grievance it has gotten worse. Thus Dr. Hammond, who has openly vowed to "get rid of Dr. Bronston," has now further increased Dr. Bronston's work load under the threat of discharge.

The handling of this case by your Department has been extremely lax, to say the least. Therefore, unless the Department of Mental Hygiene is prepared to take immediate and responsible action upon the grievances filed by Dr. Bronston, who is being subjected to the most callous treatment by the administration, we will have no choice but to regard the grievance procedure as having been waived by the Department and we will seek protection in the state courts.

Very truly yours,
EUGENE G. EISNER
Mr. John J. Lagatt May 3,
cc: Dr. Frederic Grunberg Deputy Commissioner
New York State Department of Mental Hygiene
44 Holland Street Albany, New York 12208
Dr. Jack Hammond, Director Willowbrook State School 2760 Victory
Boulevard Staten Island, New York 10314
Dr. William Bronston
Staten Island, New York

Meanwhile, there was no transaction on a day-to-day basis that was not in a state of collapse. I intensified my pursuit to try to find out what my buildings needed to function. Because of this continued effort, my consciousness about the operation of the institution reached its highest level. Pressed as always with the constant medical emergencies, my role had to expand continuously to cover areas of responsibility that were strictly routine administrative matters. I had always relied on the building supervisors to take care of such matters as food supply, laundry, and maintenance. I finally saw that these people had no control and no power. The central control of those vital services was oblivious and indifferent to building needs and allocated resources in such an arbitrary fashion as to make it look like a favor to a building if things were supplied or delivered.

The building supervisors, not realizing that they had the option to demand, rather than beg, for essentials, were kept in a state of supplication and personal indebtedness. The truth of the shortage emerged as the supervisors of my buildings began to turn to me to make the phone calls and issue the memos to support their well-documented needs. In addition, they were feeling the heat of the situation and wanted to keep from getting caught in the cross fire that was taking place.

Every day I would have to get on the phone to the head of the nursing supply and service departments and put my authority on the line to get resources for our residents. I do not believe that they responded because I was a doctor, but because these petty bureaucrats, moldy with their tenure in Willowbrook, were afraid of having a TV camera or other inquiry burst in on their operations. I never realized how many details, how huge a logistical problem existed in providing for a building. I could just imagine, without advocacy, how insufficient the conditions were in the other twenty-five buildings and what that meant for the people inside.

May 19, 1972
MEMO TO: Deputy Director
FROM: Dr. William Bronston

Building 22 has had a significant shortage in vital equipment. This includes suturing kits and sterilizeable suture removal sets. In addition, we have been unable to obtain suture material of the appropriate sizes to do the kind of face and scalp laceration repairs which are horribly too common in this building. I have been notified by the LPN that we have been back-ordered for two weeks.

There is no excuse for these deficiencies and I would appreciate, and strongly urge, that you investigate so that preventive planning will prevent such situations arising.

Thank you for your immediate attention to this matter.

WB:DD:22
cc: Mr. Palcic

August 16, 1972
MEMO TO: Pharmacist
FROM: DR. Willliam Bronston

RE: Antiseptic Soap

The practice of withholding antiseptic soap, in order to emphasize the need to avoid loss of the bottles interrupts needed treatment and must be altered. There is no need to assume that our concern for the loss of bottles will be greater if the soap supply is interrupted, over and above informing us of the problem by memo. Please maintain a continuous supply in accord with the medical prescription. Do not penalize patient care as your practice does.

WB/lb/76
cc: Dr. J. Hammond.
Dr. M. Jacobs

August 21, 1972

Mr. A. Fontaino—Bldg. 1 Supplies Dr. W. Bronston, Bldg., #23 Detergent supply for Building #23
We have been keeping careful tabs on the status of the odor and cleanliness of the building. It has just come to my attention that, although not for the first time, there is no Hospital Disinfectant Concentrate (Vestol) in the building. I believe we receive 12 gallons every two weeks and that this is to be used in diluted form. Nevertheless, conservative estimates on the part of the ward workers indicate that we use 1/2 gallon daily on wards A, B and D and a little less on ward C. By these calculations we use 26 gallons every two weeks. Today we are totally out of Vestol, an inconceivable situation that such a crowded building with the kinds of hygiene problems that we have should sustain. We are now left to wait until Monday, a full seven days away for the next delivery. What usually happens is that the ward staff buys and brings in their own soaps and detergents to use when the state supply runs out. I am sure that you are familiar with the fact that this practice is universal in the institution and absolutely unacceptable. I would appreciate it if you would deliver 10 gallons, as per my telephone request, to building #23 immediately and increase our standing order to 24 gallons every two weeks.

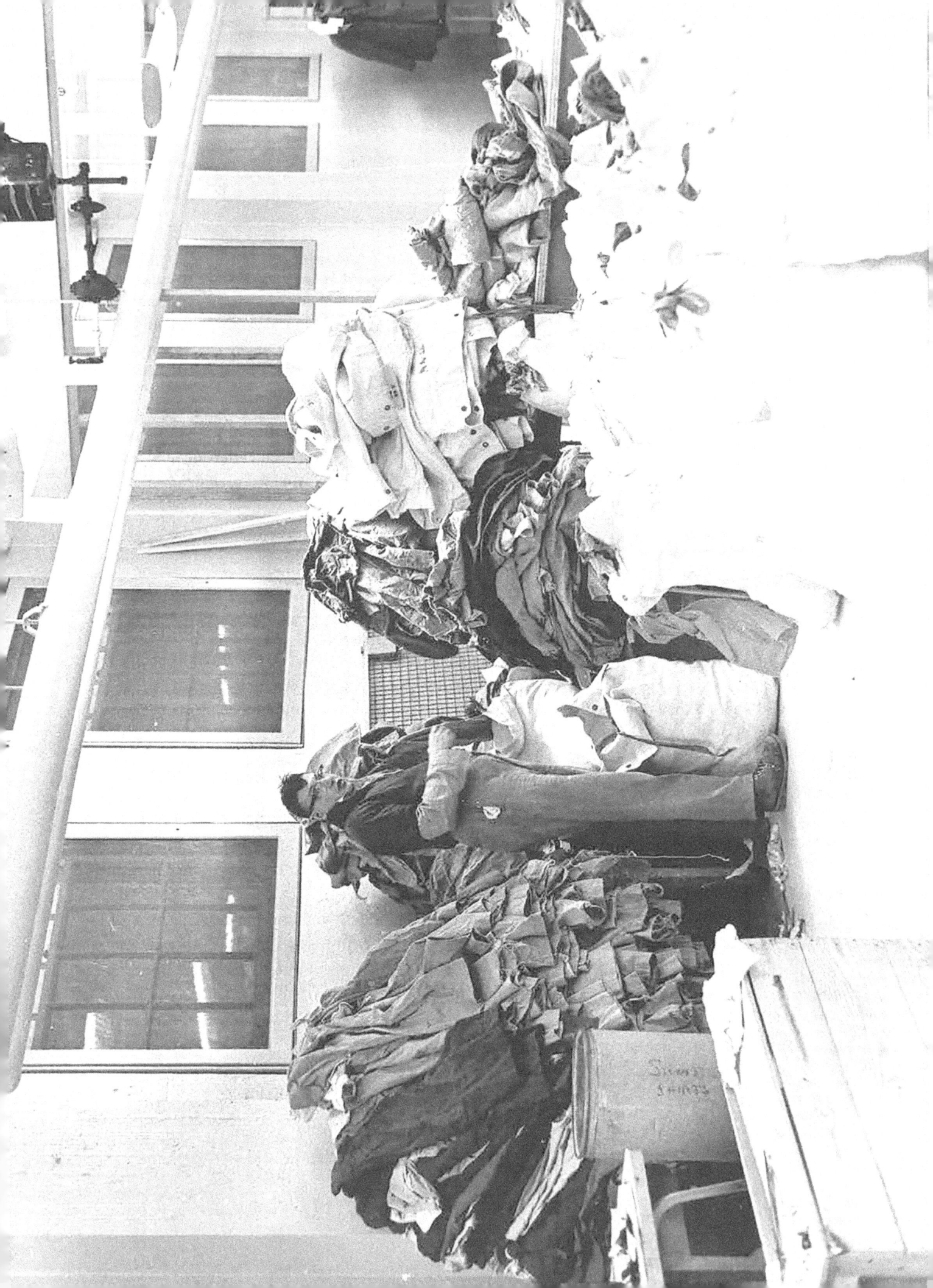

WB:vf:23
cc: Dr. Ristic, Acting Director MEMO TO: FROM:

MEMO TO: Mrs. McKenna, Laundry Supervisor
FROM: Dr. Bronston.

Soiled laundry is normally disposed of from all wards in the chute area. Time after time the people that come to collect the laundry have refused to get it as we do not leave it outside the side door staircase or even out of the building. The side door is heavily trafficked, both by residents and workers, and stacking the laundry there results in an unbearable smell and a public health hazard. To drag the bags of wet, soiled laundry out-of-doors for the women in this building when you have men picking up the laundry is inappropriate. Please instruct your pickup team that the laundry will be in the chute room for them to pick up.

WB:vf:23
cc: Mrs. Tetterton, bldg. 23
Mrs. Hairston, bldg. 22 Mrs. Bailey, bldg. 23 Mrs.
Hardin, bldg. 22

MEMO TO: Fred Carroll, Food Service
FROM: Dr. William Bronston, Bldg. #23
SUBJECT: Use of Pork

Today we had a serious outbreak of diarrhea in Bldg. 23. Thirty residents were reported with loose stools from early this morning. Such incidents happen at least twice-a-month in the building and seems to be regularly associated with the use of pork. I would appreciate if you would check a lot of pork sent to this building yesterday and substitute other meats in the future, excluding pork from this building permanently.

KB:/lkb/23

Then there were the tragedies among the people who, innocent of the storm over their fate, caught in the pitiless crushing environment, gave up pieces of their lives day after monotonous day. My memo submissions with the various administrators aimed, not only to document the infractions, but to forcefully and vividly explain the implications and to clearly set a record of the constant malfeasance. I knew that sooner or later all of these medical notes would become crucial parts of the final indictment of my workplace. It was also key that I acted as much as a model of integrity for all the coworkers to stimulate a sense of possibility for them to also resist the complicity imposed on them at every turn. The cover-ups that were the norm had to be exposed by personal example. The universal fear that stifled even the most basic dialogue had to be shattered to fracture the monolithic retaliatory unspoken threat everyone labored under daily.

MEMO TO: Dr. M. Jacobs, Administrative Assistant
to the Director
FROM: Dr. W. Bronston

This is in response to your inquiry about David M.* My conclusion that this youngster had been beaten was confined to the unmistakable nature of the lesions on his body.

I have seen more inflicted trauma than I care to recall during my employment here. Brutalization is so widespread that it reaches epidemic proportions. I hold the administration fully and solely responsible by their indifference to the plight of the employees on the wards who remained untrained, unsupervised, overworked. The perception that the people whom we serve are subhuman simply by virtue of the way the residents are forced to live clinches the base with which they can be treated like animals.

Given such inhuman circumstances, to persecute any worker, except in the rarest cases, before the people strategically responsible have been dealt with, and the fundamental conditions which lock a backward viewpoint of the retarded are altered, is to scapegoat and to deflect attention from the real problem.

WB: vf*

August 21, 1972 MEMO

TO:
RE:
FROM:
TO: Dr. M. Ristic, Acting Director Dr.
FROM: William Bronston, Bldg.#22
Clothing supply

Today 15 women from one ward ate lunch in the cafeteria completely nude in building #22. We have been keeping fairly close scrutiny on the adequacy of clothing supply in the building, rating each day according to the amount of gowns and dresses on one hand, and underclothes on the other, for each of the three shifts. This last week there has not been, at any time, enough clothes to provide coverage for a 24-hour period in relation to our census. Despite the fact that the bags of clothes that are delivered weigh what might be considered an adequate amount to contain the appropriate clothing, the laundry people in the building have reported more than 1/3 of these bags are filled with rags that are totally unusable.

I bring this situation to your attention because of its obvious significance to providing minimum patient care in the building. I would appreciate it if the situation were thoroughly investigated and corrected for our sakes.

WB:vf;22
cc: Mrs. Laub, bldg. #1

MEMO TO: Chief Supv. Nurse
FROM: Dr. W. Bronston

Three residents received lacerations in building #23 today. In each instance there was only one worker on the ward when the accident occurred. During this last week there has been at least one ward in both buildings 22 and 23 every day with only one worker on a ward. This situation is absolutely intolerable. This situation has existed for many months with only one worker required to assume the responsibility for wards with over 50 residents. The number of severe lacerations requiring suturing in buildings 22 and 23 is outrageously high and is a direct result of overcrowding and understaffing, a situation which you have been crystal clear about since the filing of the Federal Class Action in March.

I am not satisfied with your reply that you did not know that the coverage was at the unacceptable level. It is your job to find those things out. As per my verbal communication with you over the telephone today, I will not hesitate to bring charges against you as the responsible person in Willowbrook to see to it that the basic minimum coverage to assure the safety of the residents occurs.

WB:vf:21
cc: Dr. Ristic, Acting Director Eugene Eisner
Robert Feldt.
Bruce Ennis
Anthony Pinto, Benevolent Society Supv. Bldg. 22

CHAPTER 17

Photos: The Radiator

SEEING TAKES TIME. WE live in a fast society—thirty miles per hour, at least. What we see is so often like a billboard: colors, shapes, a quick message among an avalanche of quick messages—numbing. It doesn't take long to withdraw from all that for most of us. There is only so much one can sort out, understand, emotionally recognize, respond to, use.

For a health worker, seeing—really seeing—is critical. Each time an opportunity arises to see, every sense must be alert. Every bit of experience and stored knowledge must be somewhere close at hand. Each time that one only half sees, is blind to what one sees, misinterprets, makes false assumptions, or has incorrect expectations, a life is at stake.

I don't want to romanticize the doctor or add to the mystique and awe in which medicine is held in the minds of people. Seeing is not any more than a good parent or a loving and dedicated worker does all the time, naturally.

But this is a problem for the professional who is trained to be detached and alienated from people— "objectivity" is the cover term. It is a real chore for the professional to be natural, alert, and insightful, and identify with people, rather than functioning in a role, in a status pose flowing from authority, from fail-safe aspirations, possibly from even downright dislike of people and human service work.

If the feeling of identification between server and served is underdeveloped, sabotaged, or absent, seeing is arduous. Seeing, really seeing, requires feeling. It is the difference between human understanding and object spectating.

It is intensely hard to see in the institution. All the deafening language of images built from the physical remoteness, steel doors, barren rooms, overcrowding, accepted suffering, and degradation make it almost impossible to see, to feel, and identify with the victims as peers, citizens, friends, people.

I guess it was the minute-to-minute struggle to "see" that made work so exhausting. don't think that anyone can naturally identify with the people trapped in the institution without constant, conscious effort to redefine everything and fight back the tendency to withdraw and close out what is really there to be seen and done.

On all wards, there is nothing soft. The stone floors, wood and fiberglass chairs, Formica and chrome tables, steel and glass windows, iron beds. Hardness. Coldness. Hardness unyielding. No place soft. No place for warmth, solace, sanctuary, energy to support life, no place but one—the radiator.

There, for the lonely, the searcher, the instinctual migrant, is a place four feet long and three feet high—an iron cover plate radiating something drastically different from all the rest. One has but to be passively close to feel warmth, a sensation, a tingle on the skin, on the nerve endings of one's being.

It took me a long time to realize how important the radiator was to a community of people who had nothing. Once I saw the people huddling there, it still took time to really grasp, to feel the profound meaning of the radiator.

At first, I was outraged at the burns that I saw. People drugged, with a slowly diminishing ability to feel, sought the radiator for a retreat, a sleeping companion, a mother fragment, then, burned, were unable to move.

Couldn't the workers watch out for people next to the hot plates? I didn't realize how powerful was the pull to crouch and curl up there, a pull like that which draws all life to the warmth and energy of the sun. The sun, which was here cut off. Here, there was only the paint-peeling unmodulated sheet of hot metal left.

Can you imagine how empty, how deprived life can be, how empty of warmth? How can we not really see? How can we let the radiator be the sun for so many? There is always some sort of radiator, some obvious substitute for the real thing around which the lives of the public hostages cling. We have to look with more than just our eyes.

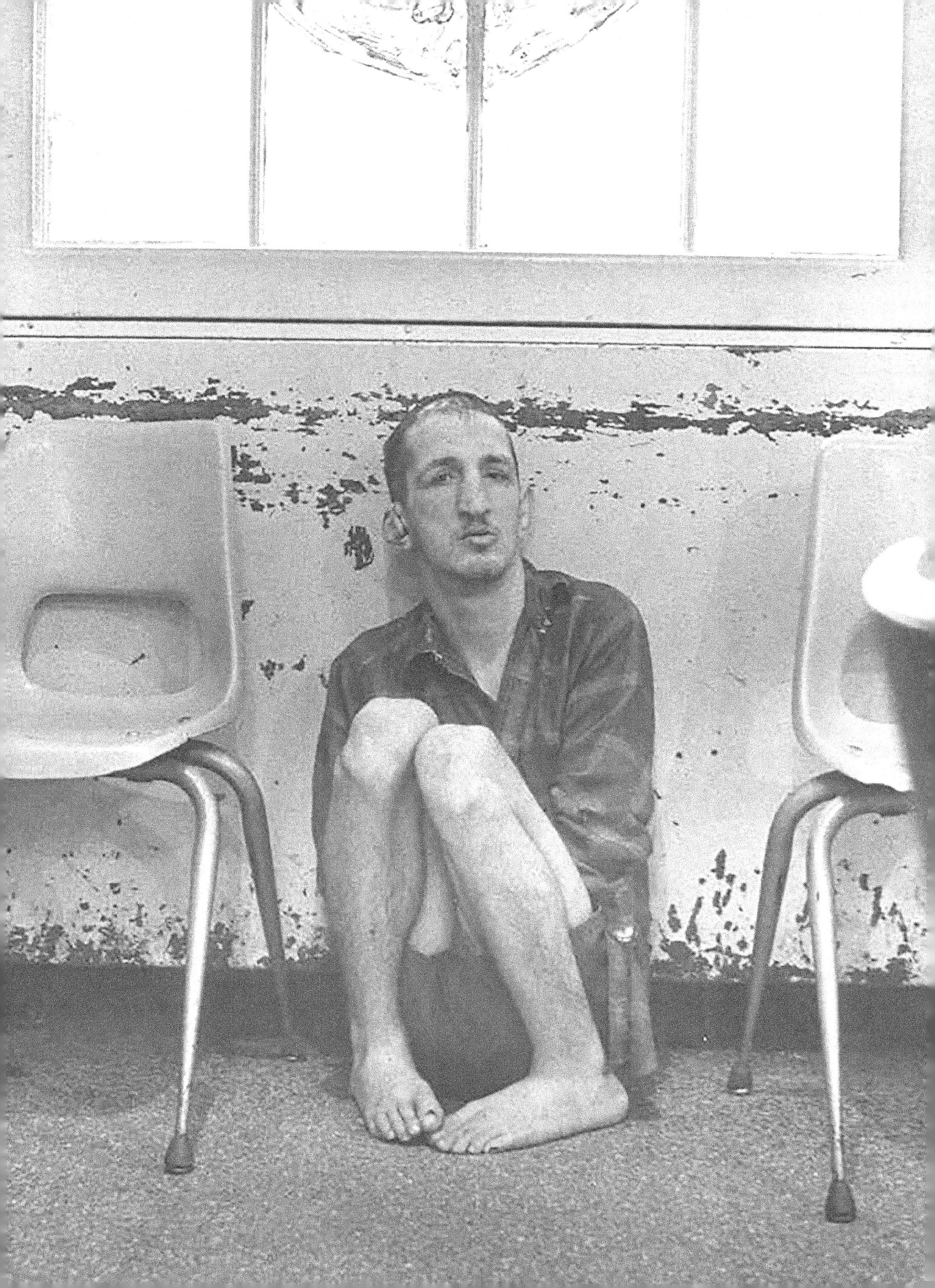

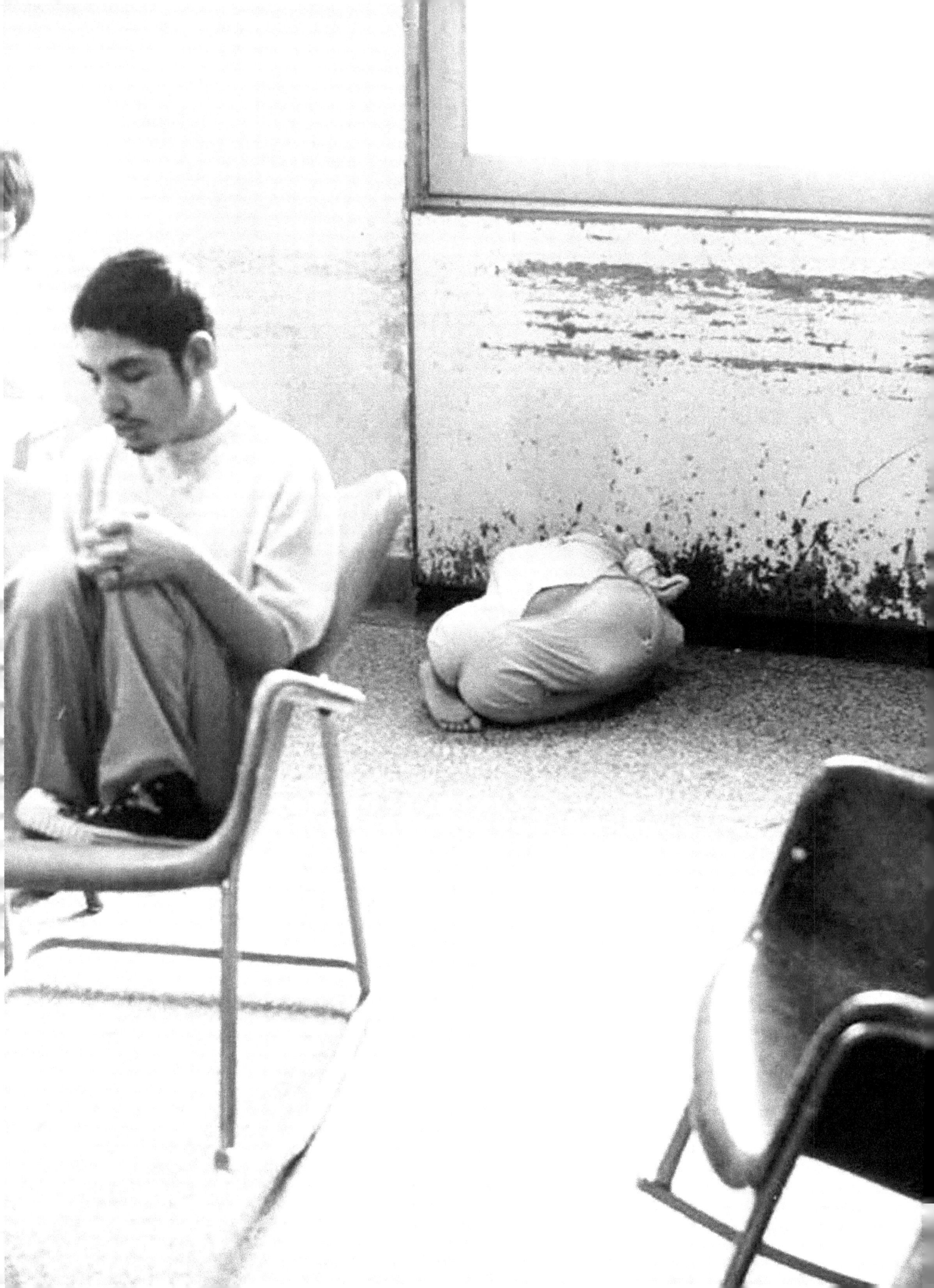

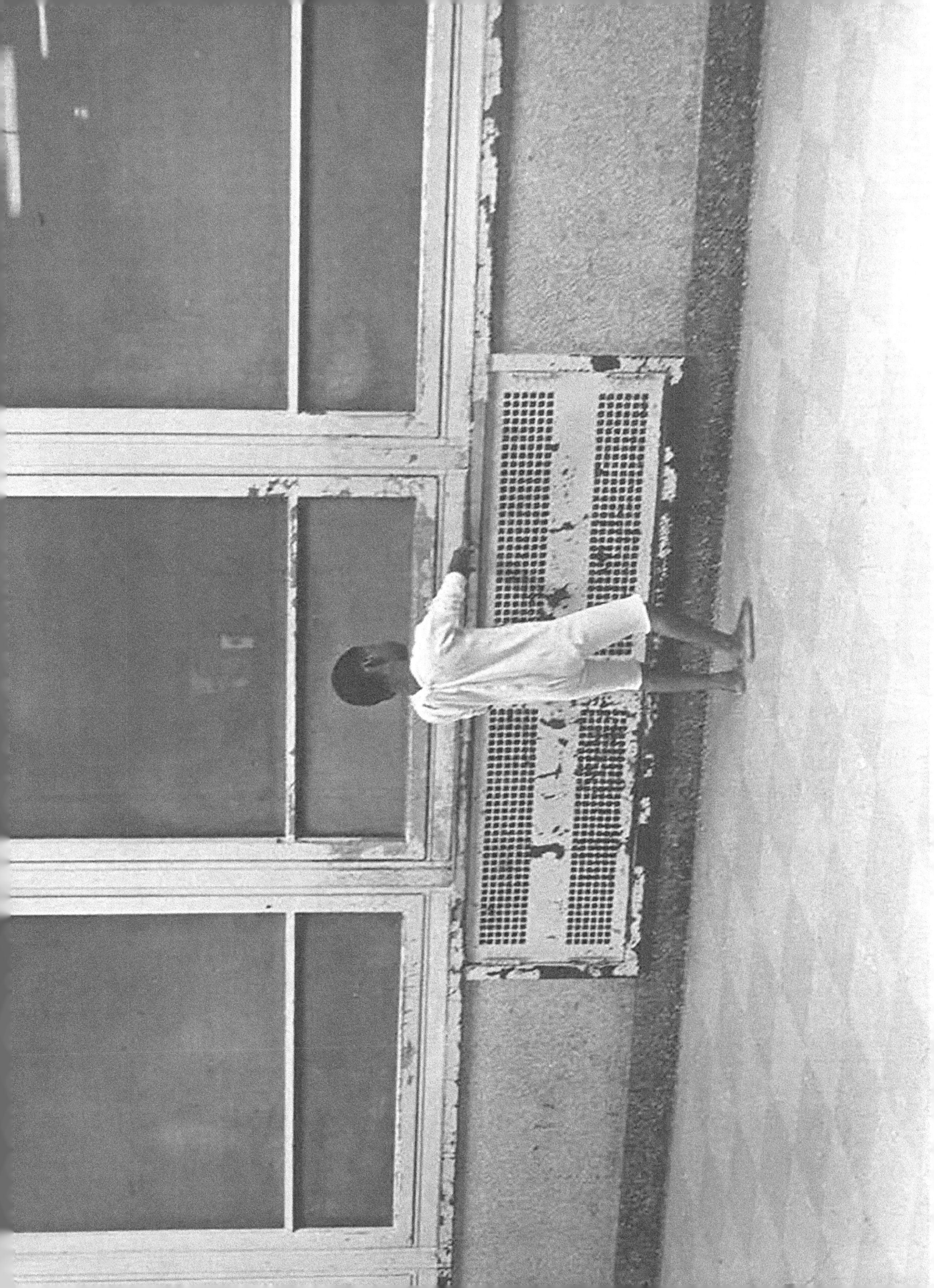

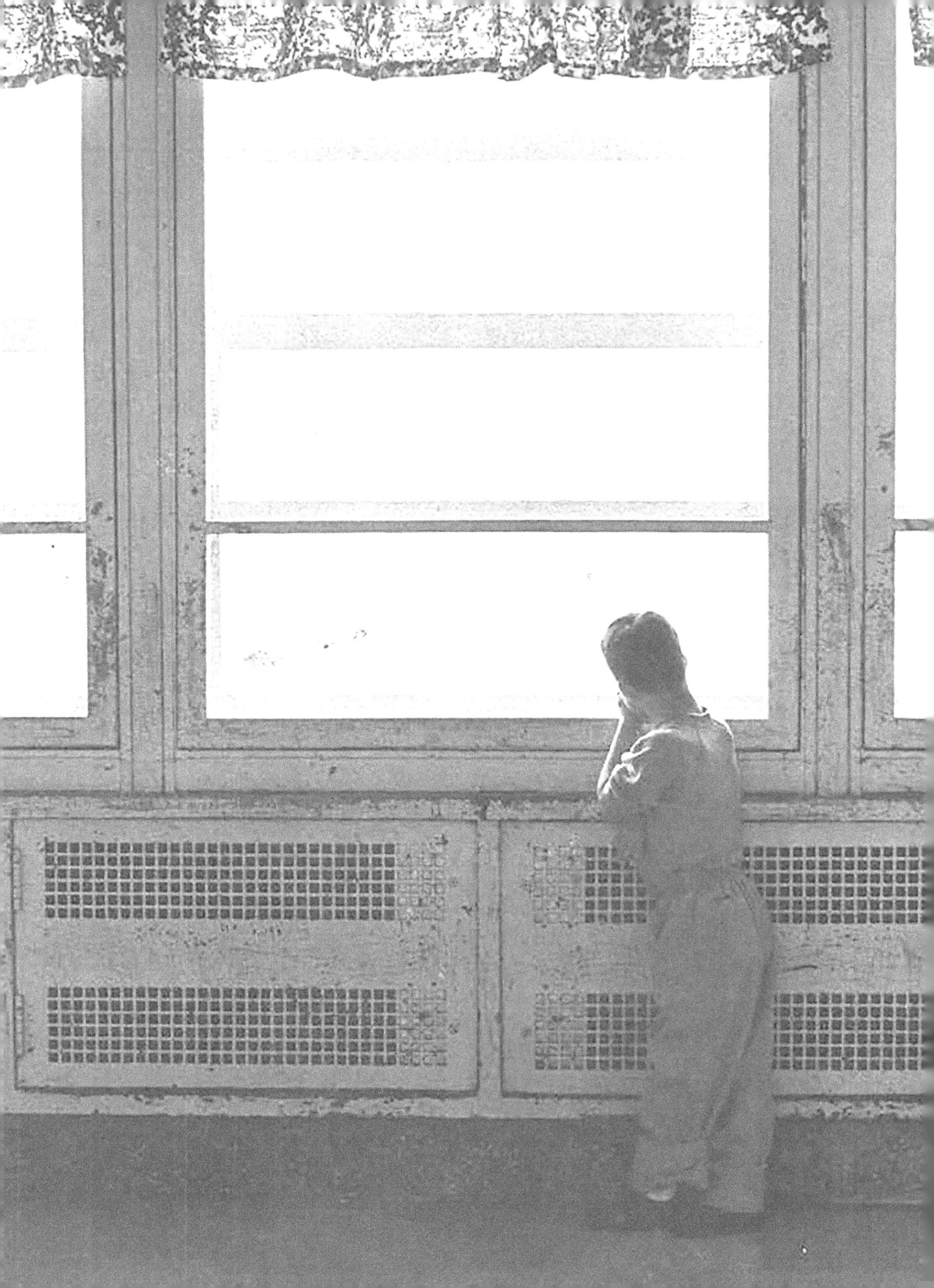

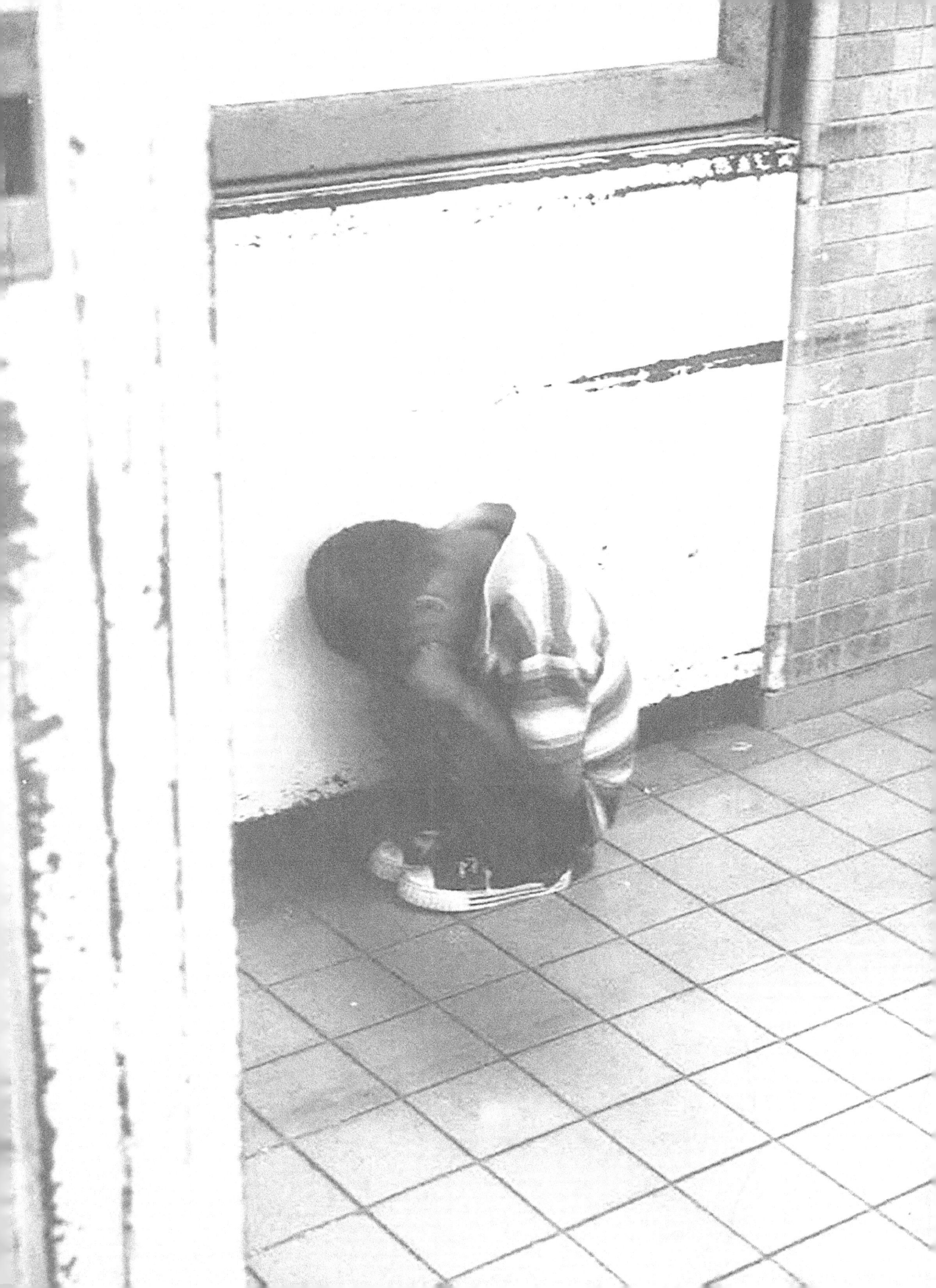

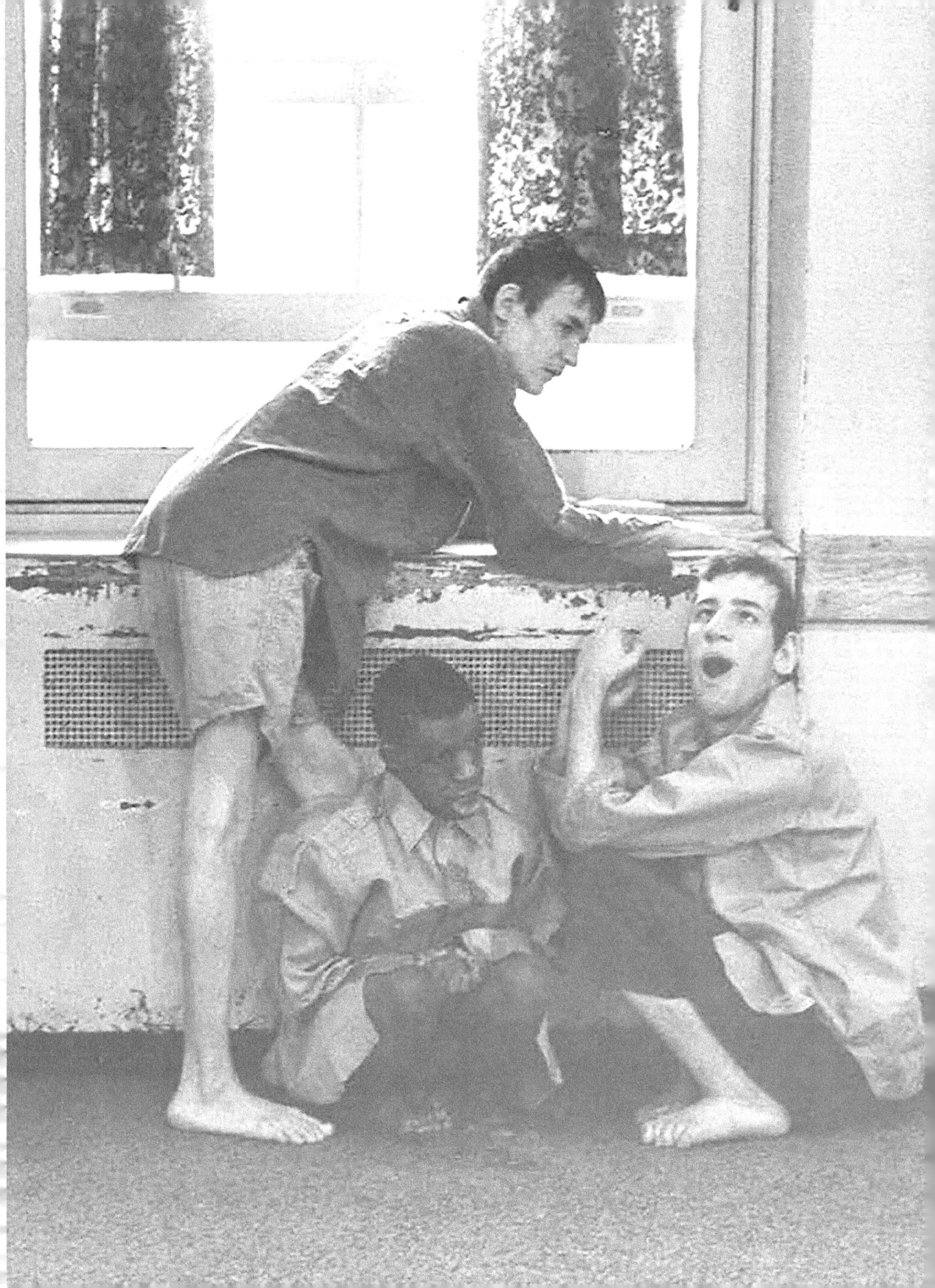

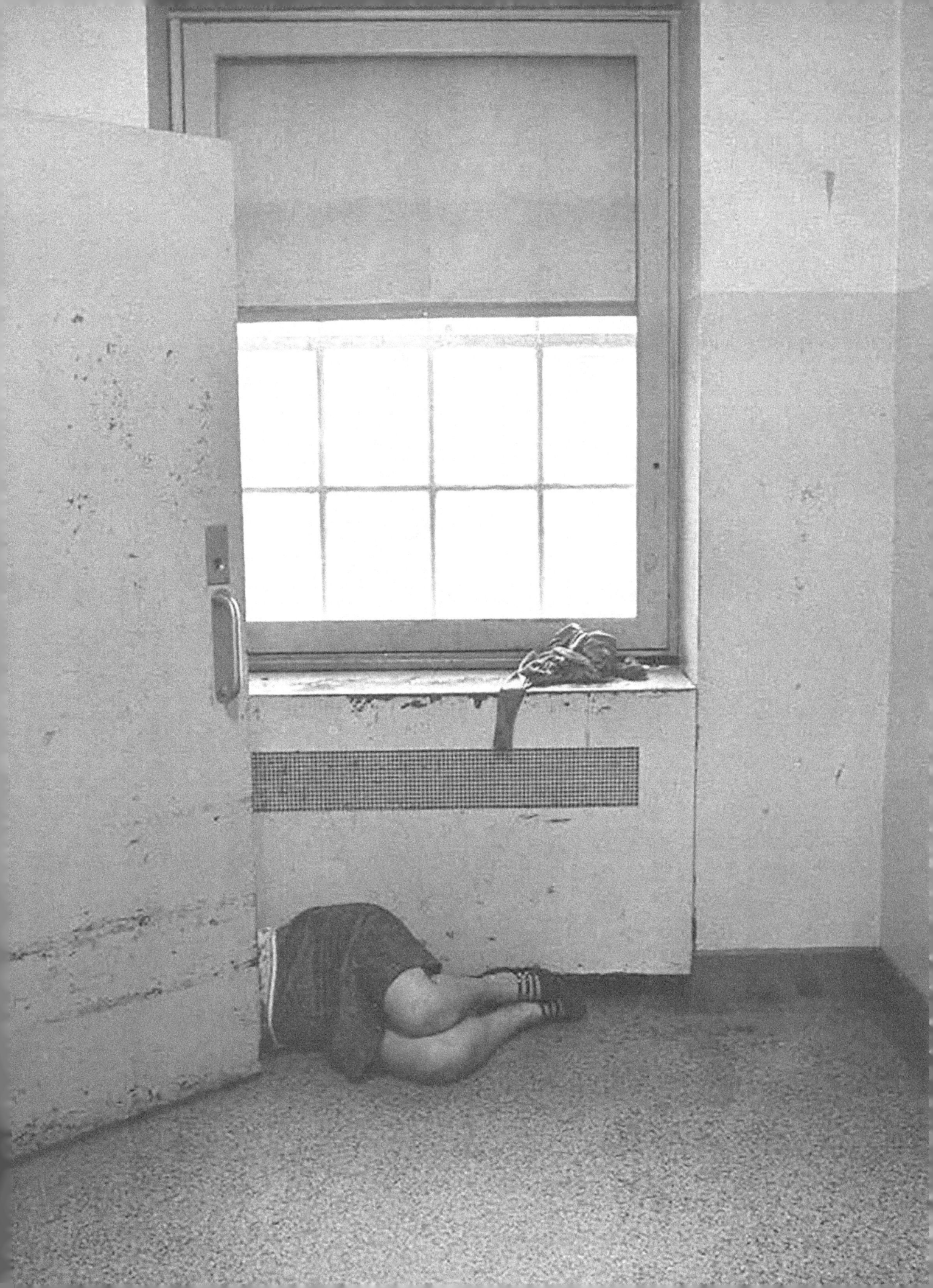

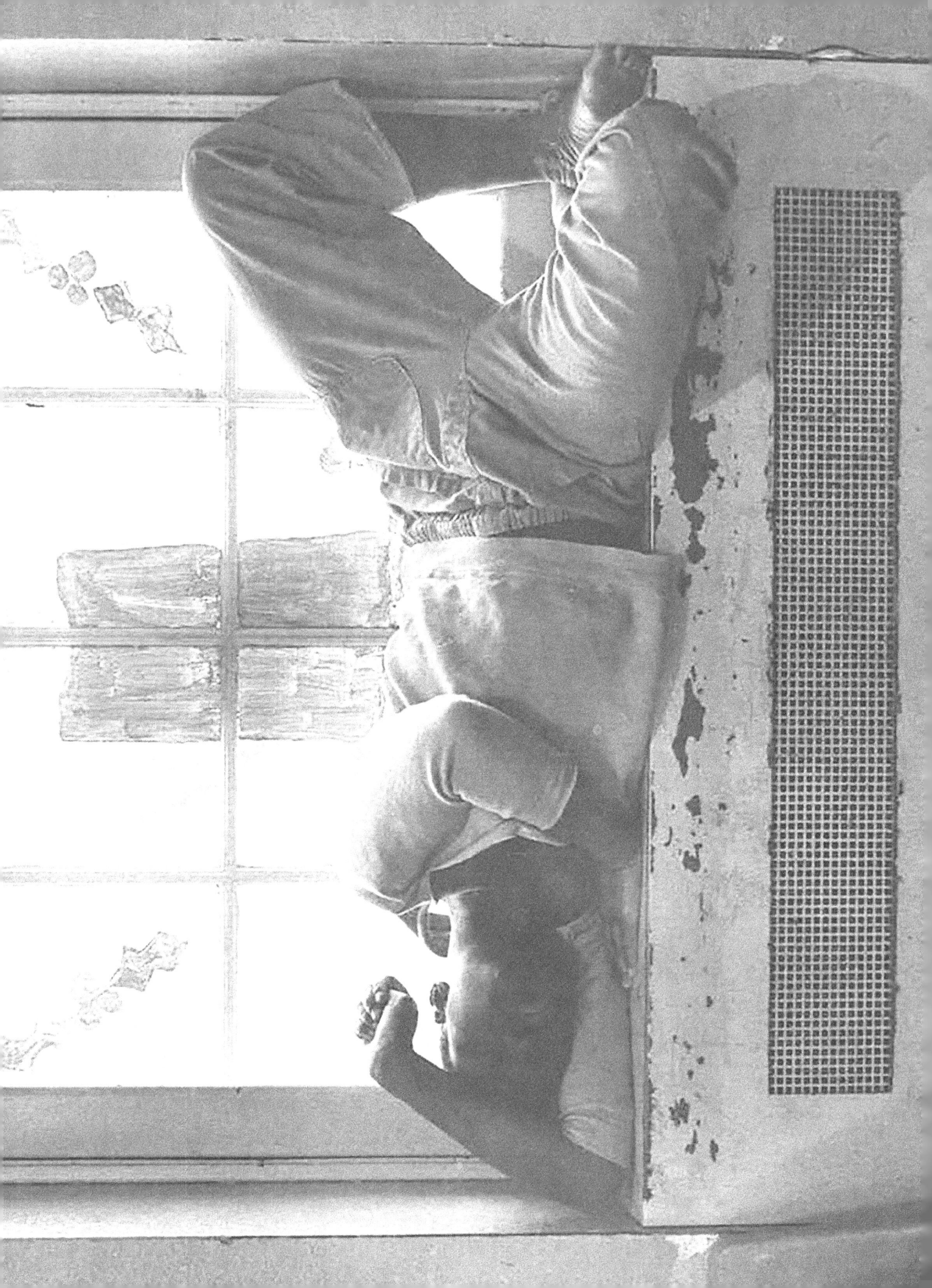

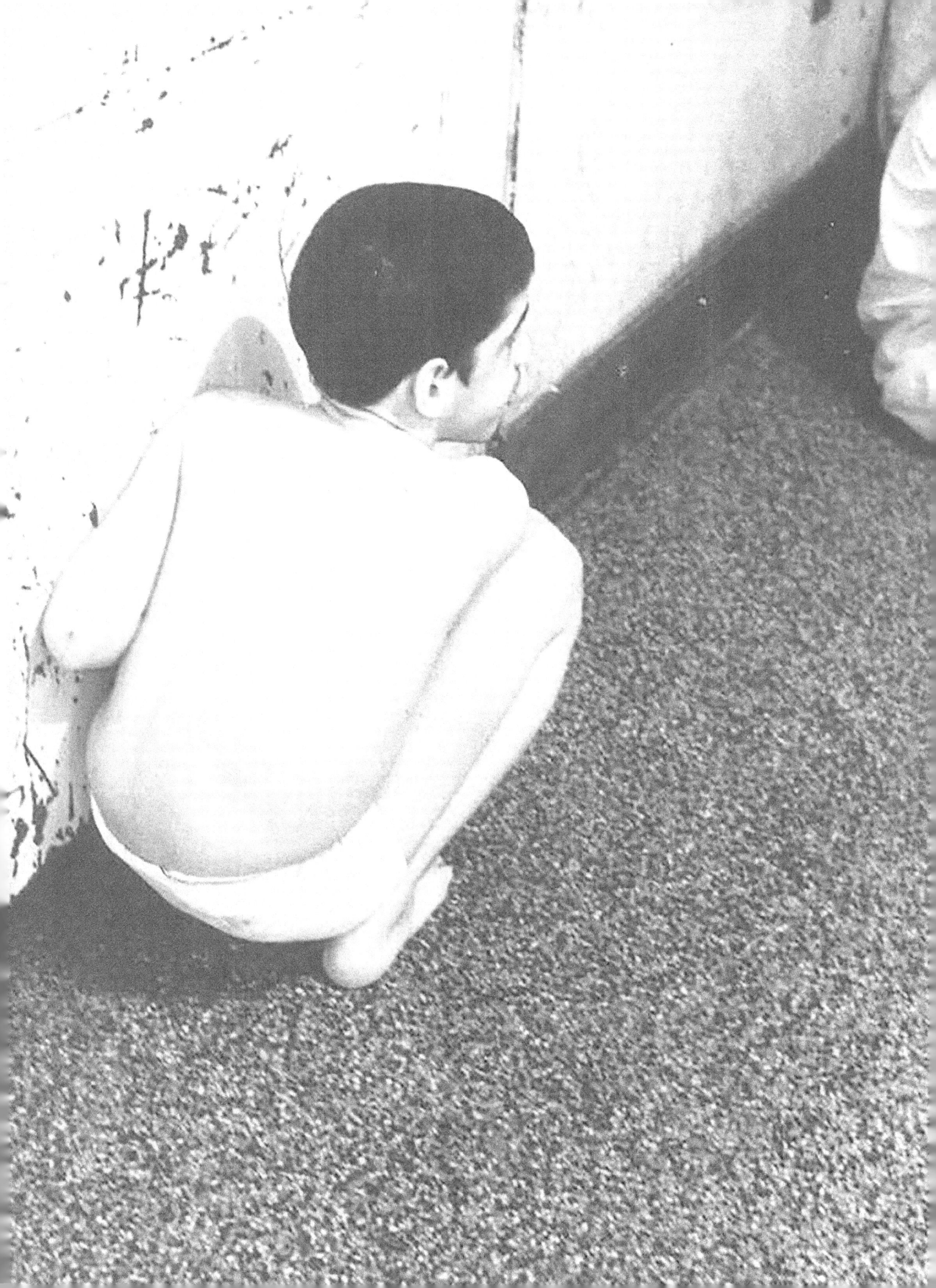

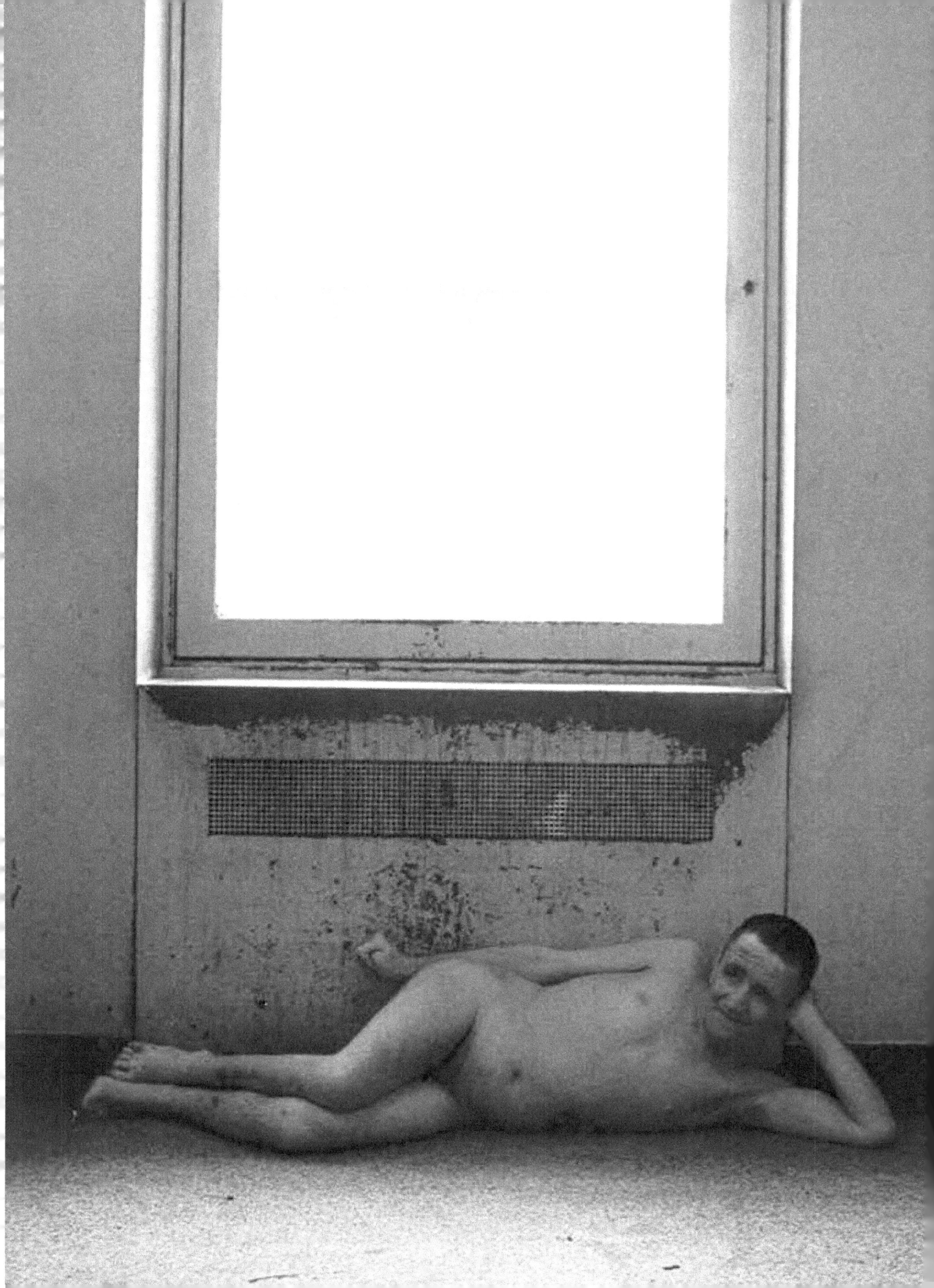

CHAPTER 18

Shake-Up: The Department's Hope

Dr. Hammond, who had been propped up since the TV exposé, graced with telegrams from the governor and the president of the United States congratulating his handling of the situation, was fired in July 1972. Frederick Grunberg, the Germanic iron heart of the department, commissioner over all the mental retardation empire in New York, would later be the next to go. Deciding to get out of the spotlight, he would take a comfortable position as professor of psychiatry in a medical school close to the headquarters of the department. It would be no victory that these two staunch lovers of institutions were thus removed from the situation, since the department had but to scan the line of willing and able applicants to carry on the work of their predecessors, hopefully with more charm.

It had taken a little time to locate the right man for the helm of Willowbrook. Dr. Miodrag Ristic's story is quite interesting in itself. The new director came from Yugoslavia. He was a young man, diminutive compared to the portly Hammond, neatly dressed, and boyishly handsome. He had been recruited from another institution in Cambridge, Minnesota—a little smaller, a little cleaner, but essentially doing the same kind of job. Dr. Ristic had been the medical director there and left rather unexpectedly—coincidentally with a number of parent protests calling for an investigation of the medical practices in the institution, where some deaths had occurred associated with excessive tranquilization. The governor of the state had been asked to mount an inquiry. The Minnesota State Association for Retarded Children had gotten into the controversy—and Willowbrook needed a new man. It was perfect.

It is not really important to say more. Ristic's coming is only important in understanding how personalities come and go. It is the system, not the system's leaders, that must be understood. The chiefs of the system are men who respect social control, who have abiding loyalties for their peer bureaucrats, and usually reverence and awe for political power. They are men whose eyes are always cast upward, never looking downward at what their feet tread upon in their career aspirations. Suffice to say that Dr. Ristic fit right in and served the department well. But as surely as anything in this world, I knew neither he nor any of his successors would last long without a drastic fix. The names and the faces change, come and go in an unjust system, but their kind persists in leadership positions. Such will be the public's burden until justice is done, until human service and respect become the state's commitments.

Nonetheless, there was Ristic, bright and in charge. He had been on the Willowbrook scene for some time and had been appointed deputy director a few months before Hammond's departure, in order to effect an orderly transition of power. Business as usual had to be faced every day. The dogfight intensified. Ristic instinctively understood enough to make a point of replying to the memos, in which I was determined to lay bare all the circumstances of Willowbrook's methodical delinquencies. In his replies, he formally perpetuated the rigid control and the standards of conformity that were the marching cadence of the department.

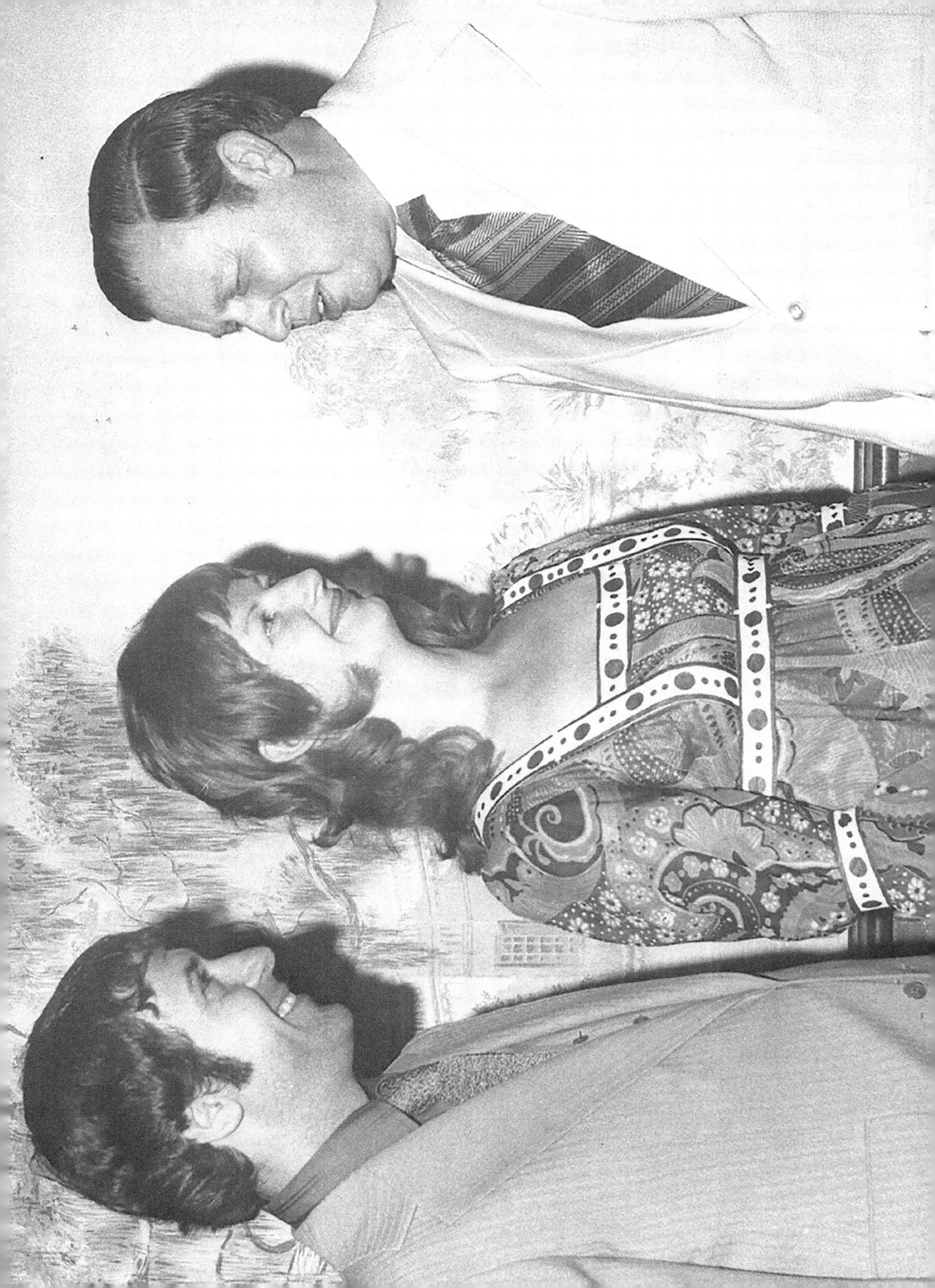

The hearing on any of my grievances never took place. A new set of conditions evolved. It was key, however, to keep on the offensive, to challenge the department's power to define what was happening. Had CSEA been a genuine union organization among the workers, able to understand the issues, or honest enough to do something about the conditions, this would possibly have been a turning point.

Alone, my approach to holding on had to be aggressive, never letting any situation go by without documenting and interpreting it clearly. I had no illusions of what the course would be if we so much as communicated indecision. We had no idea when the federal court would act on opening the class action suit that was still pending. We could not be sure the court would ever act at all. There was no alternative but to keep working, and waiting.

Once Hammond was gone, Gene and I met with Dr. Ristic to see what he would do, even though he would not officially be appointed as director-superintendent for several months. Gene counseled that we reach an agreement without waiving the right to pursue the grievances if things did not work out. After the meeting, we documented the deal.

Law Offices   EISNER & LEVY   351 Broadway   New York, New York 10013 / WOrth 6-9620

Eugene G. Eisner   Mary M. Kaufman
Richard A. Levy   Counsel

October 10, 1972

Dr. Miodrag Ristic Willowbrook State School 2760 Victory Boulevard Staten Island, New York 10314
Re: Dr. William Bronston (Three Grievances)

Dear Dr. Ristic:

First, I would like to take this opportunity to congratulate you on your appointment as Director of Willowbrook State School. As a person who has become intimately acquainted with the problems at Willowbrook during the past year, I know that your task to overhaul the archaic system at Willowbrook is a formidable one.

I have been somewhat surprised not have received any communication from you since our meeting of August 10th when we came to an agreement with respect to the three grievances that Dr. Bronston had outstanding against Dr. Hammond before he left; namely, (1) excessive work load, (2) refusal to permit Dr. Bronston to meet with parents on Willowbrook grounds, and (3) administrative harassment. You will recall that at the conclusion of our meeting (which was a resumption of our meeting of July 25th) you were to send me a letter confirming the fact that we had worked out a "detente" along the following lines: excessive work load—It was agreed that Dr. Bronston's work load, covering Buildings 22 and 23, was clearly excessive. Accordingly, you assured Dr. Bronston and myself that you were in the process of hiring new physicians and that as soon as one was hired you would assign another doctor to one of the buildings. In the meantime, you agreed to assign two registered nurses and one secretary to the two buildings to temporarily relieve Dr. Bronston's tremendous work load.

Refusal to permit Dr. Bronston to meet with parents on the ground—You agreed that Dr. Bronston could meet with parents (a) on his own time, on the premises, and (b) during working hours, on the premises, so long as Dr. Bronston does not call such a meeting, has made his "rounds", and keeps himself "on call."

Administrative harassment—It was generally agreed that the administrative harassment of Dr. Bronston had virtually ceased since Dr. Hammond's departure from Willowbrook. However, it was further agreed that we would all keep a watchful eye to prevent any recurrences.

In addition to the foregoing we had a long discussion about the "hate sheets" that had been distributed on Willowbrook grounds by administrative personnel in January of this year. You agreed that the hate sheets were despicable and you stated that had you been the Director at the time of their distribution you would have condemned them and disassociated yourself from them. Furthermore, you agreed to send a letter embodying this agreement.

I trust that I have accurately stated the details of our discussion and agreement. I would, appreciate hearing from you to confirm same.

Sincerely yours,
EUGENE G. EISNER
EGE/wto

On the heels of my early talks with Ristic, two outstanding nurses were assigned to my two buildings as assistants. Having two such clinicians to share work with was an incredible luxury. Both had worked up from the ward ranks of Willowbrook. For the first time, I had people that I could talk with who understood medicine and health care. The pleasure was short-lived. Within two months, both workers were exhausted and frustrated at their inability to make headway in establishing a system of care in the overcrowded buildings. Instead of being able to teach and catalyze the desperately needed services, they each became as deluged as I was in crises. It was as if the more ability we had to solve problems, the more problems arose.

Circumstances in the treatment room provided an ongoing situation of potential crisis. Workers there performed two basic procedures. The first was measuring and distributing medications, the bulk of which were tranquilizers and anti-epilepsy drugs. The second was providing treatments such as soaks, bandaging, skin care, and the like. The physician ordered both medications and treatments for each resident as needed, but it devolved to the nursing staff to carry out the written orders. The only way to know if these had been done was through the records kept by the nursing staff. Because of the severe shortage of staff, as well as their minimal training, documentation of medications and treatments was unreliable. Also, during the job freeze the year before, the head of the Nursing Department had issued a memo directing workers to stop recording treatments in all buildings, and this procedure still lingered. The workers performed under devastating time pressures, dispensing a steady stream of treatments all day long and most of the night. And yet, over three shifts, I knew that medications and treatments were missed. But unless I sat and watched each of the hundreds of transactions, I could not tell who or what was omitted.

Given my two new coworkers, I decided to discover and reveal exactly what was going on by doing a timework study. What this meant was simple. On one day, we could calculate exactly how many treatments and medications were ordered given out. We would clock the procedure under ideal conditions, with the most skilled staff doing the work. Given the total time and dividing by the number of procedures, we would have a baseline to calculate the time required per procedure and thus would know exactly how long it really took to do everything.

We picked Building 22 to do the study. The nurse was immensely excited to have the opportunity to check out why she could never get her work done. When we finished, the data was damning. What was so alarming was that the administration insisted that one worker in the treatment room was sufficient to do all the work, and yet, they never cared to see if, in fact, that was true. The workers, fearing that their failure to finish basic work would result in their being disciplined, hid the omissions everywhere. Not only did this make malpractice systemic, but also, it was downright illegal.

The nurse put a report together and submitted it to the administration. It showed conclusively that no fewer than two workers had to be assigned to the treatment room during each of the three shifts to accomplish what was ordered; fewer than two made it physically impossible to carry out the orders. Following are excerpts from that report:

TO: Chief Supervising Nurse
FROM: Staff Nurse, B-22
PURPOSE: Time Work Report—B-22 Treatment Room

I have been in Building 22 since August 3, 1972 and daily I encounter and become entangled in a tremendous amount of work. Thus, I decided to examine the situation by doing a time-work study for the treatment room. Not calculated in the time-work study is the time required to fill out forms for the weekly requisition for regular and control drugs and surgical supplies, in addition to the time required to deal with acute spontaneous problems that arise daily.

Below is the time work study for the treatment room in B-22.

Building Census—214 Residents

Each day patient medication contact (morning and afternoon shifts) 409

Average time to make up and deliver medications (A.M. & P.M. Shifts) approximately

360 minutes = 6 hours. (Timed at full speed) Time to chart medications for day shift—1 hour Total number of treatments daily (A.M. & P.M. Shifts) 97

Average time for treatment per patient—5 minutes = 485 minutes = 8 hours. (Timed at full speed) Total treatment and medication time—15 hours. This does not include counting the narcotics and dangerous drugs.

As you see it is impossible for one person working an 8 hour shift to manage these responsibilities in the treatment room. Moreover, Dr. Bronston informs me that among my regular duties will be included case findings that will surely increase the number of treated cases, further straining our situation.

I hope this information will aid you in thinking about the staff needs of this building. An additional aspect is the low coverage on the ward which disallows the ward workers from helping in the treatment process. Therefore, it is, in my opinion, if optimum nursing care is to be given to the residents of B-22, essential that two L.P.N.'s should be assigned to the treatment room.

Yours sincerely,
Betty Hairston, Staff Nurse DD:22
cc: Dr. Ristic
Dr. Bronston

Naturally, the situation was not rectified. We received no reply, and true to form, the outlaw practices continued despite all we could do.

For over two years, with the deepest resentment and revulsion, I had cooperated with the institution's practices of over-tranquilizing and restraining residents—the practices of social control. I knew that what was being done was wrong, but I knew of nothing else to do, short of stopping these inhuman practices. I told myself that such unilateral action would have not only alienated and frightened the ward workers, whose goodwill and understanding were vital to change, but also would have brought premature reprisal by the administration.

At last, a family whom I had befriended and supported confronted me about their daughter's straitjacket. "You sign her into that thing every day, don't you?" I tried to explain, but my words turned to ashes in my mouth. There was no real explanation! I was horrified and ashamed that after all that had gone on, I was still mindlessly, routinely abusing people. The time had come to take the next step to assert decency, to free myself from this oppression.

August 29, 1972

TO: Dr. M. Ristic, Acting Director
FROM: William Bronston
RE: Restraints

Sunday, August 27, 1972, I was confronted with two wrenching situations with regard to restraints. First the family of Mary S., a multiply-handicapped resident of B-22, visited. On the 24th of this month their daughter had been severely bitten by a peer incurring lacerations on her face and scalp. The physician who sutured the lesion missed another cut that required closing. We discovered this untreated lesion oozing pus on the back of her neck. The family, needless to say, was speechless with fury. I told them that Mary had been kept in the strait jacket since 1968, which originated when she injured a peer. I promised the family that I would remove Mary from this inhuman restraint, as I agreed with them that she should not be punished because of lack of personnel on the ward.

The second incident required that I over sedate and seclude Beverly C. because of her severe acting out behavior. As you already know, Beverly was brutalized by a worker in B-23, and knowing the speed with which the administration moves in these situations, I felt it better to remove Beverly from the building for her own protection when in truth the worker should have been immediately removed.

Signing the restraint orders and being forced to resort to methods that are totally odious to me just to cope with the state's inertia, takes its daily toll on my patience and judgment. Having to day in and day out do things which injure patients, their families, and the employees requires a hardening and an ability to rationalize abuses of which I am not capable. I will no longer sign any more restraint orders. The list of regularly strait jacketed patients who mutilate themselves and their peers has been available to you for many months. In the event that any residents are injured in the future, I will personally inform their families of the true reasons for their daughters 'and sisters' injuries and urge them to take legal action in the matter. The state's inertia in this matter, full well knowing the consequences of indifference, negligence, and systematic dehumanization of residents and workers alike, is beyond my ken and represents an extreme savagery inconsistent with our present civilization and science.

WB:DD:22
cc: Dr. Miller
Dr. Grunberg Mr. Eisner Mr. Feldt.
Mr. Pinto Mr. Ennis

TO: Dr. Ristic, Acting Director
FROM: Dr. W. Bronsto

While on duty Saturday night, August 26th, I was shocked at the enormous number of B-22 residents in the hospital. It was not surprising to me that they were ill and needed care. What got to me was the number of workers out of B-22 in the face of our worker shortage in the building. Nineteen of our residents are in B-2, the medical-surgical building.

In reviewing our staffing pattern over the last two weeks, there have only been an average of 11 actual ward service personnel in the building for both the A.M. and P.M. shifts respectively, which means that the patient ratio is 1 to 18. With the full building census, including our ladies in B-2, it would climb to 1 to 20. The people in the building are exhausted and their morale is very low. The frequency of accidents in the building has climbed significantly. The situation speaks for itself—we must have more ward staff. The last new ward worker to be hired that came into B-22 was hired on July 6, 1972.

What the hell is going on?

WB:DD:22

A week later, the new director's reply reached me.

Form 26-D.M.H.

ALAN D. MILLER, M.D.
COMMISSIONER

WILLIAM VOORHEES, M.D.
FIRST DEPUTY COMMISSIONER

ROBERT PATTON
SECOND DEPUTY COMMISSIONER

STATE OF NEW YORK
DEPARTMENT OF MENTAL HYGIENE
DIVISION OF MENTAL RETARDATION
AND CHILDREN'S SERVICES
NEW YORK CITY METROPOLITAN REGIONAL OFFICE
2 WORLD TRADE CENTER, 56TH FLOOR
NEW YORK, N. Y. 10048

ROBERT W. HAYES, M.P.H.
DEPUTY COMMISSIONER
FOR MENTAL RETARDATION
AND CHILDREN'S SERVICES

SIDNEY LECKER, M.D.
ASSISTANT COMMISSIONER
FOR CHILDREN'S SERVICES

September 5, 1972

MEMO TO: William Bronston, M.D.
RE:
FROM: Miodrag Ristic, M.D., Acting Director
Your memos of August 29, 1972

I have received two memos from you dated as of the above date. Let me first deal with the question of restraints. As you know, seclusion is not to be used again at Willowbrook State School. Situations that have in the past necessitated seclusion must now be handled by alternative means. I bring your attention to the standard 2.1.8.6 of the Accreditation Council for Facilities for the Mentally Retarded, dealing with physical restraint. In brief, the standard states that physical restraint shall be employed only when absolutely necessary to protect the resident from injury to himself or to others. This is shortly to be the official Willowbrook State School policy on the use of restraints. But right now, as your supervisor, I advise you to abide by this criterion in using physical restraint.

As you know, continuous employment of any member of the staff of Willowbrook State School is contingent upon their non-negligent discharge of their duties. It is the duty of a physician to use due care, skill and knowledge in the management of his patients' problems. This implies that you should use all means available to you, in the light of the circumstances of a particular case, always exercising that skill, care and knowledge which is appropriate to your position. A flat statement, "I will no longer sign any more restraint orders" appears to indicate that you take a certain position as a matter of principle, regardless of the circumstances of an individual case. Should a resident come to harm because of your failure to apply due care, skill and knowledge to the circumstances of his individual case, this might be presumptive evidence of negligence. Since I myself may be held negligent for not bringing about the procedure for dismissal of a potentially negligent physician, I strongly urge you to forego this rash resolution of yours, and to consider each case on its own merit.

The list of patients in need of physical restraint has, indeed, been available to me for three or four months. All I can say is that we are making the greatest progress possible under the circumstances, and that our diligence in this respect is being evaluated by the Federal District Court. I think that before you start excoriating your superiors for inertia, you could at least note that the courts have not seen fit so far to prod us to move faster than we have done so far, because the courts seem to realize that we are doing all that is humanly possible, under the circumstances.

I do believe you are sincerely distressed about the deplorable condition of residents in your buildings, and I will not do anything about the highly emotionally charged language of your memos. However, please be advised that the use of profanity is a chargeable offense, and do not use four-letter words in your communications to other employees of Willowbrook State School, as this may result in disciplinary action.

> Miodrag Ristic, M.D.
> Acting Director/th

Miodrag Ristic, MD, acting more elegantly than I could paraphrase, showed how business as usual could be carried on behind the regulations that appeared to deny the old way. It is easy to see how an outsider would concede to the logic of the administration. What was not obvious was that there were no "individual cases" the same way that there were no individualized programs, no individualized life space, and no individual identity on the wards. Ristic knew that. "Restraint when absolutely necessary" meant that in Willowbrook, straitjackets and excessive tranquilization would continue—but with a rationale, and Ristic knew that too.

In a twist of reasoning, Dr. Ristic had cast himself as the victim. According to his reasoning, he would have to discipline me in the name of resident care and to avoid negligence on his part. An image from Ecclesiastes sprang to my mind: "I saw under the sun in the place of judgment, wickedness and in the place of justice iniquity…I turned myself to other things and saw the oppressions that are done under the sun, and the tears of the innocent, and they had no comforter, and they were not able to resist their violence, being destitute of help from any."

I stopped all restraints. Ristic's threat was empty, his logic gruesome and indefensible.

In the hopes of further marshaling facts and solutions to the conditions, I mounted weekly meetings among the staff of Buildings 22 and 23. Minutes were taken during these meetings and distributed to every worker in each building. Since at least two people had to stay on the wards at all times by my order, the duplication of the minutes was crucial to be sure that everyone knew and could relate to what was going on. Copies of the minutes also went to the administration so that the usual "We didn't know" response could be voided.

These weekly meetings were astounding in terms of what came to light. I hoped that as the staff heard one another and shared in the information, they would be better prepared to see why they were hamstrung in their jobs. Until the private guilt and frustration could be dispelled, the staff would not understand the value of cooperation.

EXCERPTS FROM CLINICAL STAFF MEETINGS FALL, 1972
Buildings 22-23

1) The head of Willowbrook's dietary department accepted our invitation to be at the meeting and discuss our problems. They oriented us about how the department of Mental Hygiene set up an overall menu for a year in advance for the $1 million budgeted; how the Willowbrook menu is then built, six weeks in advance, based on what there is to choose from and what would make a balanced diet (3,000 calories per day per resident). They said that changes in the actual menu resulted from warehouse delivery delays, back ordering, use of planned food for institution picnics and special affairs, or lot of food rejected by health inspectors. They described hew the dietary department had to deal with meals differently depending on the special needs of the building—e.g. cafeteria style, roller trays, provide clean up, or just prepare food for residents to pick up.

Question: What about special diets?

Answer: We do not have properly trained staff to make up special diets.

Question: What do we do about special diets?

Answer: We will look into it.

Bread must be used too often to supplement inadequate supply of food to fill the residents.

Beans had been served three times last week in both Building 22 and Building 23, resulting in widespread diarrhea. Spinach had been served three days in a row with similar consequences. Many residents who could eat normal foods must eat the puree generally served to the buildings.

2) The laundry problem was discussed with the head of Central Laundry, who told us:

The laundry washes 1.2 million pounds per month when it should only service one-half that amount. Right now there are only 16,811 sheets in the whole Willowbrook system, which is not enough. There are 13,100 bath towels in Willowbrook's inventory as of 8/2/72. Thousands of new towels and sheets disappear from the inventory when added, which results in widespread shortages to residents and hardships to ward workers. We started talking about these losses.

Ideally, B-22 needs 3,000 sheets per week or 430 per day, which, would provide extra for 100 non toileter's in the building. Each non-toilet trained person should have 28 sheets per week and 14 pillowcases. Since deliveries come every three days for the buildings, B-22 should have 1,290 sheets to operate and 430 should be on a shelf in case substitutes are needed.

Feces should be shaken out from soiled laundry before putting into the bags so that the laundry can be put into the machines faster and returned faster. If a laundry worker has to shake out the soil, delays occur.

Condemning rags must take place accurately, otherwise rags stay in the system and are returned with good clothing bags, causing more shortages. Donation clothes that are of no use should be removed from system and not be put into the laundry.

Question: Why do the supervisors have to make out clothing and laundry requests when Building 1 knows what our bedding, towel, and clothing needs are and could send a regular supply? This way request would be cut down to just special needs and changes in the order.

Answer: We don't know, we will look into that.

Question: Why are there shortages in shoes and shoelaces?

Answer: I am ordering more shoes that don't have to be tied but have elastic tops, they haven't come yet.

Question: Have you tested to see if these elastic top shoes will be kept on the residents who always take them off, before ordering?

Answer: How can we get clothes for everybody?

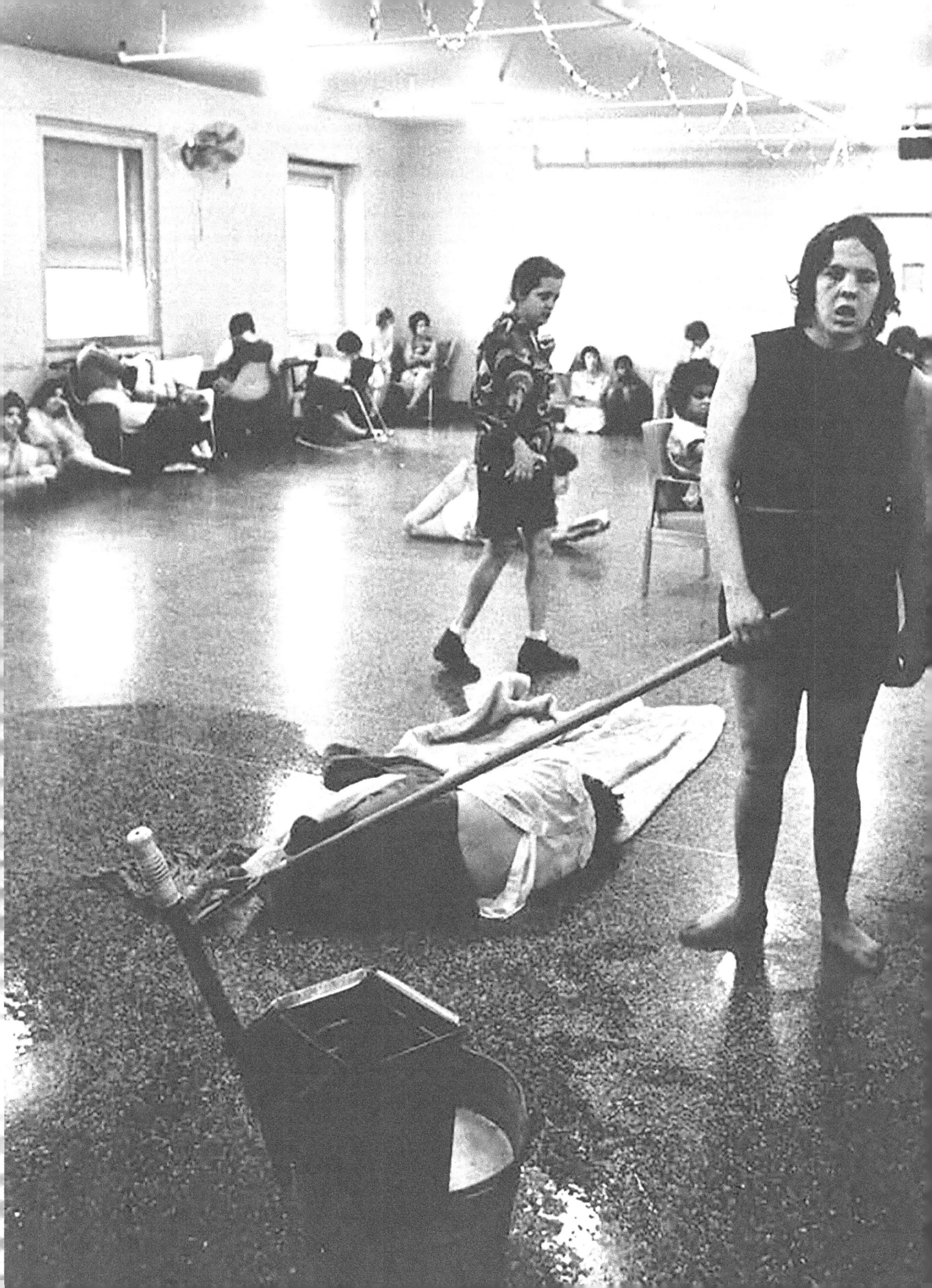

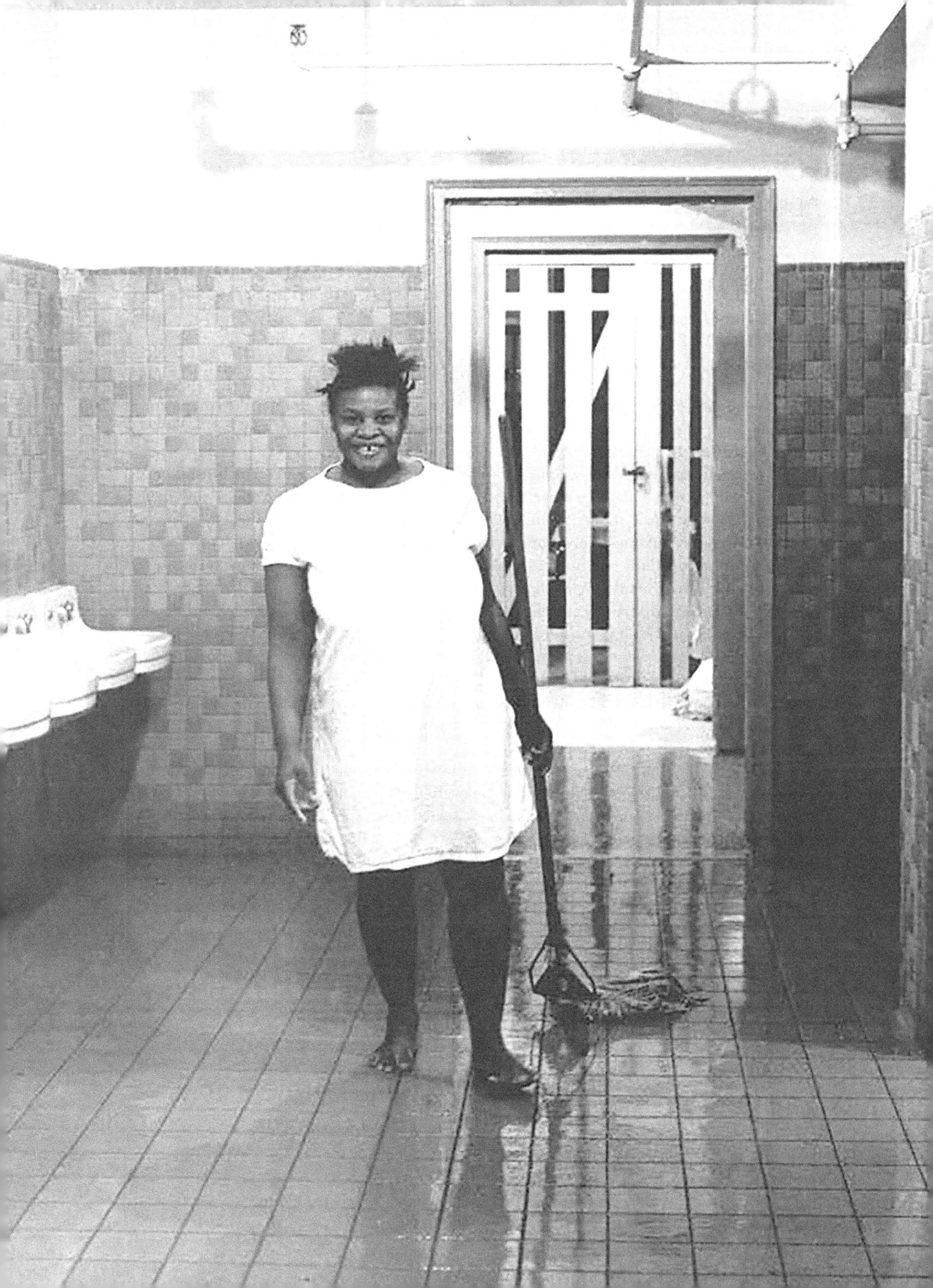

A new store for residents who need clothes is opening. For those who have a need, I will try to meet that need. Don't send residents who tear clothes.

The residents tear clothes when they are ugly, as in the case with state dresses. When pretty clothes are put on residents they rarely tear them. The residents know when they don't look good. If we had panties, shoes, shoelaces, and nice dresses we could do a lot more.

Are we going to get staff to assign to the linen room? There is no laundry worker at all in B-23 so we have to take people off wards to barely keep up.

TO: Deputy Director of Administration
FROM: Dr. W. Bronston, Bldg. 23
RE: Building Maintenance Supplies

This week the building supervisor and I carried out a detailed inventory of the equipment in the building. The reason for this is that we have been plagued by a terrific shortage of basic material to keep the building clean.

We need mops, sweep brooms, push brooms, toilet brushes, deck and scrub brushes, pails, wringers, dustpans, dolleys, garbage cans with covers, squeegees. The total requirements, although a very small monetary outlay, would dramatically improve the basic sanitary conditions in the building despite our drastic shortage of staff.

Our building is filthy and unfit to work in or to live in. I hope that you will expedite the delivery of adequate supplies immediately.

We also experience a severe shortage of furniture. In addition to the lack of chairs, we need tables on each ward before any kind of activity can be mounted. Twenty tables are needed. There are two more items needed which would immensely improve the existing situation. One, nonskid rubber mats that could be placed in each of the eight shower stalls that would cover the entire shower stall. At the present time, the workers are using sheets on the floor to aid in avoiding slipping and falling in the shower. We had a few rubber non-skid mats but they were very small and inadequate.

Secondly, the laundry situation in this building is outrageous! The fundamental reason is that we do not have a single person assigned to dealing with laundry sorting and control for the whole building. The room where the laundry is sorted is barren, and the laundry is sorted in a huge mountain on the floor. Wooden wall shelving built into one of the basement rooms would help immensely with the sorting. We have asked the carpenter shop to do this. However, they have stated that we should specify dimensions. It is my belief that a skilled carpenter should come over and spend the time with building supervisor so that an appropriate structure can be built.

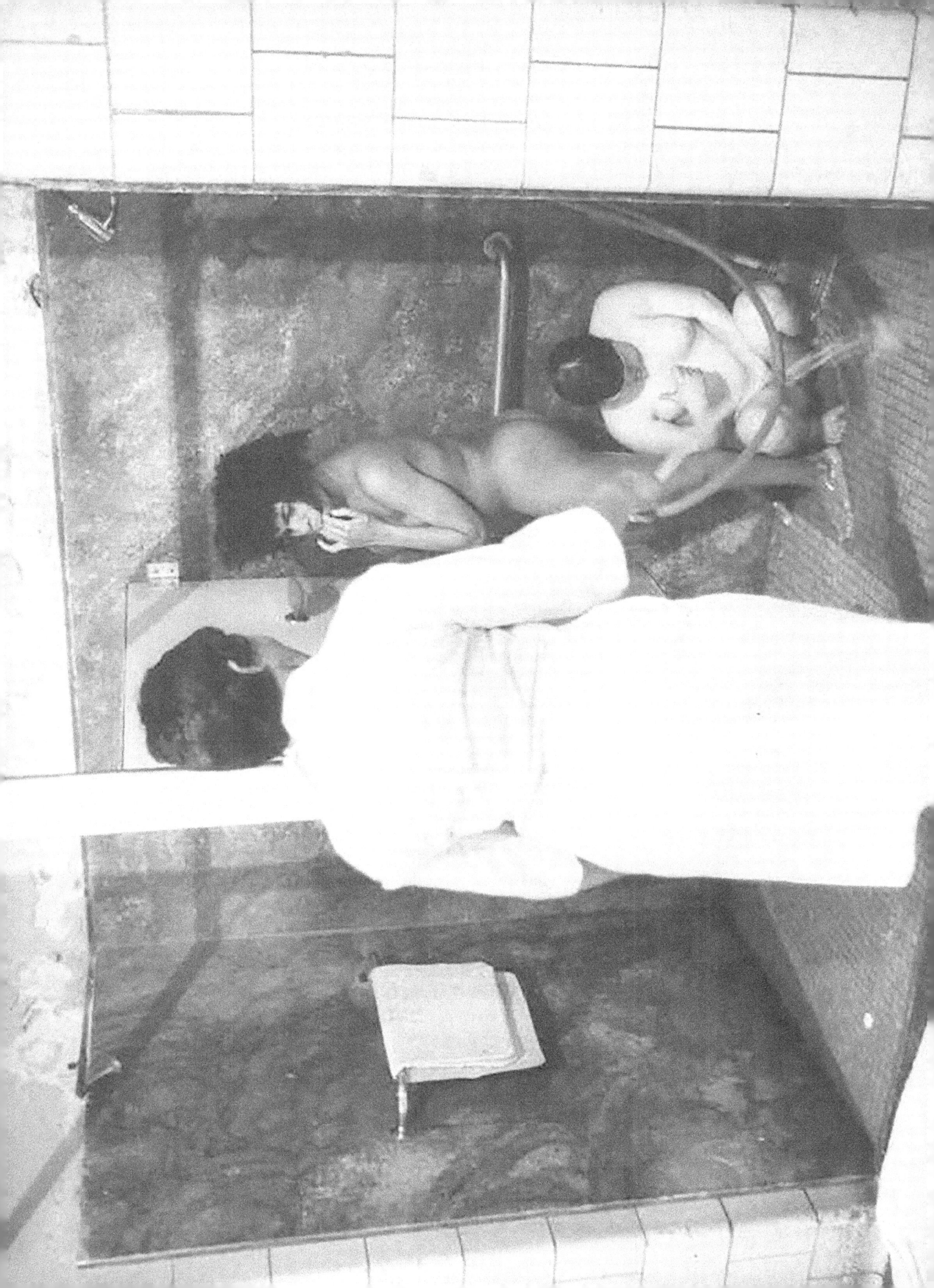

Finally, Bldg. 23 experiences great difficulty in obtaining any food to be used for snacks between dinner and breakfast. The kitchen staff disposes of all leftover food immediately after dinner and withdraws the margarine and surplus milk. If an order was given to leave all surplus food until the breakfast on the following day, at which time they could be discarded, then snacks would be available.

These recommendations have all been thoroughly discussed with the building supervisor and the day shift, from whence the majority of them arise. Morale in the building is desperately low and basic services in the building are halted for lack of adequate materials.

I hope that you will move to help the building in these basic interim ways.

> William Bronston Clinical Physician
> WB/lkb/20
> cc: Dr. Ristic
> Mr. Irwin Beir Miss Bailey

I continued to transmit concrete information to the administration. It required gritting my teeth, knowing that nothing would be done despite pouring time and energy into detailed communications. It had to be done. Somewhere along the road, and my rationale was that all these documents would become transparent and documentary evidence of the administration's gross negligence—sooner or later. The work would not be wasted, I told myself over and over. Each time I finished report or correspondence, I felt relieved. Somehow, getting the stuff on paper freed me from the constant pressure of being the sole possessor of facts. The lives of 420-plus human beings depended on continuing to squeeze the administration every day.

TO: Miodrag Ristic, M.D., Director
FROM: Dr. William Bronston, Bldg. 23
RE: Outline of Discussion held 11/16/72

Following our lengthy discussion on the evening of 11/16/72, I would like to outline some of the areas that we touched on, by way of a reminder to you.

There is no hot water in the treatment room, the showers on Wards A & D run cold almost every night and the showers on Wards B & C rapidly run out of the warm water and turn cold.

The next point is the "wake-up" procedure for the residents at 5:30 A.M. It is often harsh. The residents may have to wait for three hours from the time they get up until breakfast is served to them. I would advise that the wake-up process begin at 6 A.M. and extend gradually through the wards.

The 5:30 A.M. wake-up is directly the result of understaffing and the residents suffer unnecessarily.

We experience a real shortage of blankets. Blankets are sent to the laundry daily if they are soiled. They are only returned on Wednesdays from the laundry. Furthermore, we do not have adequate quality blankets for the poorly heated dormitories. The bulk of our blankets are old and thin from laundering and initial poor quality.

Two additional points which I would like to add to the memo which we did not discuss are:

(1) State soap causes skin disorders and does not adequately clean or deodorize the residents. We buy, by using our "luxury money", 25 bars of commercial soap per week. I believe that every

resident should have their own bar of commercial soap every week for skin hygiene. Who will make up the difference between 25 bars and 186 bars? This requires $12 more a week for the building. We also need 1 can of deodorant per week for the residents. We now get 15 cans per week by using the luxury money. The PX charges $1.10 for a small can of Arrid. (2) Relates to the dining room equipment. Close to half of our building is capable of eating in a normalized way and should be encouraged to do so. Specifically, this will require 100 dish sets, tablecloths, serving dishes and utensils. I have spoken to the building supervisor and we encourage the eating process to build dining skills among the residents.

I would appreciate your consideration of these simple and fundamental needs in the building.

WB/lkb/23.
cc: Mr. Alizarin
Mr. Bier

January 30, 1973
TO: Dr. Ristic, Director
FROM: Dr. W. Bronston, Bldg. 23
RE: Incidents of Severe Burns

I have come across a significant number of incidents where residents in Bldg. 22 and 23 are discovered with serious second-degree chemical skin buns. Angela E. was severely burned over her left chest and side. Sylvia D. and Alice B. were presented with severe burns over their buttocks, to mention a few in the last couple of days. These burns are caused by the concentrated floor detergent.

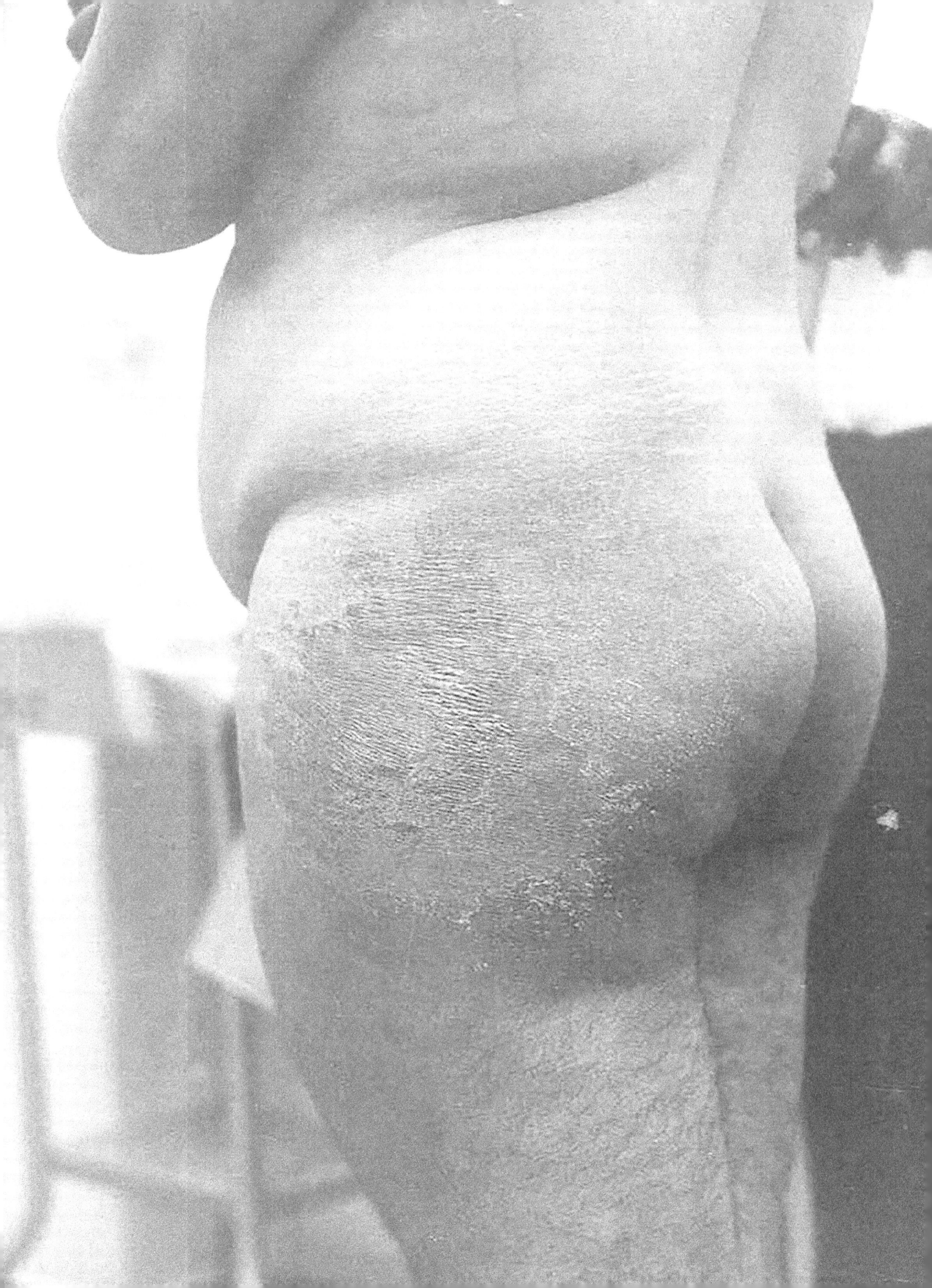

It is my strongest recommendation that the concentrate not be provided to the buildings but that a properly diluted mixture, ready for use, be obtained centrally. Furthermore, every effort must be made to alter the habit of residents sitting and lying on the floor without garments and with absolute indifference to whether the floor is being mopped or not. I have already discussed with you the massive problem of residents walking barefoot resulting in a universal skin problem that leads to serious complications. I cannot explain why there seems to be an increase in the problem but, in fact, it exists.

I hope you will see this as an easily remedial basic problem that should be corrected immediately.

Dr. W. Bronston Clinical Physician

MEMO TO:
RE:
FROM: Dr. Bronston, Bldg. 23 Ambulance Service
TO: Deputy Director Clinical

I appreciate the information memo you sent to us regarding ambulance service and feel obliged to share with you my concerns about ambulance service. I consider an adequate ambulance service as important as basic emergency equipment in each building. The fact that nothing of any real consequence has been done to bring the ambulance equipment and ambulance service to minimum functioning capacity is very upsetting. The ambulance service at Willowbrook is no more than a horizontal transport. The people that operate the ambulance are without any training nor do they possess the attitude necessary to intervene and assist in emergencies that require the ambulance. Specifically: the people that drive the ambulance refuse to bring patients downstairs from upstairs wards, requiring the ward workers to do this in makeshift ways, always at the expense of patients' safety. The use of mechanics and engineers to man the ambulance on the weekend, who have no training nor orientation toward emergency medical care, is absurd. The lack of ambu bags and positive pressure respirator units in the ambulance is a serious deficiency and contributed to the death of at least one resident in recent months. It seems to me that an adequate ambulance service as any other emergency medical necessity, should be given the highest priority and requires attention above that which the administration has traditionally granted to this vital need.

WB/eb/23
cc: Dr. Frew.
Mr. Elizazrian

At one point, Dr. Ristic summarized the position of the administration and plainly set forth the bread-and-butter leverage that any employer—even the state— exercises to retain control.

CONFIDENTIAL
January 11, 1973 235
MEMO TO: Dr. W. Bronston
FROM: Dr. M. Ristic
SUBJECT: Your January memo

I am really astounded that you should take the time to write a four-page memo. A memo written on State time and typed by a State employee is not an act of a private citizen exercising his right of free speech, but an act performed in the course of your employment and, therefore, subject to review by your supervisors.

In your typical fashion, you seek to divert the attention from the matters at hand to the broad picture. I am determined, however, to keep the record straight. You have criticized Dr. Hammond on the Op-Ed page of the New York Times without attracting any official strictures. You have testified for various plaintiffs against the Department of Mental Hygiene and Willowbrook State School without incurring the slightest inconvenience to yourself. In point of fact, the memo of December 29th was delayed so as not to reach you at the time of your testimony in the Federal Court, lest you should feel intimidated.

We expect no thanks for our tolerant attitude, as we are only doing what is right. You, on the other hand, must not expect that your private activities should make you immune from supervisory scrutiny and corrective action when you are in error. The fact, which you cite, that both the late Dr. Hammond and I have tolerated your critical comments, shows that we are not unaccepting of feedback from our subordinates, even when it is unfavorable to us. It merely proves what latitudinarian limits have been set for you.

Please be advised that organizations serve people, and employees, while drawing pay, are expected to serve the organizations directly and people indirectly. On their own time, of course, they can do as they please, as long as they stay within broad limits of the laws of a democratic society.

Miodrag Ristic, M.D. Director/lk

CHAPTER 19

Lest We Ever Forget the Cost

WE WAITED, WAITED, FOR action to begin on the class action suit. Each day brought on more casualties because of the delay. The stakes were ultimate relief for the wretched souls whose every day was a living hell, while the political battle went back and forth.

In the year 1972, the twelve months during and following the exposé, nine young women died in Building 22, the most crowded and bereft building in my charge.

This represented ten times the death rate for the city of New York. What were the words, the memos, the hearings, the photographs, the meetings in comparison to these lives lost—merely a fraction of the death toll of New York State institutions.

January	Ethel Z.	Found dead
February	Alice S.	No diagnosis
May	Nancy S.	Choked to death vomiting during seizure
July	Katie H.	Pneumonia
August	Dorothy C.	Pneumonia
	Geraldinee K.	Cancer
September	Vilma A (twelve years old)	Hepatitis
October	Josephine C.	Head injury
	Ronnie G.	No diagnosis

October 13, 1972

MEMO TO: M. Ristic, M.D., Acting Director, Bldg. #1
FROM: Dr. W. Bronston, Bldg. #22 & #23

I have been informed of a serious incident that occurred yesterday afternoon in Building #23. Carmella D. choked on a piece of food at the dinner hour and required emergency attention. A frantic call for help went out from the building to the head nurse who, rather than responding personally, referred the call to another R.N. in Building #23. The physician on call was sought from the inception of the emergency. He did not arrive on the scene until after a second physician arrived an hour later to assist in the resuscitation procedure.

The frequency of negligent behavior in relationship to the residents in Building # 22 and #23 is appalling. I demand that a full investigation of this matter be carried out and that action be taken against the guilty parties.

Last week in Building #22, Dr. R. contributed to the death of Josephine C. by ordering a contraindicated medicine while she was in status seizures and did not come to see her. He was notified again of her extremely critical condition at least 30 minutes before he finally did arrive only to pronounce her dead. Josephine C. died subsequent to a head injury from a fall, which led to her seizures and aspiration. That did not have to happen.

In both cases, the patrolman arrived significantly ahead of the covering physicians. In both instances, untrained ward workers struggled heroically to care for the residents and to bring the gravity of the situation to professional attention.

I would appreciate a copy of the report of your findings and the action that you take.

October 27, 1972

MEMO TO: Dr. Bronston
FROM: Miodrag Ristic, M.D., Director

This memo is in reply to your memo containing accusations against the two doctors.

Please be advised that both doctors have submitted satisfactory explanations, in writing, and that there will be no further action in this matter.

Miodrag Ristic, M.D. Director

Then, this arrived.

Form 26-D.M.H.

ALAN D. MILLER, M.D.
COMMISSIONER

WILLIAM VOORHEES, M.D.
FIRST DEPUTY COMMISSIONER

ROBERT PATTON
SECOND DEPUTY COMMISSIONER

STATE OF NEW YORK
DEPARTMENT OF MENTAL HYGIENE
DIVISION OF MENTAL RETARDATION
AND CHILDREN'S SERVICES
NEW YORK CITY METROPOLITAN REGIONAL OFFICE
2 WORLD TRADE CENTER, 56TH FLOOR
NEW YORK, N. Y. 10048

ROBERT W. HAYES, M.P.H.
DEPUTY COMMISSIONER
FOR MENTAL RETARDATION
AND CHILDREN'S SERVICES

SIDNEY LECKER, M.D.
ASSISTANT COMMISSIONER
FOR CHILDREN'S SERVICES

October 27,1972

William Bronston, M.D.
168 Cebra Avenue Staten Island,
New York

Dear Doctor Bronston:

The New York State Civil Service Commission carefully considered your appeal from your 1971 Unsatisfactory performance rating at its meeting on October 17, 1972.

After reviewing all the information presented, the Commission found the record supports the original rating. Accordingly, your appeal was dismissed.

Very truly yours,
Robert A. Quinn
Deputy Administrative Director

CHAPTER 20

Photos: Living Death Alone

ALL THAT IS NECESSARY to kill life is to deny growth; to deny a future; to relegate life to a perpetual, monotonous, suffocating, and repetitive present. Life energy, the struggle to grow and change is the most powerful human force we know. To stifle that force takes incredible and constant repression. Global denial of life exists in the institutions. It is so all-pervasive and essentially uniform that, to the casual observer, it may be altogether unapparent.

People who come from the outside to see the institution would walk about and invariably be unable to bring themselves to see the evidence before their eyes. "Why the looks of lifelessness, hopelessness, despair, emptiness? It must be mental retardation. That's why these people are here in the first place!"

Not true.

"How filthy. What an odor. How deafening the echoing noise." The "things" of the institution— the lesser crimes, the objects that we respond to—dodge the central reality. What the visitor cannot log is the state of the hostages, the death of the spirit— each in his or her own decline.

This is not mental retardation.

This is not emotional disorder.

This is not developmental disability.

This is not illness, God's will, or any other trumped-up etiology.

This is a phase of monetized extermination, *public extermination* of the unwanted, the devalued, the powerless, the institutionalized of our country.

There, to a greater or lesser extent, children and adults are marked for death by the systematic denial of their lives and their innate capacity to grow and change.

Some go quicker than others; most live on, mimicking life for decades.

Here is the most outrageous of all the crimes of the institution, the crime against humanity.

Look carefully, slowly, at the living death—the consequence of massive and systematic repression. The toll to our society, to fellow citizens rendered to this state of existence has yet to be fully documented and even minimally responded to by the public. It will continue as long as any people are seen and treated as less than you and I.

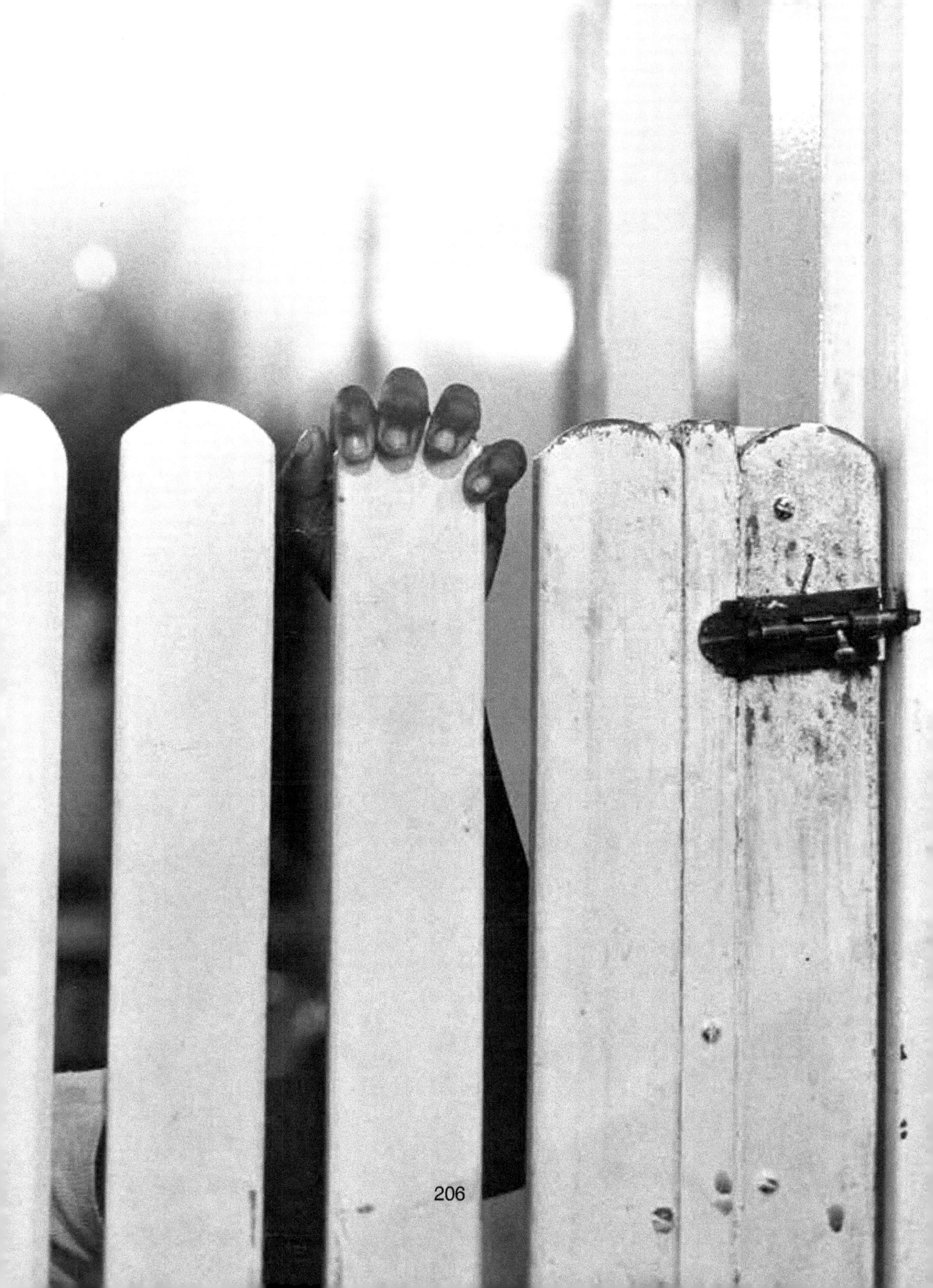

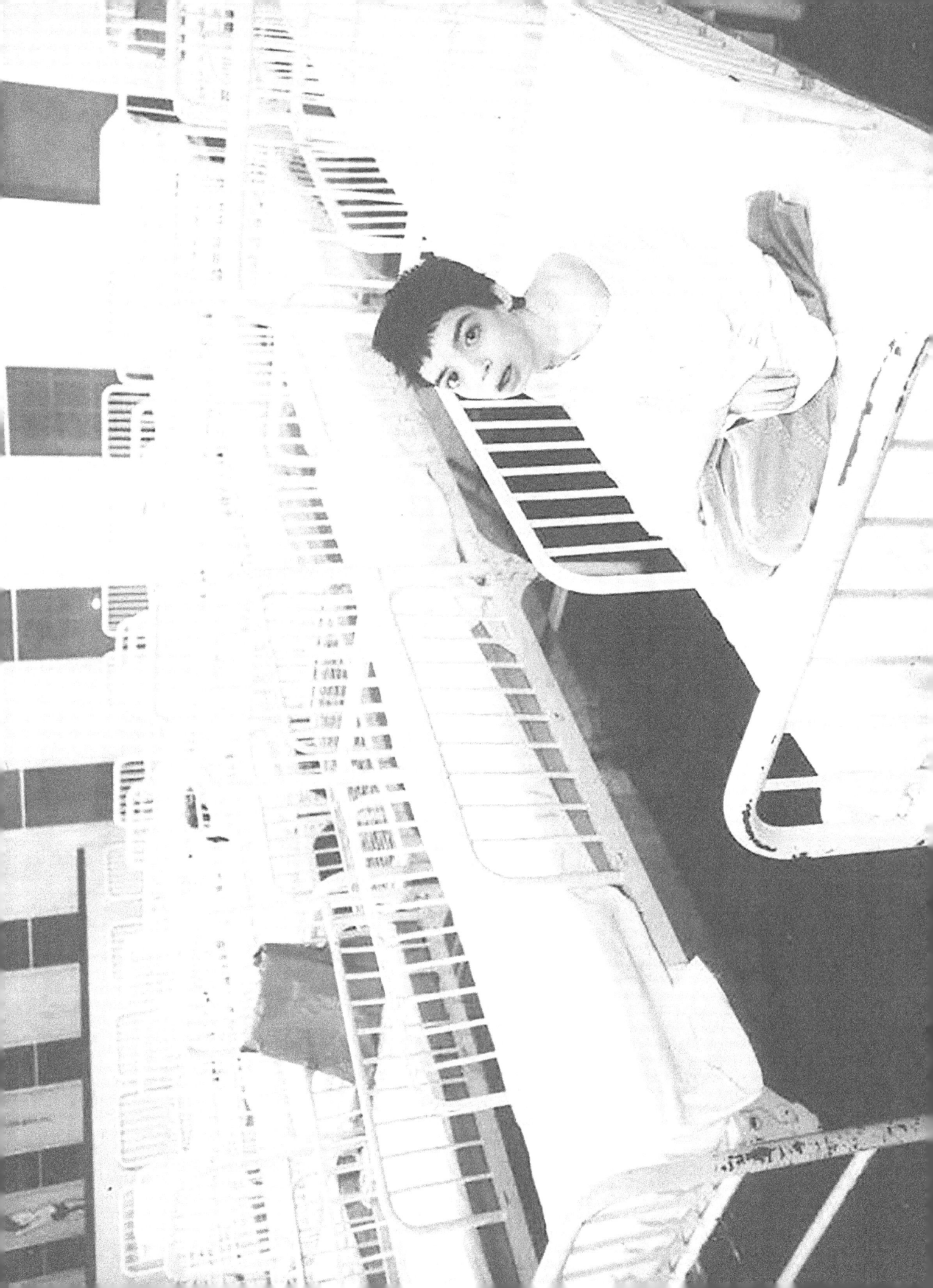

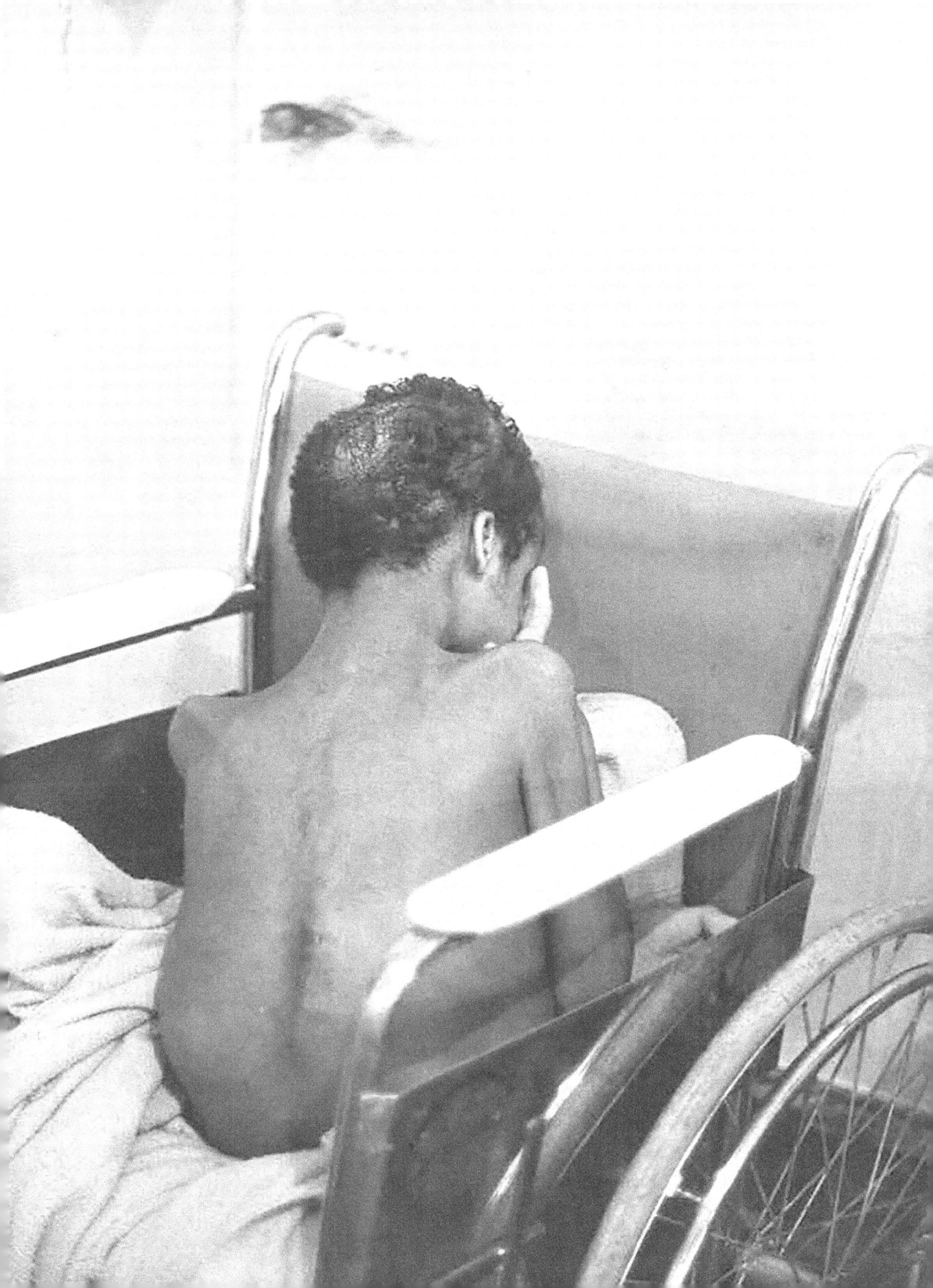

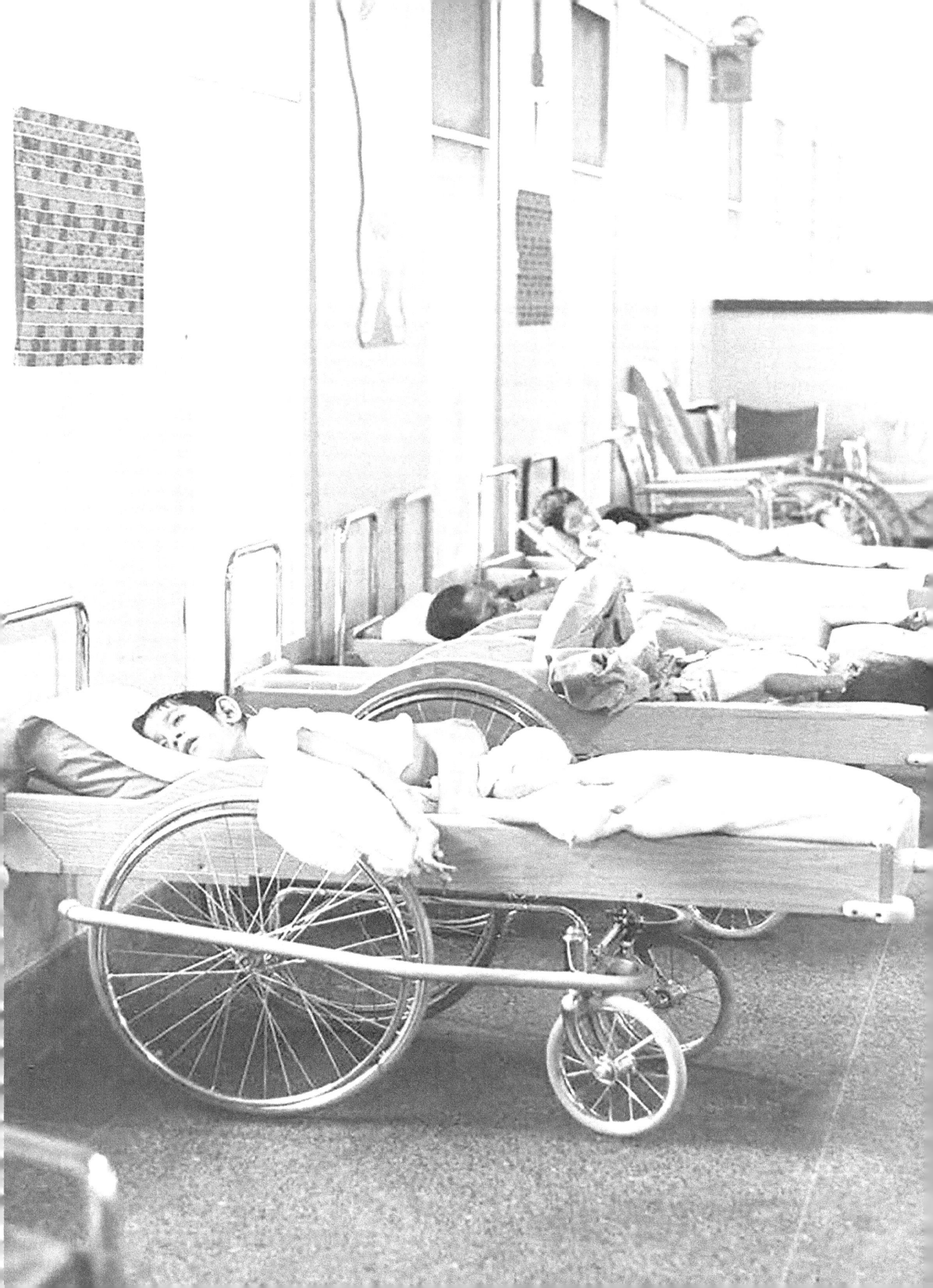

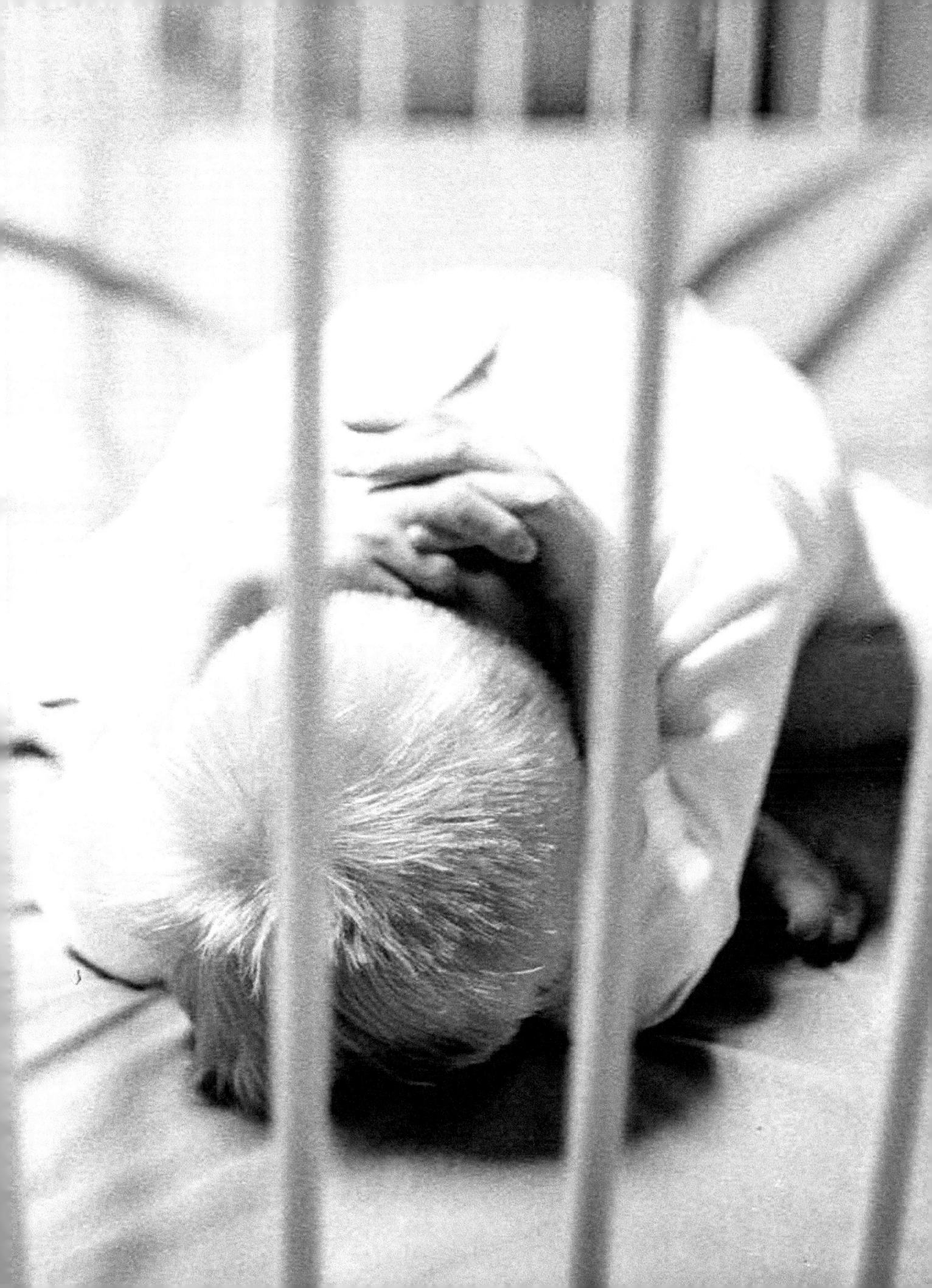

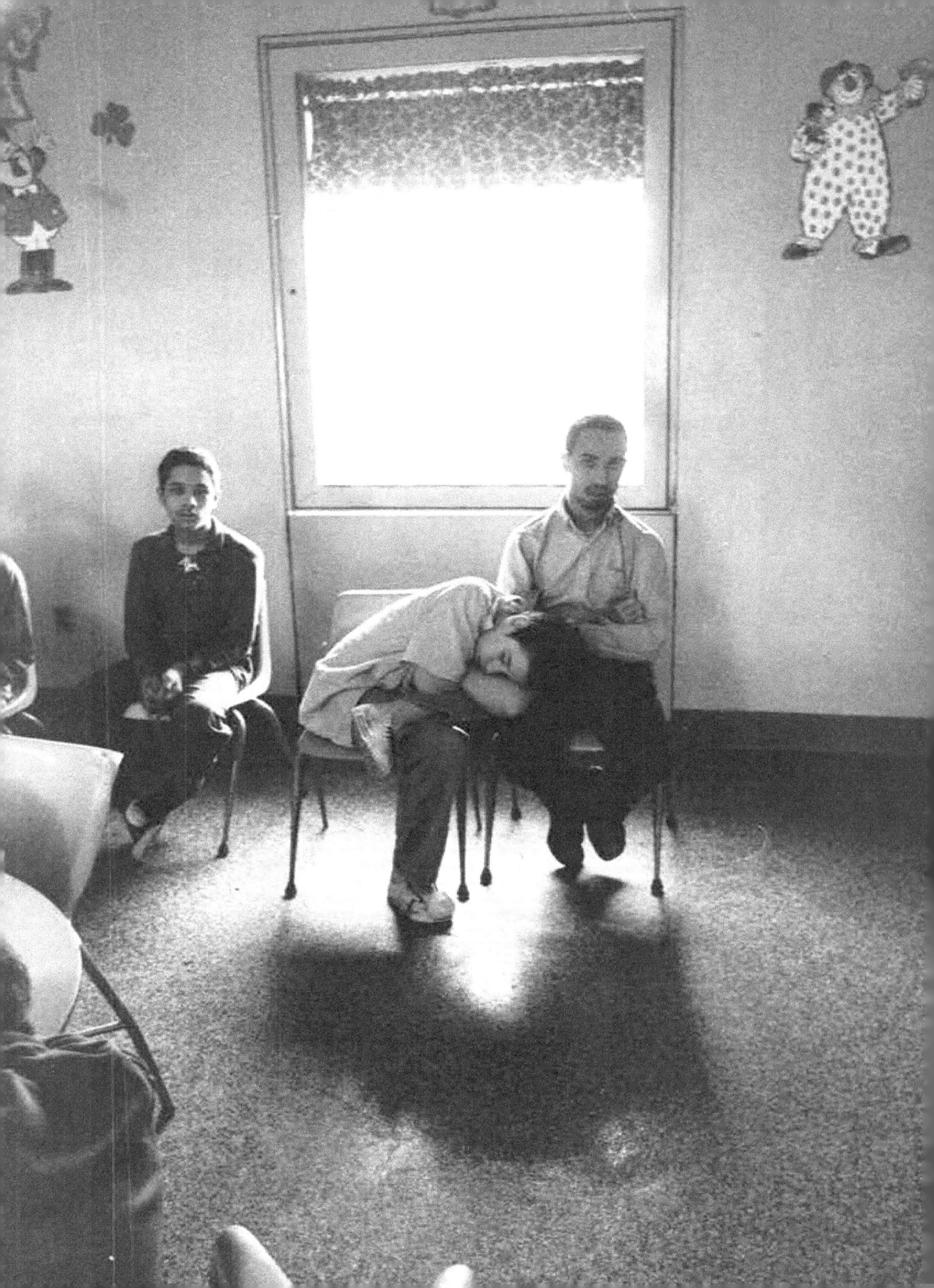

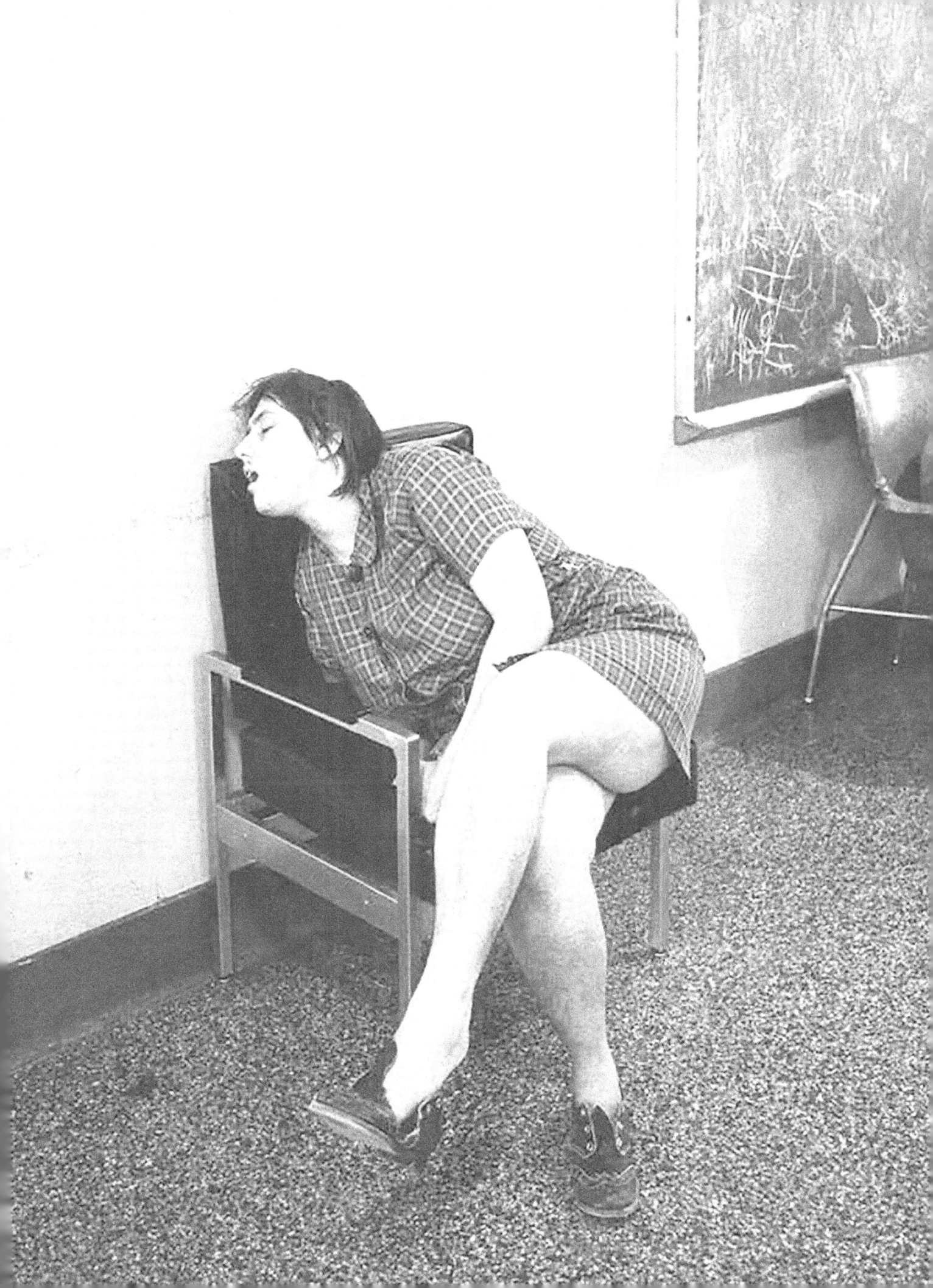

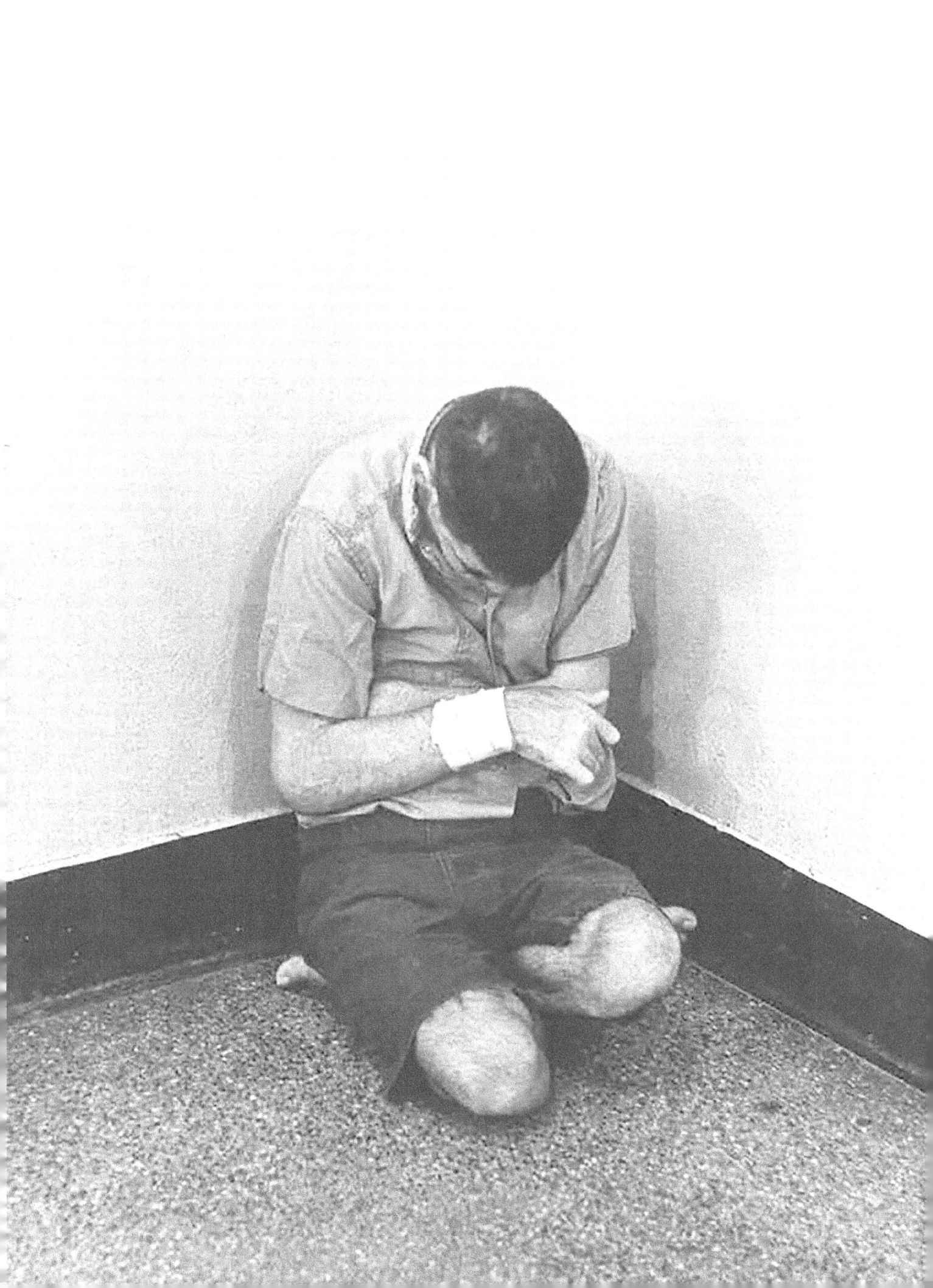

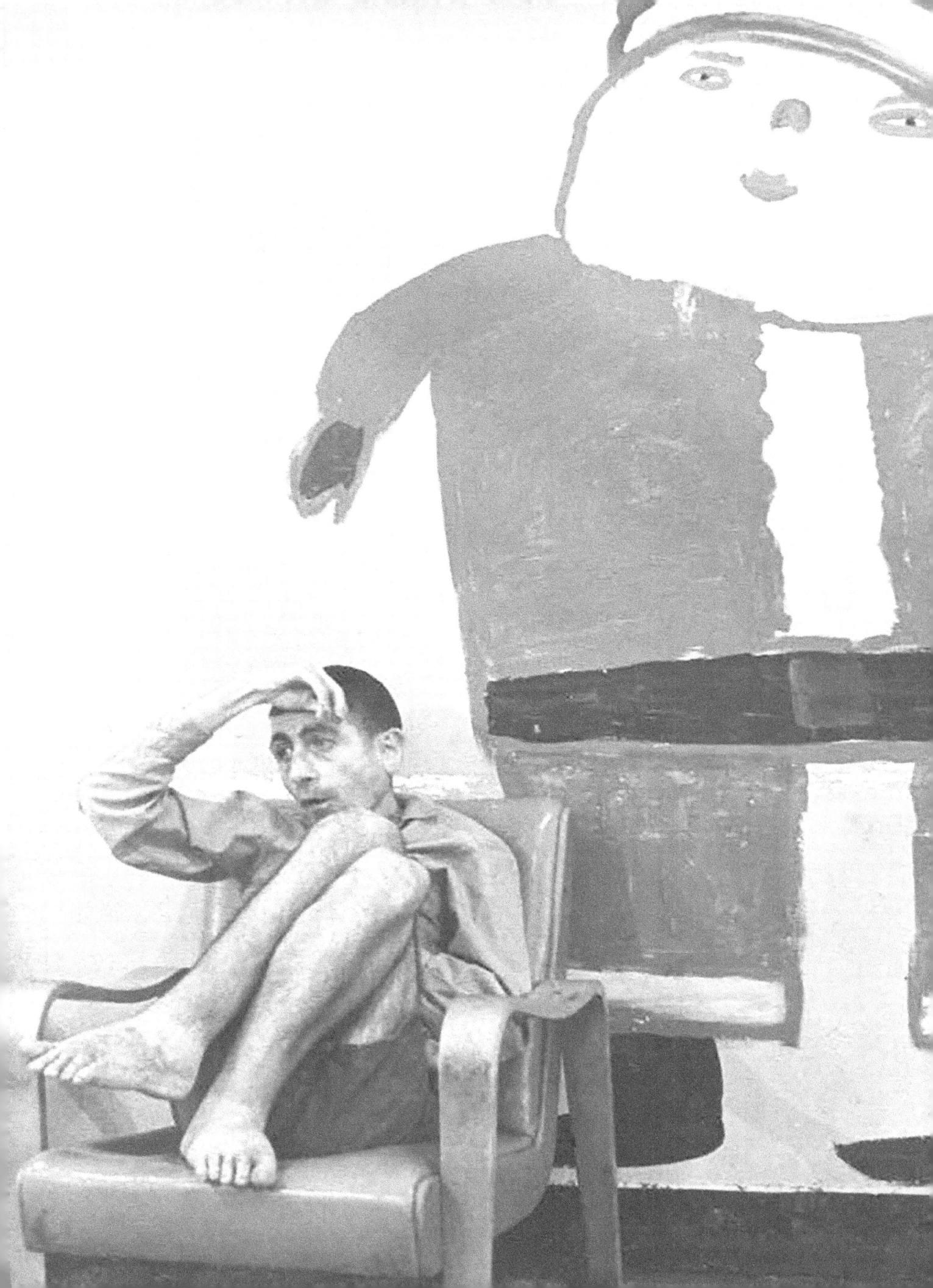

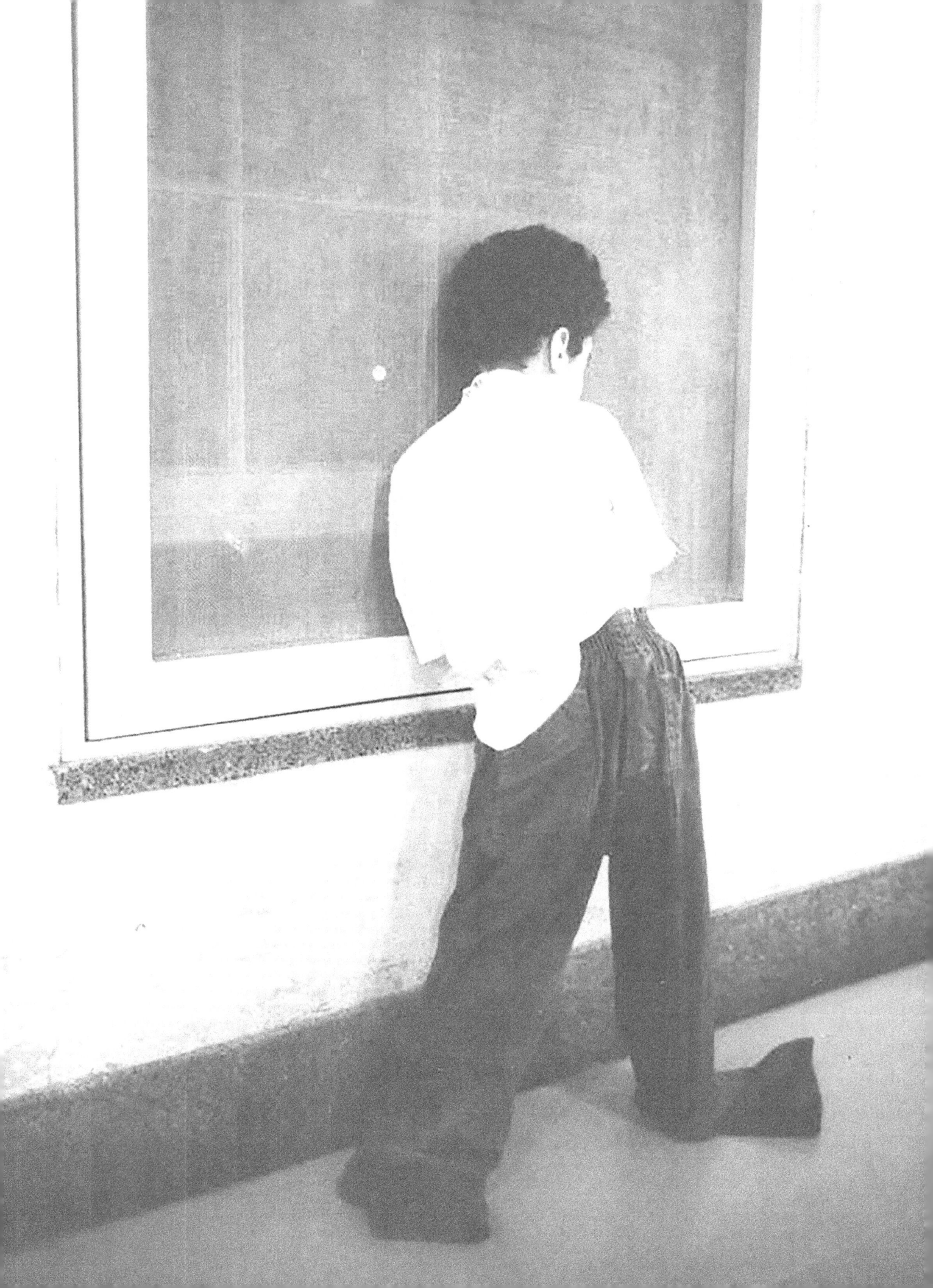

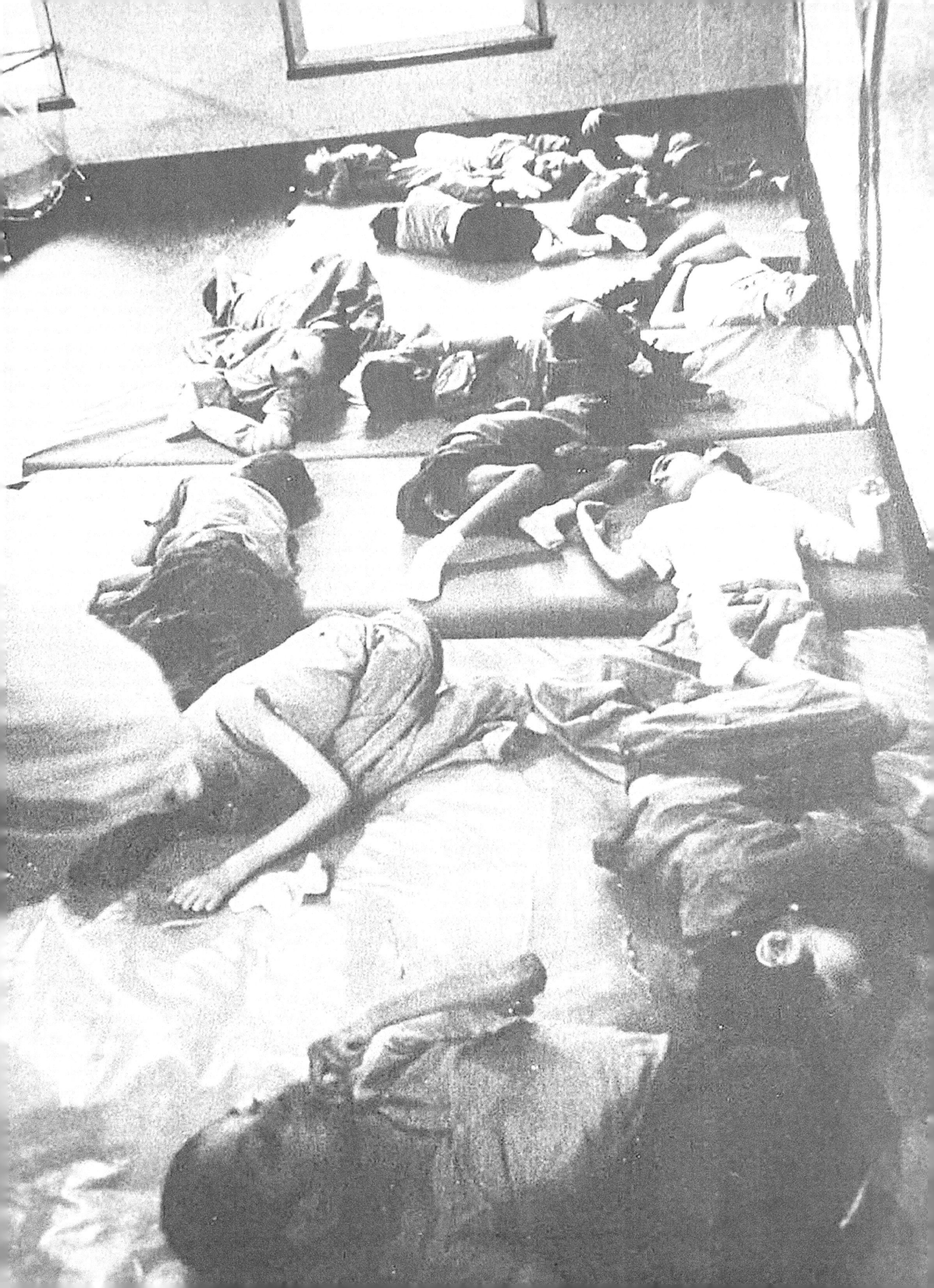

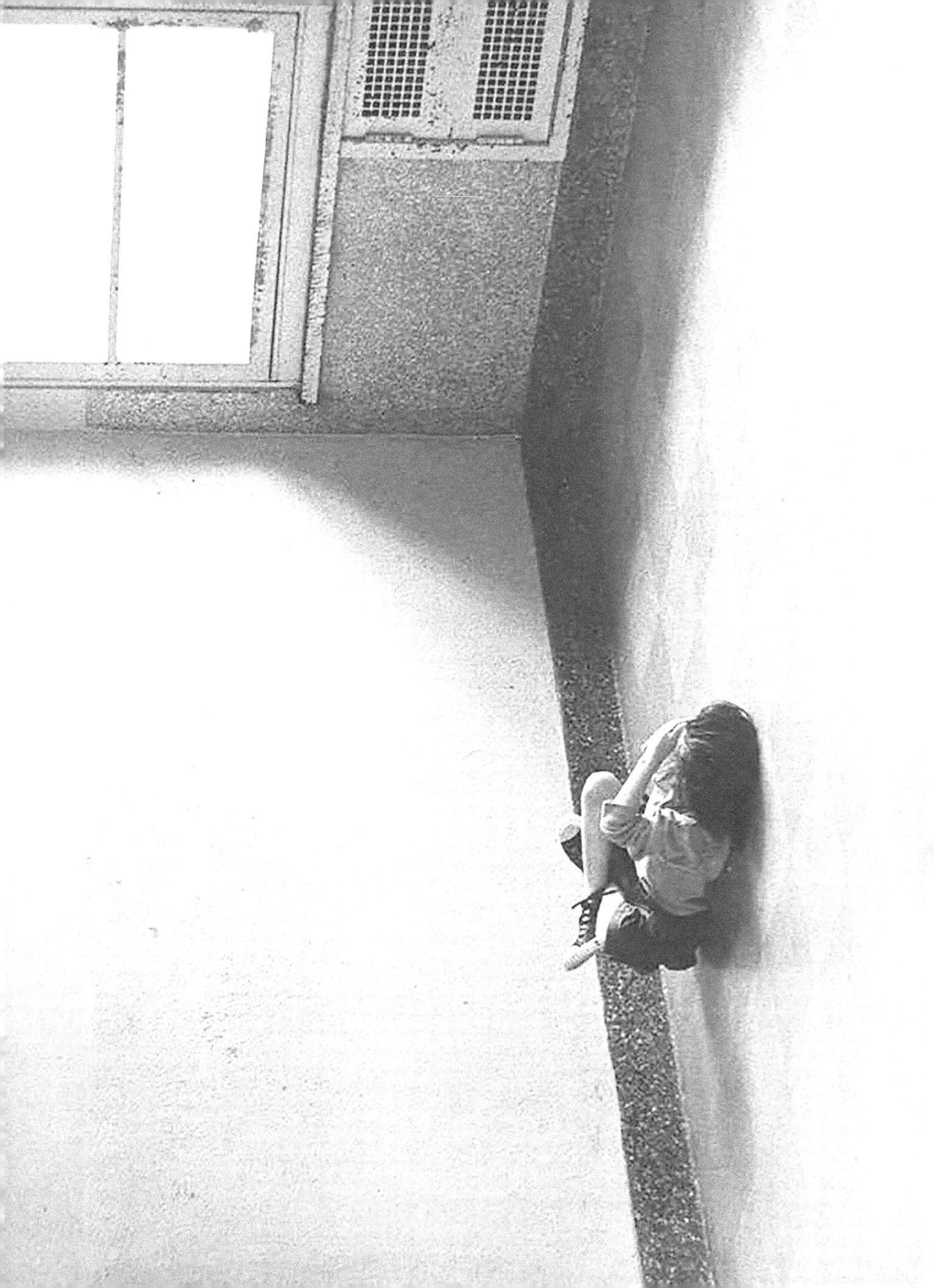

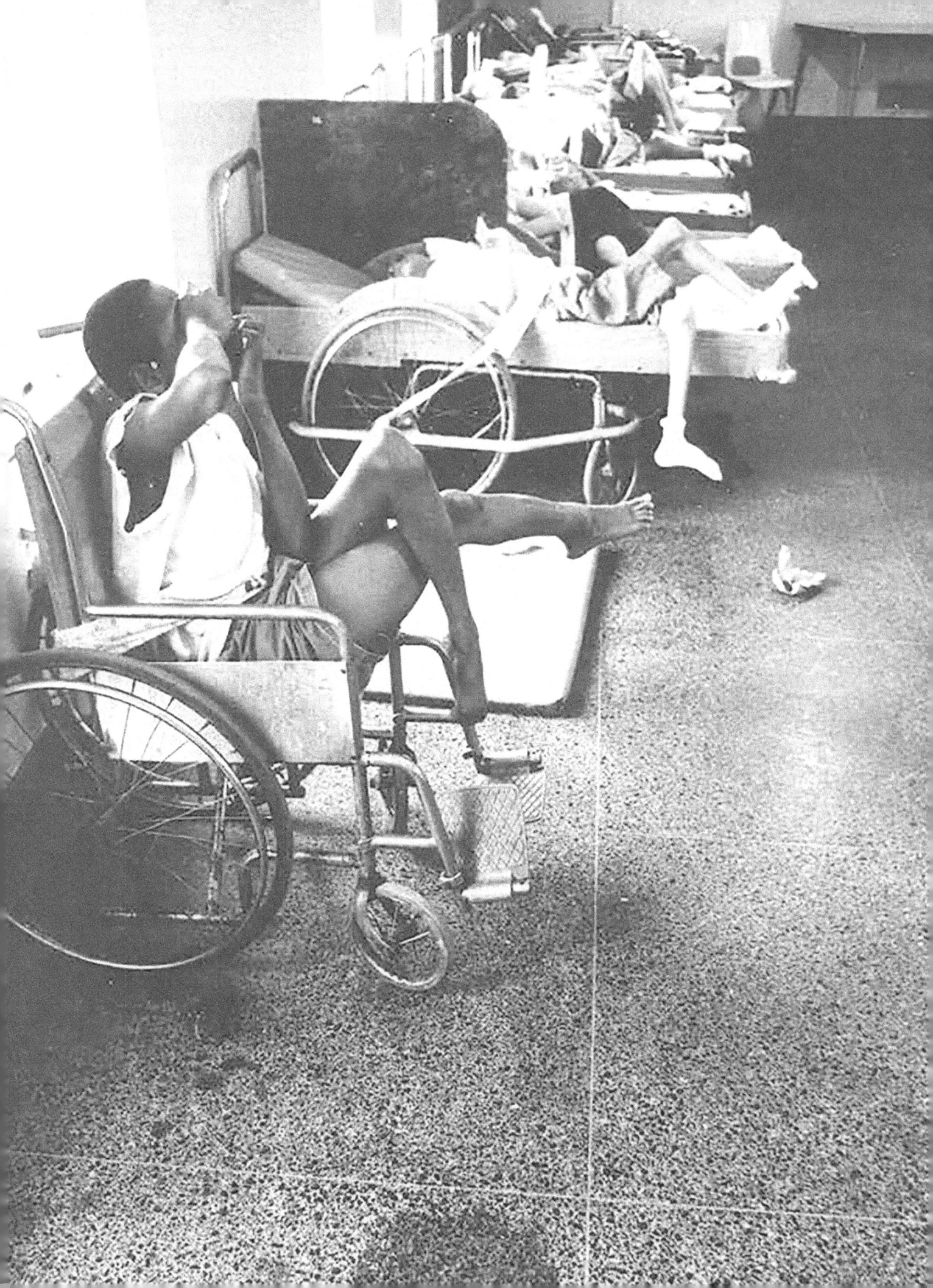

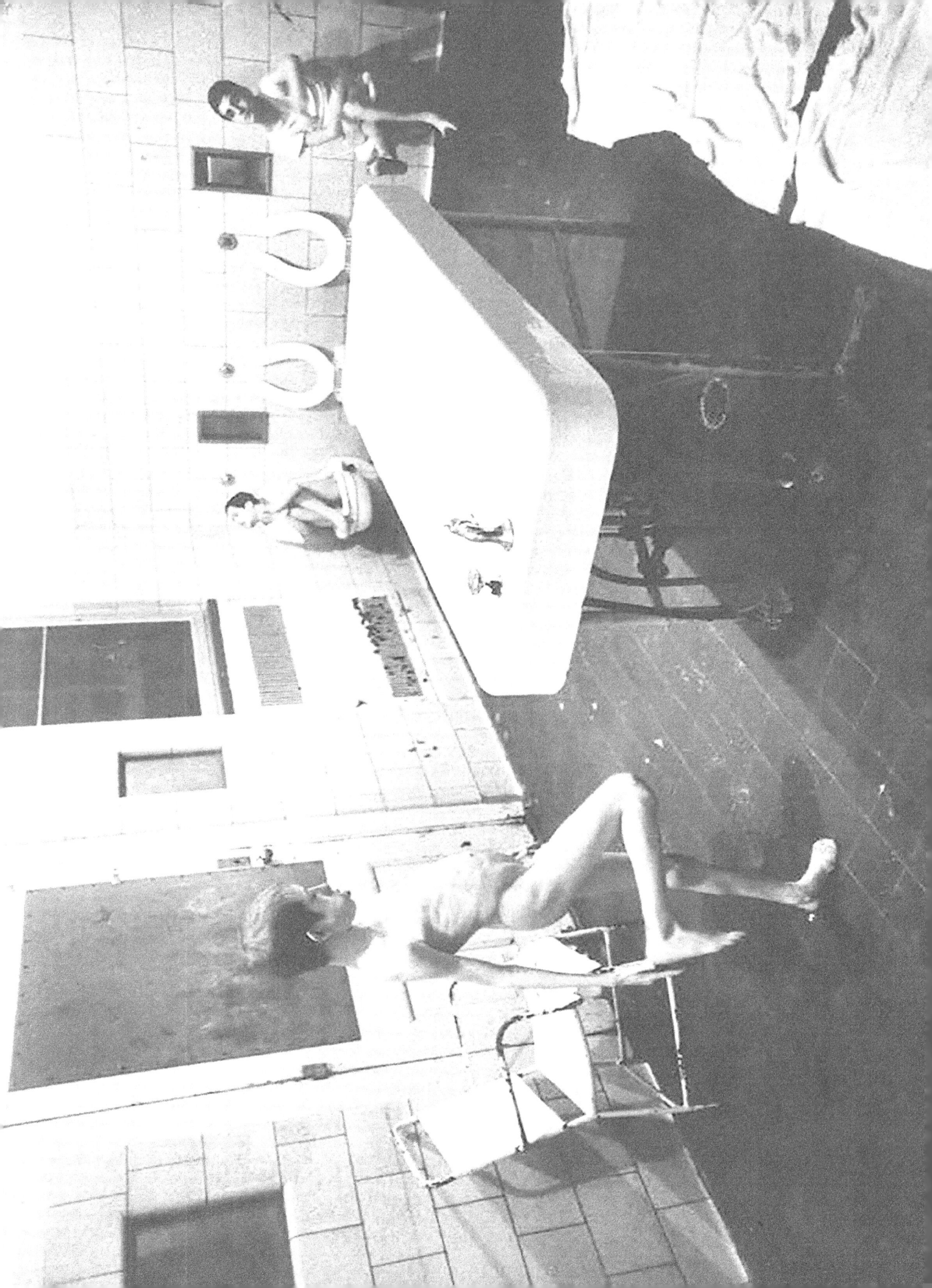

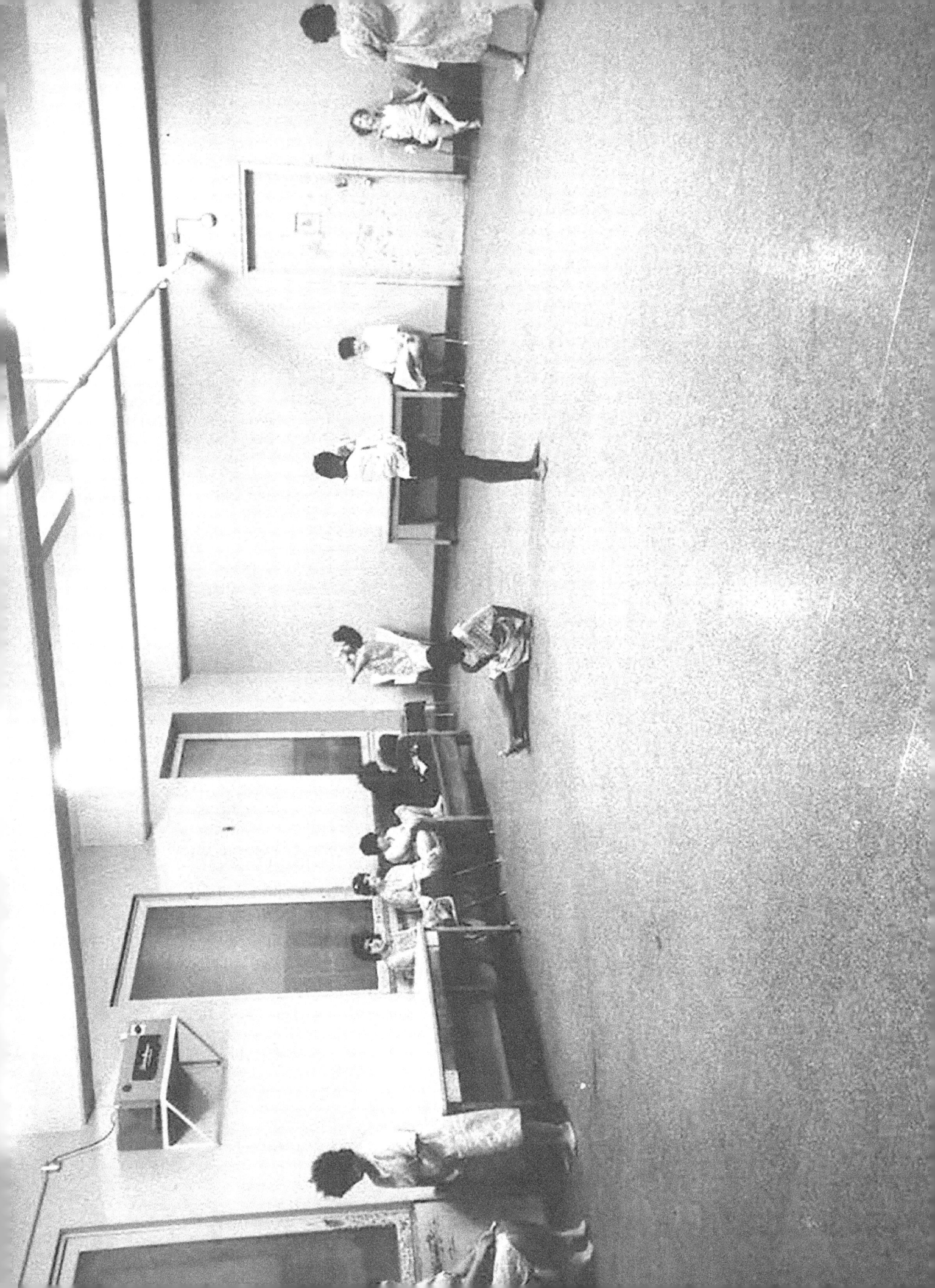

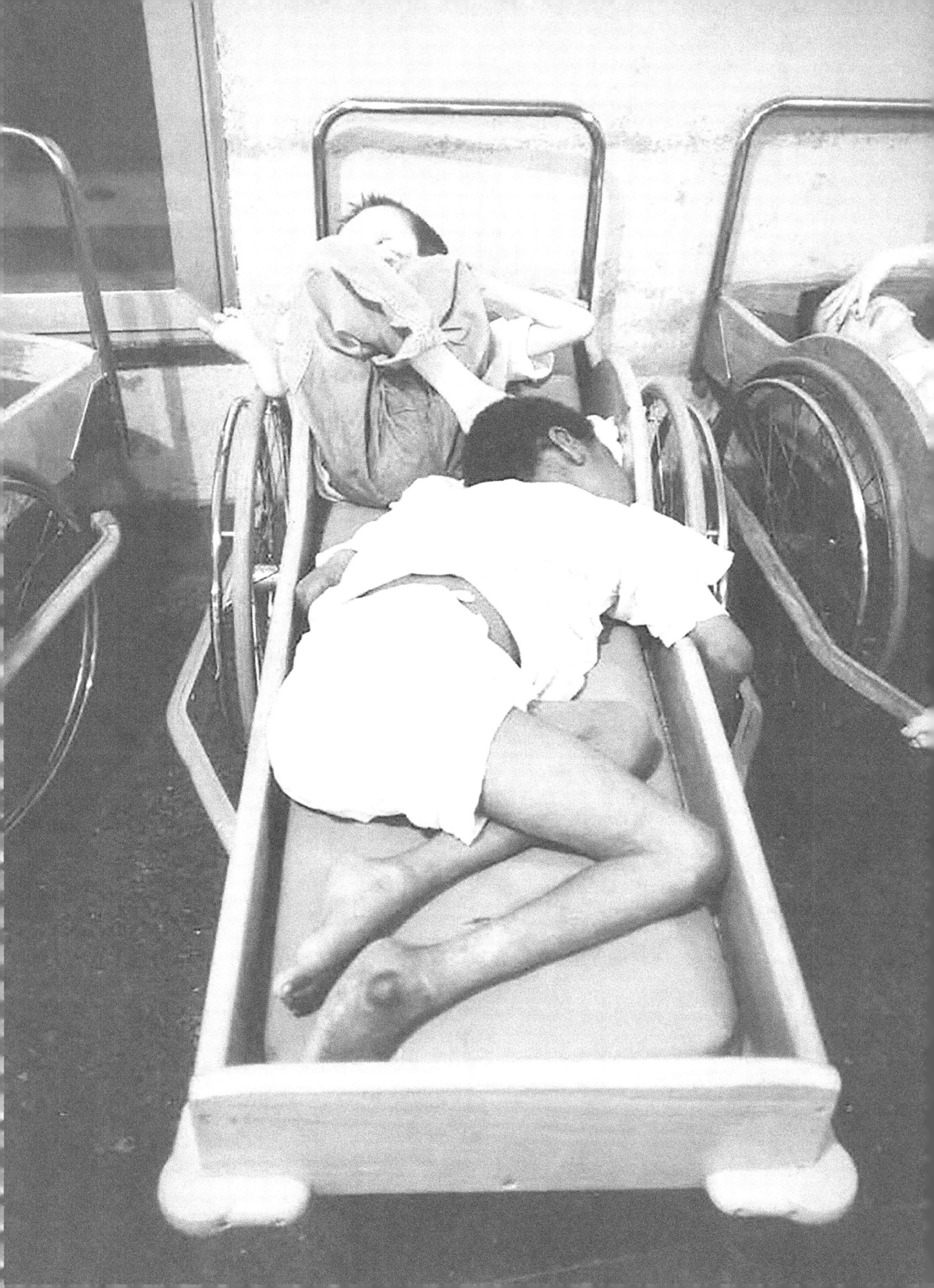

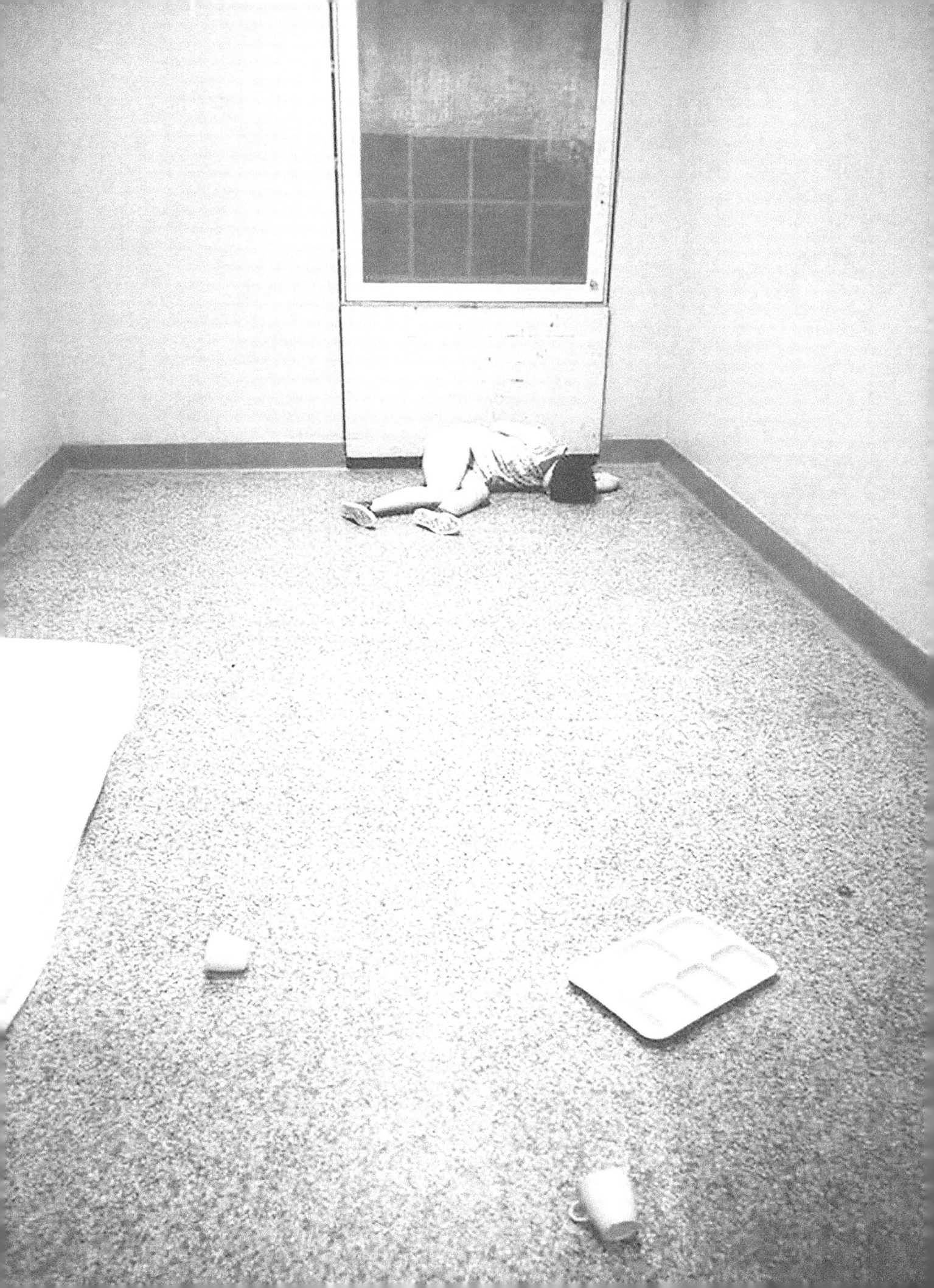

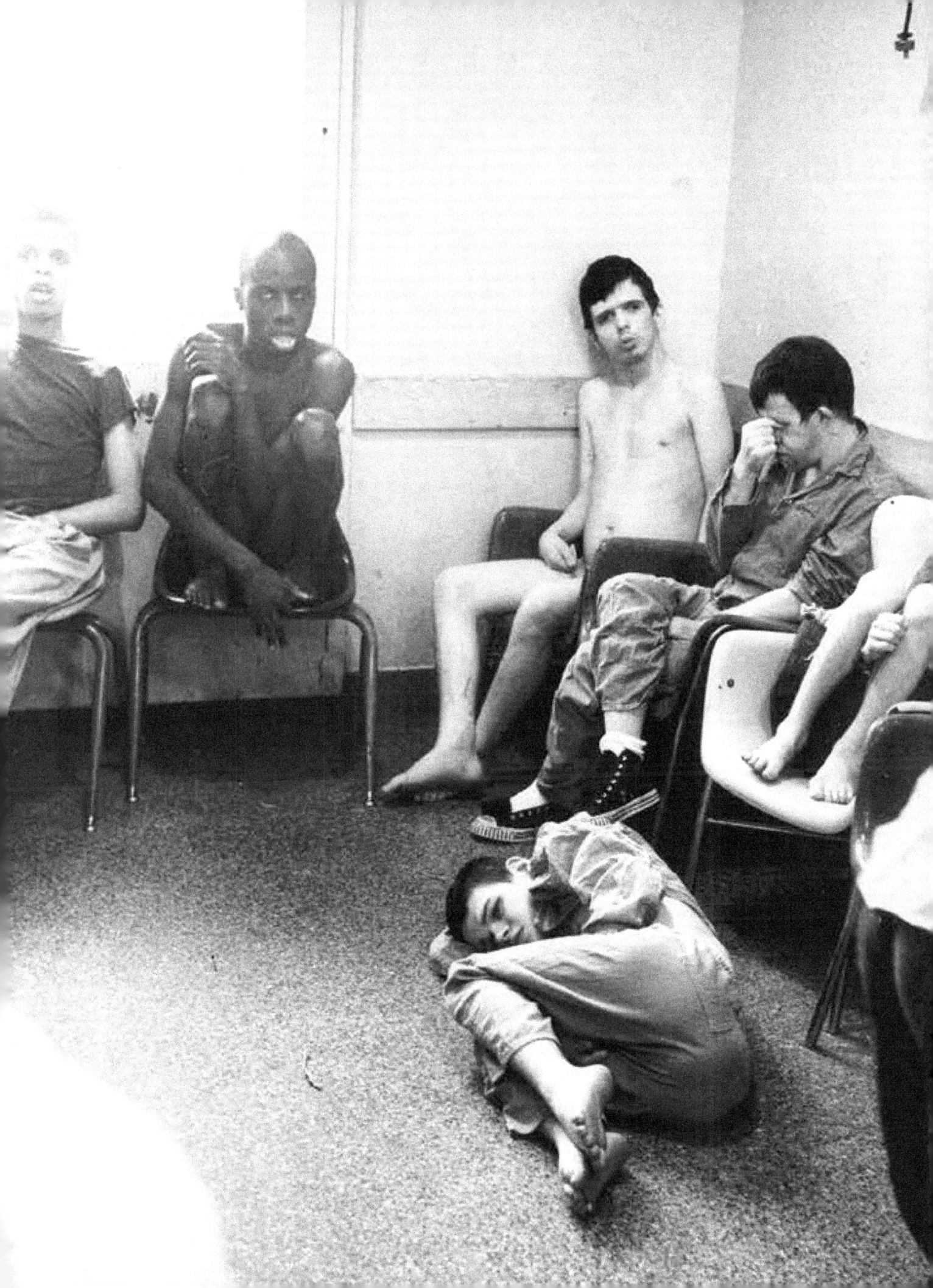

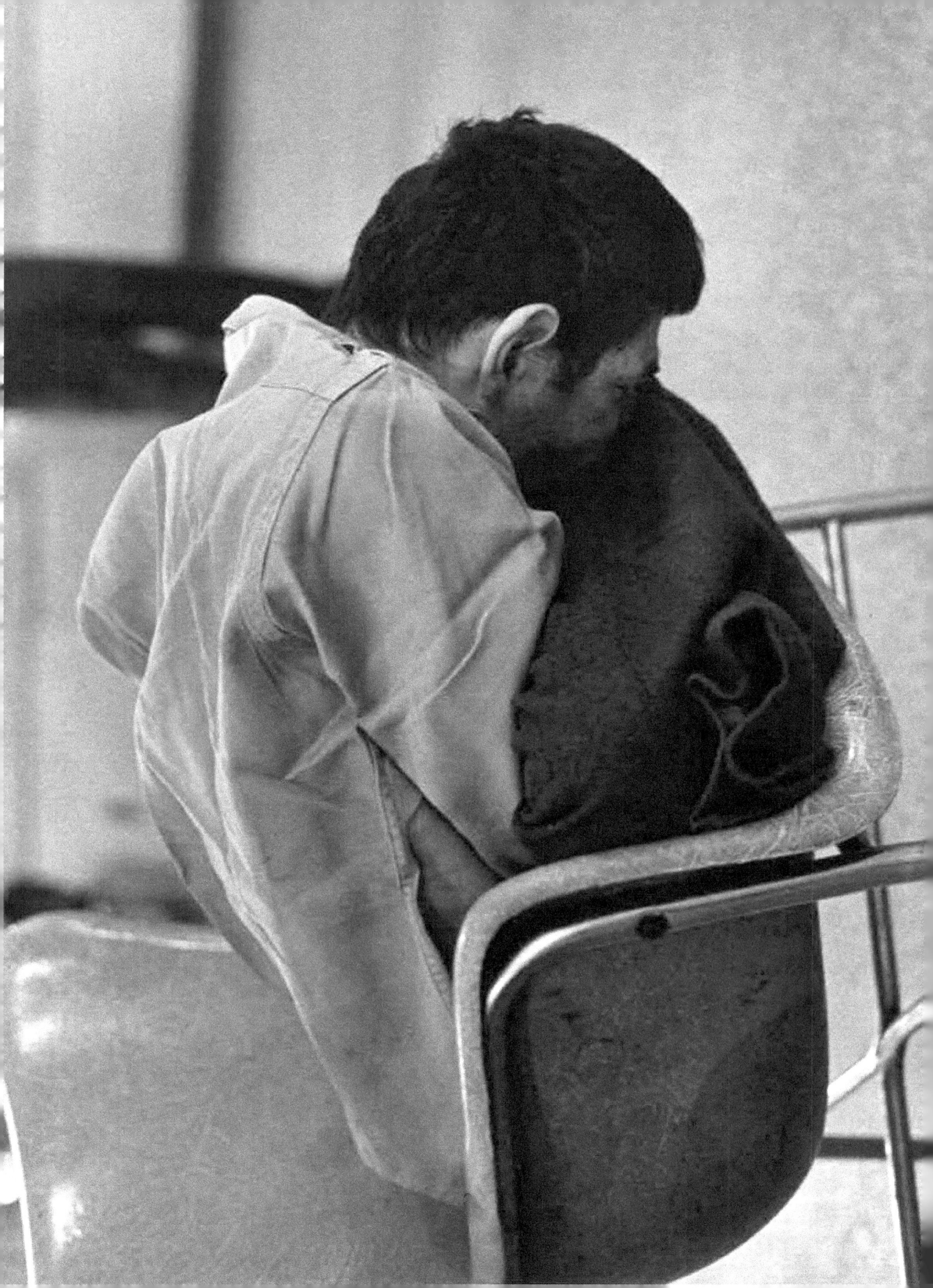

CHAPTER 21

The Passing Over of the Torch

AT LAST! SUDDENLY THERE was finally the opportunity to hand the defense over to another force, a force that could take hold of Willowbrook and allow a respite for the valiant parents and those of us who were raw from the horror. It had seemed as if it would never come, but the long legal wait was over. The Eastern District Federal Court—nine months after the initial class action trial briefs were submitted—announced a hearing to decide whether conditions in Willowbrook warranted an emergency intervention by the federal court; whether, in fact, constitutional violations of the rights of the class did justify federal supervision over state affairs. No longer—whatever the outcome—was the bureaucracy stung by "agitators," "misfits," "emotional parents," "pinkos." Now it would have to openly defend itself to the United States.

I was assigned the responsibility of summarizing and interpreting conditions, as well as the structure of the institution in my testimony before the federal judge, Orrin Judd. Even though the earlier documentary materials submitted in the filed complaint dealt in part with conditions, the affidavit which follows brought the entire picture together. After two and one-half years, what had been fragmentary in my own mind— experiences here and there in the institution, guesses, observation— finally could all be put together into a confident whole.

UNITED STATES DISTRICT COURT
EASTERN DISTRICT OF NEW YORK PARISI, et al.,:
Plaintiffs,
-against-
NELSON ROCKEFELLER, et al.,
Defendants. x
STATE OF NEW YORK)
) SS.:
COUNTY OF NEW YORK)
Civil Action No 72 Civ 357

AFFIDAVIT

I, WILLIAM BRONSTON, being first duly sworn, depose and say:

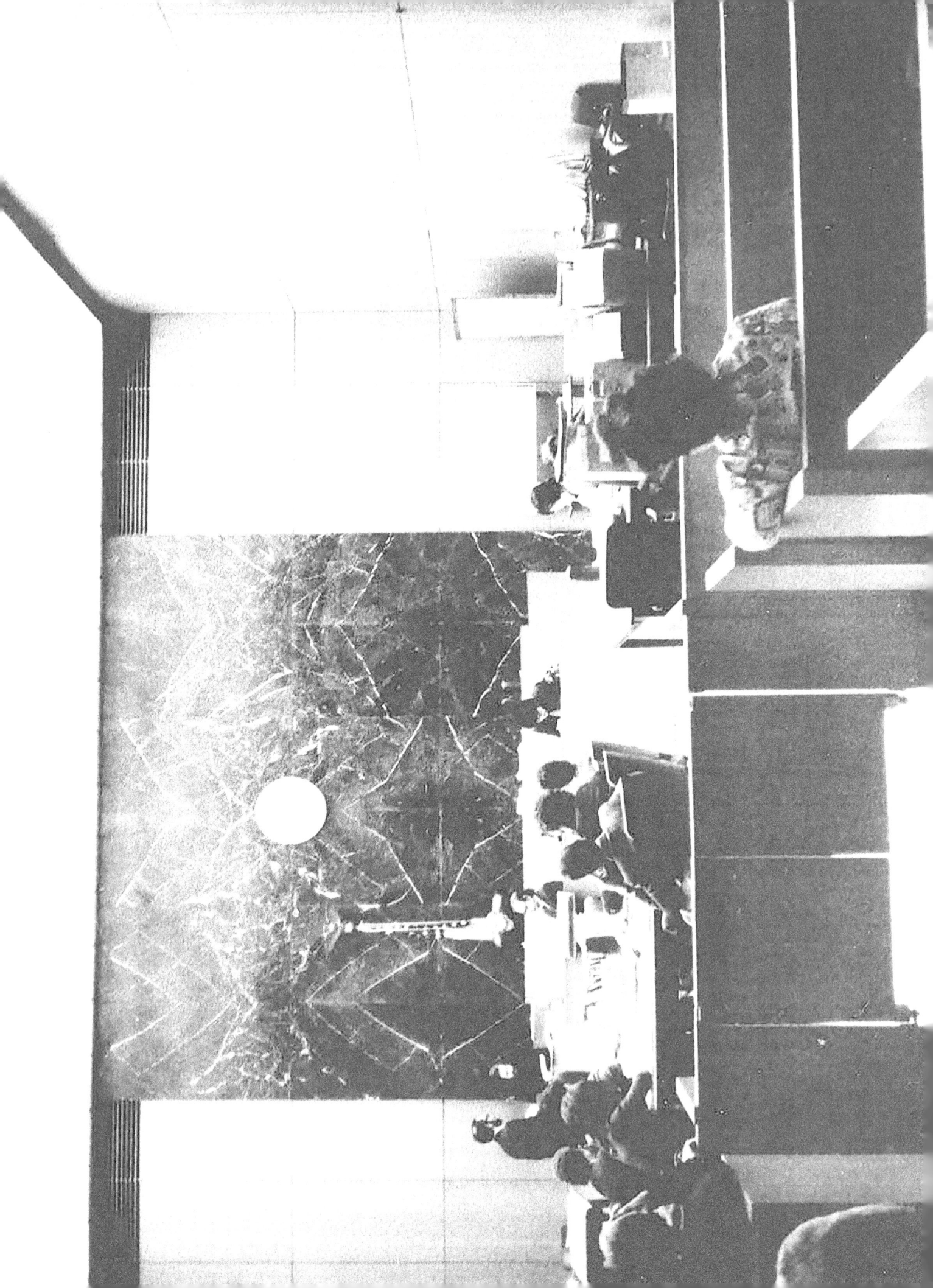

The following is a general review of the organization of buildings at Willowbrook State School with some notes on the dynamics of the population within them:

The so called 'Baby Complex' is comprised of Buildings 12, 14, 16, 26, and 28. These buildings consist of four wards with up to 50 children in each ward. No more than a token attempt is made to sort out these various groups of children. Here the basic distinction between so-called "bright and low-grade" children is inevitably made by the ward staff, and program tracking begins. Children are selected to participate in programs primarily on the basis of their IQ score. This IQ testing is rarely repeated more than once in the course of the first 20 years of the patients' residency. The selection for programs is made by a variety of people and based on a variety of circumstances. Anyone from the ward staff to the building M.D. may decide to put the child into a program. The goals of the program are never spelled out, and the program efforts are confined to the one or two hours per day that the child actually spends in the activity. Rarely, if ever, are the achievements of the child shared among all the caretaking staff.

Whether a child is considered "bright" or "low grade", the majority of his or her time is spent on the ward doing nothing. The so-called "low grades", or children for whom the institution has no workable strategy, spend all day on the ward. In addition, the children for whom Willowbrook has no services are also lumped in with the so-called "unsuitables" (e.g., blind toddlers). These children are relegated to what are called "ward activities".

An essential fact must be held in mind in order to understand building differences and the value of "programs" throughout Willowbrook. This is that the institution is a closed system with essentially no exit. Thus, the superficial, fine distinctions made as to whether this or that resident belongs in school, in OT, or PT, etc. exists within the overall context of the reality that the final common pathway for virtually 98 percent of the people in Willowbrook is to die there. The fate of these children as they grow older, is to be moved to the two-story adult buildings. A child who shows no "promise" and has little parent advocacy can be dumped (before reaching the maximum age or size for the baby complex), and that person goes to the "back buildings". In this transitional period from early childhood to young adult, there is a feeble attempt to provide some attention, in a formal way, to a low percentage of the residents; but again, with absolutely no intention, nor explicit plan or goals, to coordinate the child's experience in order to give it direction.

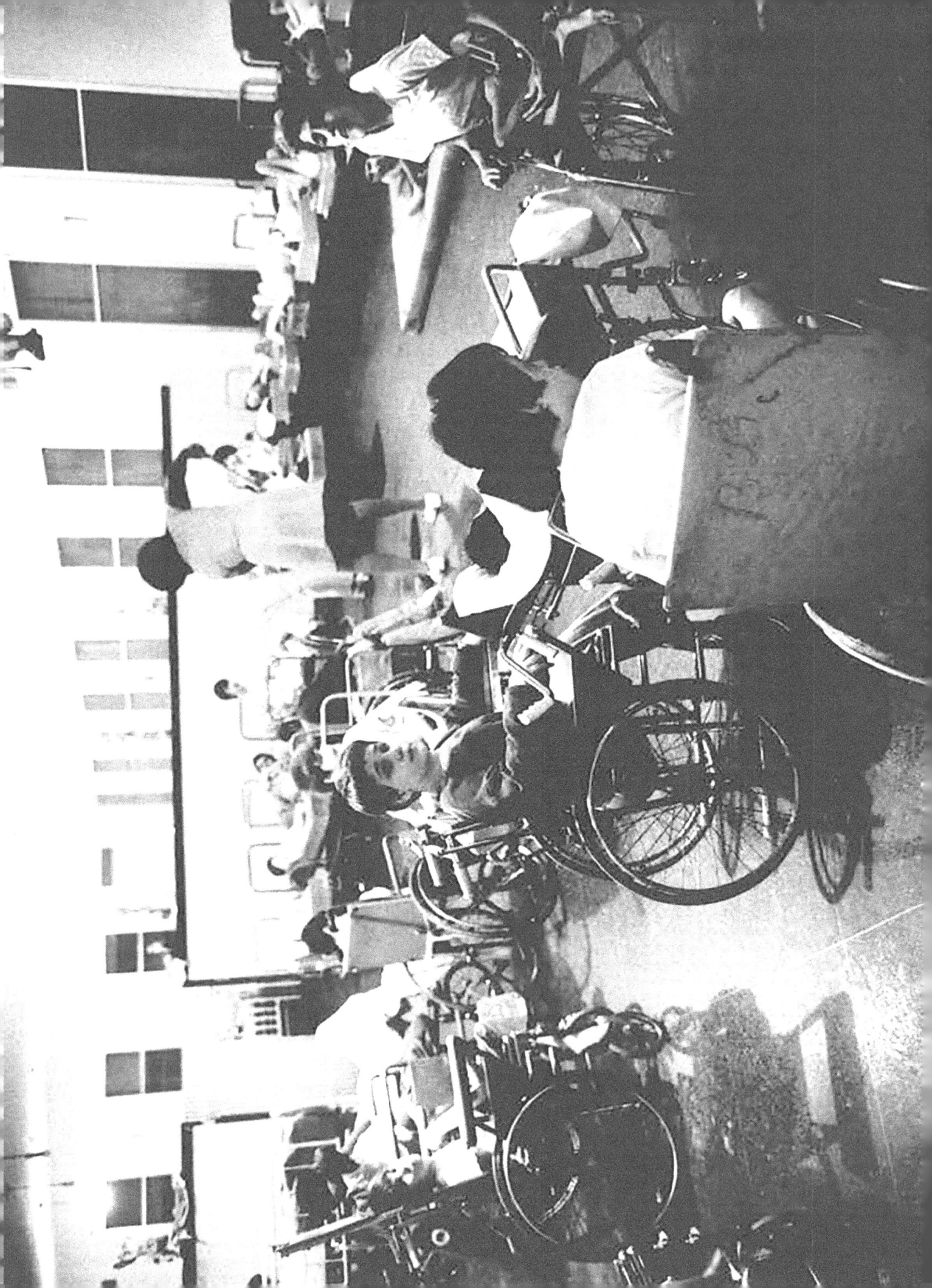

A very few go into some sort of school in the Field Buildings where they are lodged or into Building 3, which is specifically reserved for the more advanced children who are capable of attending school. The classrooms in the one-and two-story field buildings are usually located in the basements and service about 20 people each. Altogether, possibly one-fifth of the people in the institution are touched by a period of school during their tenure.

The process for moving a person to another building is an ugly affair. Generally, residents are not moved for positive reasons but are shifted and dumped out of buildings as a result of management problems or dislikes (of one sort or another) by the staff. As the children grow and advance through the various adolescent and adult building placements, the true strategy of Willowbrook becomes sharply apparent. Services of any kind become scarcer, overcrowding becomes more severe, the physical wards and buildings become more gloomy, and the overall quality of the staff and the interest of the administration wane. I think much of this is related to the reduction of the parents' advocacy efforts as time passes. The bad situation becomes a matter of acceptance by the families.

Since there is absolutely no individualized planning or evaluation performed at Willowbrook, the buildings are perceived in a very gross way in terms of their dominant population. The employees experience the buildings in terms of how much work there is. The buildings where those with motor disabilities are placed represent the most oppressive and dangerous to work in. For the most part, the work force is composed of women. The wards in these "spastic buildings" house at least 45 people who are bedridden. Every manipulation requires lifting, tugging, or equivalent physical exertion. There are rarely more than three staff on these wards, as is the case throughout Willowbrook, and this effort day in and day out is terrifically exhausting and frequently associated with occupational injury. Thus, the obvious strategy of the staff is to master the situation and organize the effort in such a way as to minimize moving the residents. Once out of bed and hoisted onto the thinly padded "cripple carts" (a horizontal wooden plane on wheels with a low lip about its edges), the residents lie about most of the day sometimes 2, or even 3, to each cart. If a wheelchair is used for those persons with the ability to sit up, the wheel chair becomes their day-long depository. All bathing is done in an elevated shallow tile slab sink (often seen in mortuaries) with a spray nozzle, onto which the worker must hoist the resident, often unassisted. Lacking program personnel on the wards and adequate equipment, not to mention the existence of profound technical underdevelopment, the staff on the ward (almost irrespective of numbers) will exercise crisis-care interventions and remain passive, tending to spectate over their charges. Thus, stripping the beds, mealtime, bathing (maybe once daily) are foundation efforts. Sharing the lack of hope, inspiration, and knowledge from the administration, the employees—new and old— sink into a defensive posture. As a rule, no professional is out on the wards. The vital decision-making falls to these least trained people, whose judgment is blunted by the work conditions. Thus, two facts must be kept in mind. There is not enough staff on the wards to even begin to provide for the basic needs of th`e people. Secondly, the orientation, the lack of quality control, and the attitudes among the ward employee population all tend to harbor backward and unscientific notions, coupled with patterns of work which reflect the "here to die" reality of Willowbrook residents, regardless of the expansion or contraction of the numbers of staff.

For example, in my ward 231 there are upwards of 50 extremely disturbed, severely disabled young women. Usually there are three or four workers on this ward. The floors are mopped, as are the bathrooms cleaned, by residents forced to do the work who are recruited from other wards in the building, while many of the employees stand about the ward walls with arms folded. Each worker is confronted with watching the entire ward, as no breakdown of residents into any kind of therapeutic groups exists. This requires the residents to stay seated, or as immobile as possible, all day, to ease their overseers' efforts. So demoralized, passive, and overwhelmed is the average ward worker, that changes of status for residents often flow from exhaustion and tend to develop over about a two-month period, when surrender on the part of one or two ward staff in relation to a particular problematic resident results in a series of complaints and /or accidents which communicate dramatically the need to transfer that patient somewhere else.

The sojourn of children in the young adult buildings described above depends on these factors: first, the tolerance and relative organizational stability of the building staff; second, the degree of difficulty presented by the resident; and third, the pressure of the parents on the staff and the administration. All of these three conditions rest upon fixed expectations. If the resident does not conform to what is available, struggle ensues and danger climbs for the resident. This process builds up over the years and creates the conditions that condone the ultimate placement of the person into the building where he or she will ultimately die. The normal grinding-down process of the institution has effectively reduced these 1,500-2,000 high-risk residents to bestial status or bizarre spectacles in their present setting.

The wards in these terminal buildings represent the final common pathway for over 80 percent of the people at Willowbrook. The essential element here is the fact that the system is closed with respect to exit from Willowbrook. Thus, if the "better" buildings (i.e. 2 or 3 of 27) are jammed full and a person capable of sufficient independent living has struggled through in the youth buildings, he or she is destined to be placed into those buildings where space can always be found—into buildings where virtually no programs exist and where overcrowding and warehousing has taken its toll. Maybe this young person will stay in a school program for a portion of the day until he or she is 21, but the significant life experience is the brutal degradation in the wards with 50 to 80 other adults. It is this violent daily experience that molds or remolds every person.

Jerry B., Mike R., and Daniel M. are typical of this practice. Those three children were in a model prefab building. The former two boys were in "trainable" classes on wards with 35 other children. The third boy suffered severe seizures. Because of staff attitudes about their particular behavior and performance in the building, these boys were dumped into a building and onto wards with double the census and less staff. They now can anticipate 20 or 30 years of this new environment. As I mentioned, the decision is made from the ward level with concurrence from the professional staff who rely wholly on ward input for information. Children who do not "cause trouble" last longer in the less murderous wards and buildings; that is to say, they are permitted to remain 'children' longer.

In summary, if an image were appropriate one would conjure up a swamp stream that initially settles on low land, flowing onto the swamp area with some vigor, but losing strength as portions split off into stagnant pools. The entry of the stream is the baby complex, which gradually gives up the children into less and less tolerable ponds represented by the 'back' buildings, the 'spastic' buildings, the 'young adult low-grade' buildings, and the final buildings of ultimate stagnation. The few that receive reprieves along the way and eddy into model buildings are given a temporary "stay of execution", so to speak.

Even this is questionable if one looks thoroughly at these so-called "bright" buildings, where the staff attitudes and practices are dictated by the universal principles of Willowbrook: "Don't make trouble. Don't stick your neck out. If nobody else does it, why should I?" Futility, defeatism, and staff turnover are the consequences of mismanagement, lack of planning and lack any educational/developmental science.

Orderly Chaos: How the Buildings Run

The everyday operations of Willowbrook, as one scrutinizes them more closely, reflect such remarkable deficiencies in organization and coordination that, were it not for the horror and consequences of this situation, one would simply laugh. Since the time I started work here, I have not received a policy manual nor have I seen one where services are carried out. A memo or two is sent weekly, to supervisors or physicians relating to a specific situation that has arisen but these communiques are usually extremely minor, stop-gap efforts (usually arising after the fact because of some snafu in the bureaucracy). Moreover, the situations that obsess the administration are invariably bureaucratic in nature and bear slightly, if at all, on patient care.

Each building over the years has developed its own way of running, in the face of the fairly frequent shifting around of physicians and professional staff. Who does what job, when, and how, varies. For example, whether attendants or housekeepers or residents clean the bathrooms, sort the clothes, are supervised or not, vary with each building and invariably differ across the 3 shifts.. Whether a shift report is given, how illnesses among the residents are reported, what constitutes an incident worth making out an accident form on, who among the employees gets privileges and who doesn't, and how problems get solved differs from building to building.

The stock of medications and treatment materials is so sharply at variance between the back and spastic buildings versus the baby complex and model buildings, that it is hard to believe. In the former, one may not even find instruments to examine inside ears nor basic materials for applying sutures under sterile conditions. The staffs of each building are so tuned into the expectations of the specific doctors that the use of gloves when suturing or requests for Novocain elicit gasps of disbelief from treatment employees, and excuses that no one has ever used these items before. Essentially, Willowbrook runs without an administration, with practical policy being hammered out at the building level to handle the overwhelming majority of problems and transactions.

By far, the most far-reaching and serious of these problems is the staffing patterns. I have been simply thunderstruck since coming to Willowbrook at the irrational way in which the wards are run. From this, and the way records are compiled and kept, has come the most dramatic evidence to support the conclusion that dehumanization is calculated.

The basic atmosphere of the wards, and the overwhelming work load which is part of the ward situation, net the lowest possible productivity and stem from lack of progressive leadership and a rational definition of goals and practices. I will explain the chaos of work roles and remarkable inefficiency in providing services that I have directly experienced in three buildings.

When residents must go to clinics, where, they are seen by consultants, at least one attendant must accompany them. In the youth building that I was assigned to, a worker "chaperone" is assigned from the ward on which the child lives. With five wards, it is normal for five attendants to accompany five children to a single clinic, such as the dentist, sharply depleting the ward coverage, which is the result of grossly incompetent building administration. Lunches and absenteeism-with resultant shifting about of the remaining people-also cut into the ward staff. It is virtually impossible for any given resident to receive individual attention at any time, except when that resident acts out and disrupts the ward. Because of this severe understaffing, undesirable resident behavior is reinforced by attention just as surely as if it were planned. The depletion of staff is compensated for by the use of other residents as ward staff as enforcers, to carry out all duties from toileting, feeding and controlling peers, while the employees are usually reduced to a spectator or supervisory role.

It is common for a ward attendant to be shifted into the treatment room to assist or, for that matter, to totally manage medications and treatments. It is normal for the senior workers on the ward to drift out toward the nursing office and occupy themselves with "busy work," leaving the ward further uncovered. This is especially prevalent because there are no planned or meaningful activities on the wards that require more than the most superficial effort where people simply mill about endlessly devoid of any purposeful activity. All in all this additive attrition of people and purpose has a devastating effect on the conditions on the ward, where the 50 residents roam around the stone rooms in which they are incarcerated.

During last fall, as well as the winter months, when days were pleasant, it was absolutely impossible to take any residents off the wards and out of the buildings, as there were only two workers on each ward of 50. This depressing state of affairs is further aggravated by the infinitely mixed patient population for which no single strategy, except repression can address itself to the group. Many are severely visually handicapped, some deaf, some with seizures which, though for the most part controlled, intimidate the ward staff, who are fearful of having to focus their attention on one person once out of the confines of the building, thereby losing "control" of the balance of the patient group.

Where does this attitude originate? Not in the patient care echelons, but at the highest level of the administration. Four months after assuming responsibility of two adult women's buildings, I canvassed all the wards discussing the basic status of each resident, searching for those people who would be capable of handling walks on the grounds in small, unsupervised, structured groups. A list of 111 women was compiled, and the administration was asked to approve this effort. The director personally vetoed the offer, saying that the women in these two buildings were unsuited to being unsupervised. No formal reply was forthcoming despite three repeated attempts on my part to elicit reasons for the rejection of this plan. Shortly after the sharpest note to the director, and about the time of the filing of the law-suit, a meeting was held with the administrative staff who supervised the women's complex. In addition, the supervisors from the two buildings and the nursing supervisor over both buildings attended. The women's complex administrator, a deputy director, verbally supported the idea, but the project was never pursued.

The normal fearfulness of erring and being held personally responsible (which prevails among the employees) provides the final inertia to undermine even this basic attempt to see the residents as people with varying abilities. So fragile is the effort to offer humane care for the residents that a rumor, a gloomy personal mood of a worker, a frown from the building supervisor, is enough to lay the slightest initiative low, returning Willowbrook to its usual degrading routines.

What characterizes the day shift and differentiates it from the P.M. shift, or second shift, is the presence of structure brought about by two factors. During the day, the professionals are much in evidence and the bureaucracy is in full force. Secondly, a certain number of residents are taken off the wards for other activities in the morning slightly reducing the census. The afternoon shift, on the other hand, is characterized by an almost complete lack of professional presence, absence of supervisors. The bureaucracy has gone home. In addition, the full press of residents returns to the wards for the dinner meal, undressing, bathing, and bedding down. It is on this shift that the majority of accidents seem to happen. There are no programs run in the P.M. shift. The atmosphere at the end of the day is more relaxed and casual, and the rigid pressures of the day lift, with residents acting up more and feeling freer to express themselves in every way. My direct experience with the P.M. shift comes because my work day usually extends until about P.M., which covers much of the dinner hour. On night duty I have observed the bathing process and the bedding process in numerous buildings. The usual staff of the day declines in the P.M. to such a degree that it is not at all uncommon to see one worker covering an entire ward alone. The greatest number of severe lacerations seems to cluster in the shift. When I am on night duty, these tend to be reported between 5 and 8 P.M. Then, I get scattered calls in the morning around or 7 A.M. when people first get up. When I come in on regular duty in the morning there are usually lacerations from the proceeding evening or the early morning waiting to be sutured.

Whatever can be said of the P.M. shift from a structural standpoint also operates for the night, or third shift. The night shift must pretty much get the building into shape for the A.M. In many instances they must do laundry, oversee the waking up, dressing, initial ablutions of the residents, and the morning medication. In some instances, a portion of the morning meal is fed to the residents.

If one were to increase the staff on the wards to meet the basic emergency needs, a number of situations would have to be considered. First, numbers alone are not the answer. Conversely, without adequate numbers one cannot begin to talk about qualitative change. A rational organization must exist to make the individual worker effective and feel that what he or she is doing is meaningful, dignified, and in both his and the residents' interest. New knowledge and continuous practical demonstrations are essential. Next, if the ward staff was to be increased, and it must, this would increase the need for support personnel to supply the multiplying needs on the wards. For example, in the baby complex there is always a severe shortage of diapers, clean linens, and clothing. Thus, if the wards are only supplied with two changes daily and adequate staff are there to really change the residents when they soil, additional linens would have to be provided to meet the real need. This means that careful thought has to be given to the total needs of a more efficient operation on the ward, in the kitchens, in the laundry, for transportation, clinics, etc.

When a new admission rarely comes to Willowbrook, a set of papers precedes that person by a few hours. These usually include a history of the new person with assorted notes from assorted agencies involved. The thrust of the admitting documents is to justify individual's admission, and, are therefore immensely one-sided. A diagnosis or label usually accompanies the person or is easily designated, since by the time the person comes to Willowbrook, all the limited remedies and services in the community have been exhausted. The admitting Willowbrook doctor does a physical examination, usually the only thorough physical performed and recorded throughout the person's stay at the institution. A psychological evaluation is done as a routine matter within three months. This is rarely more than two or three paragraphs. It assigns and IQ score and totally avoids programmatic recommendations. Again, the overriding purpose is to justify admission and classify the scope of the liabilities as quickly as possible. In most instances, the evaluation is done at the most traumatic period in the person's experience: torn away from family, admitted into the frenzied and desiccated human atmosphere of the institution, changes in food, routines disrupted, and placed under the control of strangers. Moreover, with the lack of alternative languages, such as Spanish, the psychologists heavily penalize children raised in bilingual or non-English-speaking homes. It is clear when reading 30 or 40 of these evaluations (upon which the residents' future is pinned) that they are an exercise in cynicism, not science.

More staggering is the lack of reevaluations. In one building, I reviewed the IQ data and found that the average period that had passed since the last evaluation was 7.4 years, while the average age of the children was between 13 and 14. During the review of charts in transferring 42 adult women between buildings, there were only four charts that were less than five years old. One 52-year-old woman who had been transferred from Letchworth had never been tested. Despite this, the obsolete and often invalid IQ test score was accepted and repeated over and over by doctors filling out eligibility forms and the like. In fact, in a memorandum from 1968, which is still in force, from an assistant director to physicians and stenos regarding filling out Medicaid forms, explicit instructions were given for physicians to estimate low IQs to be below 65 when in doubt. These admitting papers essentially form the core of information about the resident. If they are deficient, slanted, inaccurate, they still become the truth for that person in Willowbrook. What follows is the series of "progress notes," usually six to eight lines long, which log the invariable downhill course of the resident. The entries are formalized and highly repetitive, using jargon which emphasizes every negative. There is neither self-criticism nor admission anywhere that possibly the child's course reflects environmental conditions. The expectation of performance is exceedingly low and conforms to a model of behavior which minimizes care taking problems. For example, if a person is able to feed themselves, self-toileting, and self-dressing, passive and withdrawn, that person will be seen as "good, cooperative, and adjusting well," No precise depiction of the anatomy of performance, the efficiency of performance, nor the individual aspects of personality are to be found. Over the years, doctor after doctor adds dull and lifeless entries toward which the brutal environment and fixed expectations of the staff mold the resident in a self-fulfilling tragedy.

Occupational therapy and school records are variably present in scattered charts. These may range from 1 to 10 periods. They are on different colored paper and allow four to five handwritten lines to describe a semester or a year's experience. Terse, narrow questions direct the technician towards terse, narrow answers. Again, the institution's evaluations accept this inappropriate form and gear their analysis to abstract brevity. No social service reports are to be found, no warm and sympathetic or human anecdotes, no inclusion of samples of school or OT work. No photos follow the admission mug shot which would show in every case the terrible physical toll taken by the years at Willowbrook. The bulk of the chart may be confined to a series of isolated consultations requested of medical specialists for a series of isolated conditions and health crises.

So lacking in focus, so impoverished of original observation, so fragmentary and heavily laden with negative aspects of the person are these charts that they are virtually useless to anyone wishing a clear picture of a resident in question. In my opinion, the charts document the gross incompetency of the administration; for here is where the entire history of a human being resides. Many times it is virtually all that is known or recorded about a life; and instead of a documentary of flesh and blood people, it is Willowbrook's perverse universe and vision that dominates. This is nowhere more shocking than when a person dies and the chart is perused, a situation where the finality of the review is apparent. The information missing is staggering.

The outrage is the lack of any full professional entry at any level in any field. Each specialist limits himself to the narrowest concern and confines himself to the shortest time piece. Little continuity is to be found; follow-up or explanations for changes in status, be they physical, mental, functional, are altogether ignored, leaving a two-dimensional report. One would be relieved if the contemporary staff had learned the lessons of the past recording deficiencies. But it seems that the situation has led to even more deteriorated performance. The records reflect the "acceptable" professional ethic and standard of the institution and nowhere is there a break in this blind, ignorant, and slavish practice. In no way should the existing professional community presently employed at Willowbrook, especially the medical and psychological staff, be enlisted to evaluate the residents. Again, it is not only the misinterpretation of what is seen that is so ugly, but the omissions and fragmentary approach that obliterates everyone.

The Consultation Process'

Of particular concern to me are the procedures for responding to a medical problem and the snafu inherent therein at Willowbrook. If a resident presents a problem where a specialty evaluation is indicated, a referral is made. This referral is forwarded to the coordinator of the clinics and the resident is listed for evaluation in the particular clinic indicated such as eye, ENT, cardiac, dermatology, orthopedic, gynecology, urology, surgery, etc. Generally, the resident is seen for the first time within a week, as each consultant visits once a week for part of one day. Recommendations which come back may request other evaluations, indicate the "difficulty" examining the resident, or other remarks which ultimately mean delay. In many instances a treatment is prescribed despite the repeated use of this treatment unsuccessfully in the past. Strategic delays mount up slowly. Diagnoses are prolonged for weeks and frequently months. Even though the ward physician has the option of making an emergency request for specialists, which somewhat shortens the waiting period, or can recommend hospitalization, considerable pressure and peer disgruntlement result. The result has been that, though I have felt in many instances (too numerous to list here but certainly recallable) that this or that resident needed immediate attention, it was not an emergency in the traditional sense and thus the process was dragged out.

A few examples should give the feeling for this standard situation. Pat M., a girl with Down Syndrome, was followed for ten years in Cardiac Clinic. The cardiologist intimated that her congenital heart defect was not troublesome and conveyed that everything was under control, insofar as the girl would be rechecked every year or so. Despite this, the heart size became immense and the question was whether or not the girl was in congestive failure. No diagnostic tests to determine the precise anatomic location or the dynamics of the heart defect were recommended. When I pushed to have the girl transferred to Bellevue Hospital for cardiac catheterization to determine the exact nature of the problem (after discussing the matter fully with her very concerned parents), the institution cardiologist ignored my recommendation and upon rechecking the girl said she was not in trouble. I suggested that the mother take the girl to an outside cardiologist familiar to the family. This doctor immediately recommended the catheterization, and a copy of his letter was forwarded to the consultant at Willowbrook. Finally, the consultant begrudgingly gave in and gave his OK. Then a resume had to be compiled to be sent to Bellevue and consent for the procedure obtained from the mother. When this had been done and the red tape of approvals for the transfers cleared, a memo was received indicating that the girl was to go to a clinic at Bellevue for a medical check before she would be accepted for catheterization. Despite the severe cardiac disease present and the progressive nature of this disease, these delays have now extended beyond six months from the initial recommendation for the testing and corrective surgery. The catheterization has still not yet been done.

A girl, Carol K., with an unsightly two-inch mound of flesh growing between her eyes above the bridge of her nose was referred to the plastic surgeon for evaluation. This lesion had developed secondary to head-banging with recurrent infections at the sight which gradually led to the buildup of this 'horn-like' protuberance. The plastic surgeon said that the horn protected Carol from further injury and that an operation on such a retarded girl was not particularly indicated. I returned the request, reminding the consultant that this horn was very unsightly and became a barrier for people relating to the girl. The plastic surgeon suggested that I contact the general surgeon. The surgeon then saw the horn and indicated this protuberance was really a covering over a bony growth on the girl's forehead and that an operation would result in a chronic opening at that site. Unfortunately, X-rays, which the surgeon had available to him, did not bear out this sage rationalization, and when he was confronted with the fact that this was nothing more than an easily removable lesion, I received a repetition that this horn was protective. I resorted to a strongly worded memo to the administration and received back a reply from a deputy director saying that if I felt compelled to pursue the matter, I could make my recommendation and the girl would be seen on the outside. I made it clear that four months of struggling with this matter had convinced me more than ever that something very wrong was happening and that I felt strongly about the matter. I have heard nothing since for two months. Lena H., a virtually normal elderly lady, developed pain and swelling in her abdomen. Physical exam revealed a mass. I immediately referred her to Gynecology Clinic. After two weeks the report came back confirming the mass and referring the resident to the surgeon. The surgeon saw the patient after another two weeks and requested lab work and medical clearance. After six weeks of bouncing about, the lady became severely incapacitated and demonstrated the unmistakable symptoms of malignancy. At this point I admitted her to the hospital building where she soon died. The point here is not that this lesion was preventable, but that this unconscionable delay, promulgated by the lackadaisical attitude of the specialists, intensified the suffering and allowed precious time to slip by.

Two residents had been followed by the ENT specialist for chronic infected ears that intermittently drained pus. The treatments over a year period involved the cyclical repetition of antibiotic therapy and packings to the infected ear. After three rounds of this seemingly mindless cycle, I ordered X-rays of the skull looking for an underlying infection of the mastoid bone behind the ear. I found this to be the case in both instances. The diagnosis of chronic mastoiditis, as this condition is called, is the first consideration in chronic ear infections. Despite this, the consultant did not request this basic test. In fact, in all my experience with this consultant, he has never ordered an X-ray as part of the diagnostic workup, which in these cases was confined to culturing the pus. This same (and only) ENT consultant has ordered tonsillectomies despite his previous removal of tonsils from residents. So superficial and sloppy is this outside consultant's approach that I have found that the only reason I make referrals is to help me keep track of the case to insure that I remember to follow up the problem.

Kathy M. was shown to me one day with free blood occluding the pupil of one of her eyes. This had been discovered the day before and was seen by another physician who had covered the building in my absence. The girl had been sent to the eye consultant who recommended that she have a dressing put on the eye and be returned to the eye clinic on the next occasion. Now this particular condition in the majority of cases constitutes a medical emergency and is called hyphema. When I saw the girl, the dictated findings and note from the specialist had not yet reached the building. I called him at his private office and described the case. The consultant indicated without hesitation that the girl should be hospitalized and both eyes patched in addition to being given medication to force voiding fluid from her system to reduce swelling. I made arrangements to move the girl to Building 2. A few minutes later the physician in charge of Building 2 called back and refused to take the girl on the grounds that he had called the eye specialist, who said that I had not informed him that he had already seen the patient the day before.

I pointed out that I had not known she was seen and that the lesion in the eye had gotten worse. So fierce was the refusal to accept the injured girl that I was forced to enlist the aid of an administrator who related, after he had failed to effect the transfer, that the Building 2 doctor had complained that "too many women from the two adult buildings were sent to the hospital and took up more than a proportionate amount of space". I then was forced to recall the eye consultant and explain that the conditions in the patient's building were absolutely dangerous, with only two to three workers on the ward and no nurse in the building, and that the motives of the Building 2 physician did not relate to his concern for the basic safety of the resident. Two days later I found out that the injury had required eye surgery to drain the blood which had collected. Kathy is now totally blind.

These are just a minute sample of the crude, indifferent, unscientific, malpractice and inhumane treatment accorded our residents. I have no doubt that protests of these truths will be forth-coming, but an interrogation of a sample of the attendants from the buildings who accompany the residents to the clinics will bear out, in gruesome detail, the gross negligence exercised by each and every consultant.

Over and above this catastrophic situation with consultants is the impossibility of systematic follow-up on any given resident. Recording and follow-up of illnesses in Willowbrook are in a complete state of anarchy. There is no recording system for the gross diseases among the population. Only through a special research grant has the institution obtained the services of a parasitologist and the hepatitis research operation, both deeply into isolated endeavors fraught with ethical issues, oblivious of the fundamental conditions of the institution. Case finding for general pathology among the residents goes on day by day. Each building and each doctor has his or her own idiosyncratic approach, but all have certain fundamental similarities. First, the bulk, if not all, of the case finding comes from the wards with the least trained people on the wards locating illnesses. Thus, by the time pathology is presented to the doctor, who comes in in the morning for cases to be brought to the treatment room, the lesions are full blown and the resident in significant pain. It was not till I had worked and taught in a building for over a year with two nurses full-time in that building that the lesions presented, be they skin, respiratory, etc., were less than two days old. In my present assignment over two women's buildings, unless I make an intense search first-hand on the ward among the residents (which under any circumstance can only be ultra-superficial), the lesions are at least a week old. The personal frustration from this experience is difficult to communicate and only peripheral to the massive sufferings.

All of this forms a pattern that is unmistakable. The reason for this systematized cruelty that is part and parcel of every transaction—is traced to one thing. The "retarded" are defined as subhuman. The retarded at Willowbrook will die at Willowbrook; and, in distress. Every person at Willowbrook becomes a "low grade" to the professional community who are, as a group, strategically disinterested in serving such patients.

Thus, it is my opinion that an utterly new authority must be established within the institution. The malignant disdain and revulsion, in which the residents are held by the overwhelming number of medical professionals within Willowbrook, and all the administration, disqualify these people from contributing to solving the problem. At once these attitudes lead to misdefinitions and result from an era of vast medical technical cover-ups, which has crept in and now dominates the language, imagery, and evaluation procedures of the institution. It is this professional betrayal of trust on the part of those people with access to modem science and technology that generates the universal underdevelopment and myth-ridden thinking of the rank-and-file employee who carries out, if not acts out, this arrogant and feeling less perspective from above. "The retardate is an outcast from society; therefore, anything we do for him is better than he would have received anywhere else." With this attitude, parents are insulted and residents are subjected to practices that can only demoralize, disorient, destroy, and dehumanize.

The Problem of the Emergency

There exists no generally accepted approach to deal with "the Emergency" at Willowbrook. There are two EKG machines in all of Willowbrook: both of these are in the so-called Medical and Surgical Building, Building 2. There is no prepared and organized tray containing all the essential materials to respond to the basic emergencies such as cardiac, respiratory, allergic, or convulsive crises in the buildings. I have ministered over a half-dozen deaths, which I have been called to prevent but arrived to find no equipment readily available to use. To this date, despite the seemingly vigorous response by the administration and the fact that the task is placed into the most trusted hands at Willowbrook, there is still no prepared equipment in any building that I have worked in.

Violence and Defeat

Insofar as Willowbrook is essentially a closed system where a fixed community is trapped without a meaningful, graceful, nor dignified exit for residents or workers, tension and frustration are very high. At Willowbrook, normal life is impossible and these irrepressible forces are stifled, nullified by the material conditions, including subjective attitudes that thrive. Violence becomes overt under such conditions. It takes traditional forms that are everywhere visible but more frequently occur in the passive, mute aspects mediated by what is missing, what is not done and not expected. The first and most essential step toward this end is the social disenfranchisement which is the sentence of each resident once he/she is designated "retarded", and which is clinched upon entering the institution for life.

No real, present, permanent, and informed advocate exists for the resident. Loss of human dignity is not only permitted but encouraged. Too numerous to recount are the instances when a resident will implore for this or that benefit, often wracked with sobbing despair, while I make my rounds. One says her ball has been taken away; another, that her shoes are tatty or hurt her feet. This one wants to call her mother; that one relates wanting to get off the ward or out of the building because peers or staff are persecuting her. One cannot tolerate the food; the other isn't allowed to go off the ward or wants to write a letter to a parent. All these are the consequence of the total isolation that the institutional setting imposes, the homogenized and concentrated misery it contains, and the absolute lack of any mechanism to insure that requests and complaints from the hapless victims are registered and resolved in a thorough way. No one has time to listen or to care or to do anything, as the institution is presently constituted.

Residents go unclothed, are pushed about, yelled and cursed at by employees, reviled and physically scorned by the doctors and administrator who keep as much distance as possible between them and their charges. There is no future for the 90 percent. They have been brought to Willowbrook with no goal in mind, no problem to solve, and thus the mandate is to take the person out of and away from society and its protective social and legal structures.

In my earlier remarks, numerous general aspects of violence were indicated: exclusion from programs and the non-utilitarian thrust of programs which do exist; the essential lack of physical services for the motor involved people; neglect and relentless isolation for the people who are blind and deaf; degradation on the wards from filth, overcrowding, peer violence, and perpetual struggles; delayed intervention in the disease process; prolonged case handling without definitive relief; noise levels in the stone buildings that magnify and reverberate the smallest sound; lack of use of analgesics by almost all professionals (dentists extract without Novocain; doctors suture without xylocaine; illnesses are treated without aspirins, regardless of the pain involved, such as with gigantic boils, etc.; menses that cause severe cramps go by without antispasmodics; excessively painful treatments are ordered, such as using injectable antibiotics instead of oral medications whenever possible). The list goes on and on.

This can only make sense and be seen in its true light if one understands the basic assumptions that operate in closed institutions of which Willowbrook is only emblematic. Lacking any orientation toward prevention, and resorting to the multiple levels of restrictive and confining practices, almost all human relations are colored by violence. It is only natural that death results frequently.

A few examples should suffice to communicate the depth of the problem. It must be emphasized that the most dramatic consequence of institutionalization is that a creeping death of the spirit, and a psychological derangement occurs fifty-fold over before the physical death that arouses such finality. Were I compelled to tolerate one or the other (if we were forced to choose which murder to address our energies toward forestalling), I would give my full attention, without hesitation, to ending the living death which is so widespread, so tragic, and so preventable. No death by choking or cancer or kidney failure can match in pathos the agony of the lost souls who wander about the wards from childhood until senior years with dull stares, cringing, going through frenzied, bizarre rituals of hand flapping; with running spittle, endless shrieking, twirling string, regurgitating, sleeping in piles on the stone floors—in human piles—for contact, and seeking warmth with legs drawn up, covered with sores, bodies reeking with filth which repeated washing barely reduces, shielding themselves in a lightning flash when approached. This is not the consequence of mental retardation but the result of a murderous, brutal environment.

Adelaide L. was a young adult woman who had her first seizure late one night while in bed. She was reported to have fallen out of bed, hitting her head on the floor, and there was a vague report that possibly she had fallen earlier in the shower. She vomited and was reported to appear looking poorly. A doctor was called who was on night duty. He took a blood pressure and ordered "observation". In the morning a doctor came who was on day duty and noticed that the patient was asleep but responded to painful stimuli; then he left. At 2:30 that afternoon, Adelaide was found dead in her bed. Despite all indication that something ominous was happening, reflected by an unexpected seizure and vomiting, nothing was done.

Danny M., an infant with Down syndrome and a congenital heart disease, developed a fever in November and was placed on antibiotics. The medication was reordered continuously, despite continuation and progression of the illness, until March the next year when the boy was placed on the critical list. During all this time, no diagnostic tests were ordered that gave a clue as to why the treatment was not working. In March the antibiotics were juggled and altered briefly, especially since a yeast infection had become superimposed consequent to the prolonged antibiosis. The child was seen by no less than five physicians who had rotated through the building during the course of the illness. No analysis of the case was posed. The boy became weaker and was placed in oxygen with a return to the ineffective antibiotic until he expired. Over four months of treatment without a diagnosis, no explanation existed for the lack of response to treatment!

As a child, Frank G. was transferred from Letchworth in 1949. The copy of the letter sent to his parents was in the chart. It said that due to dangerous overcrowding at Letchworth, the boy would be transferred to a new unit just opened at Halloran Hospital on Staten Island called Willowbrook. The boy maintained a habit of grabbing food and cramming it into his mouth, often gagging. Twenty-three years later, last week, the young man rushed into the dining area naked, snatched a giant handful of bread and fled back onto the ward. Suddenly he turned blue and fell to the floor. The attendants on the ward tried to pull the pieces of bread out of his mouth to no avail, and Frank died minutes later. Despite three workers on the ward and the supervisor, the years of neglect and dehumanization had allowed the food-grabbing habit to remain, and the system finally caught up with the unfortunate man.

Alice H. was noted to be severely pale one day on rounds. A blood check was ordered and profound anemia was discovered. The young woman, on a ward with 60 peers, was admitted to the Medical-Surgical Building and noted to have vaginal bleeding. She was sent to a community hospital where surgery revealed advanced cancer of the uterus. Would less crowded wards, better medical control and routine professional case finding have discovered this woman's cancer sooner?

191

Patricia V. was a great, obese girl who wandered about basically indifferent to her environment. One day she was not to be found on the ward. An intensive search was made in the building turning nothing up. The ward staff insisted the resident had wandered into the steam tunnels located in the basements below the building. The attendant knew the outside doors had been locked and that workmen had been working around the steam tunnel. Despite her conviction, the building doctor and supervisors insisted she had gotten out, and shied away from pursuing the matter into the steam tunnel. Finally because of the attendant's continuing protests, the girl was discovered suffocated deep in the hottest part of the tunnel.

These sketches can only represent a few of the many deaths, a portion of the multitude of cases where lesser tragedies occur. I have worked in some of the worst city hospitals and seen health care provided all over the country, in Europe and Mexico. In the face of my past experience and acquired expectations, these incidents at Willowbrook have become more and more ominous. In each instance, I am convinced that such events bear the special stamp of death and disease—Willowbrook style—institutional style. The way things happen, the frequency and savagery with which injury is incurred, the flat almost joking attitudes among the staff upon all these occasions is absolutely new to me. These deaths are Willowbrook deaths and simply would not have occurred in the same way anywhere else. This feeling drives me, compels me to demand the fullest investigation and the most sweeping action to eradicate the complex of conditions and attitudes that permit such horror to survive unchallenged.

As I have written this section on violence and death, I have been on duty at Willowbrook overseeing the entire institution. At 4:44 P.M. I sutured a head laceration. At 5:00, I was called to suture another laceration. At 6:00, I was called to see a young man, J.T., whom the workers in the building could not awaken. The fellow was prostrate on the floor of the clothing room on an upstairs ward. Walking through the ward of 59 adult men, fully one-half were naked, the smell of urine and feces was simply stifling. The men were squatting about the wall, gibbering and moaning, the sound echoing about. 1 wondered if any of them had been "bright" boys once upon a time who, by the natural course of things, stopped being cuddly children, began masturbating, became assertive as living creatures, and had been summarily sent to this building. The floor was covered with pools of urine, and water from a soiled mop. The young man whom I had been called to see was obviously overdosed. Though he was receiving 800 mg. of Mellaril (a major tranquilizer), certainly enough to put a horse to sleep, he had evidently been given an indeterminate amount above that maintenance dose earlier in the day.

The man need only be presented in court to the judge for the truth of Willowbrook to be patently and indelibly clear. The man's head and face were reduced to a mass of swollen blobs, scar over scar; his ears so deformed from blows that they were but two balls of grotesque flesh. Both eyes had become slits surrounded by the swollen sequellae of repeated bruises and cuts over his face. The man's hair was tufted and grew in scrubby patches interlaced with scar upon scar incurred over the years of his youth in Willowbrook. Pus oozed from a recent lesion on his scalp. J.T.'s back had a silver-dollar sized crater, running pus. He cried out when I knelt down on the floor to examine him, "I don't want anymore...I don't want anymore!"

CHAPTER 22

The Trial: "Lives of Hushed and Suffocating Silence"

IN A SUPREME COURT ruling, once upon a time, the promise of the Constitution of the United States to its citizens was set forth as "independence and self-confidence, the feeling of creativity…lives of high spirits rather than hushed, suffocating silence." Somehow, maybe all of us know this in one form or another. It is possible that this quiet truth governs one's deepest feelings. How else to explain when we recoil at misfortune or exult without knowing why when we see some human goodness, when we feel a breakthrough from one level of existence to another toward well-being or human growth, toward freedom and choice.

As the court hearings began, there lay ahead a period of struggle that we had not foreseen. Entering it was probably like breaking out of the water and onto the land for those ancient amphibians millions of years ago who must have sensed a new range of possibilities without having the slightest idea of what lay ahead, what new knowledge and changes would foster evolutionary transformation. Passing from acceptance and despair into action, from anonymity into visibility, was such an emotionally blinding movement. We were to become adjusted to a new posture, upright. I will not try to share all the details, for too much happened, and the profusion of events would only be confusing. It would be like blowing apart a dandelion and pursuing each airborne gliding seedling to its destiny. Even the summary may tax a sense of coherence.

The Willowbrook court process unfolded, playing out till the end of the hearings, and then the ruling in 1975. I will try to capture the specific issues raised at Willowbrook during the span of three years and the counteractions taken by the bureaucracy. I will also touch on the panorama of like situations going on at the same time around the nation. Willowbrook was simply the largest, representing every institution. The court was every court. The promise of the Constitution had been going starkly unmet. March 17, 1972, marked the date that briefs had been filed against the state. A human emergency existed for the incarcerated thousands. No one could doubt that; it was common knowledge in the state of New York. Institutionalized people were deteriorating and had been for decades.

By mid-June, federal judge Orrin Judd, a very busy man with a full federal docket, planned a July hearing on the emergency situation. What the parents' lawyers were demanding in 1972 was immediate action—a temporary injunction before the trial to force the state to hire people, repair the toilets, look at each person in Willowbrook, and do something about their omnipresent plight. Delay seemed incomprehensible in the face of the patient situation, but delay went on. The state, pleading unpreparedness, used every technical, legal strategy imaginable, pushed for more time, postponements before the hearing, hoping they could break free from the grip we had on their institution.

Finally, on December 18, 1972, the first hearing began. During this nine-month lapse, which seemed more like five years, the situation had changed little inside Willowbrook. The state seemed incapable of marshaling itself to change anything, even with the constant, active presence of investigator-men sent to Willowbrook from Albany to do something about the laundry, the maintenance, the food, all the thousand and one collapsed and chaotic conditions as were the norm. The investigators gave the feeling of milling about the buildings like so many ravens circling carrion on a rush-hour highway.

The parent plaintiffs' lawyers had done their job well; nay, they had done a supreme piece of work, compiling nearly two thousand pages of testimony from experts flown in from across the land to assess the situation for the court. Photographs, many in this volume, were taken of every corner of the warehouse. These pictures documented forever the facts, that confined to just words, could never be fully demonstrated, nor truly fathomed. It was the most comprehensive documentation conceivable put to record before the court to prove what everybody already knew—Willowbrook was an American concentration camp. There were twenty-five more institutions just like it in New York, only a little bit smaller, just for people labeled retarded. But the court, being what it is, had to be told all this anew. Reality had to be reconstructed right there in that imperious marble and wood palatial courtroom for one respectable elderly man who had been appointed by the system he was being called upon to indict.

Would the hearing be able to put forth in a convincing way the reality that we all knew existed, or would technicalities and the remoteness of the marble courtroom dilute and prevent the reality from being recreated? The drama of the courtroom, the apprehension that permeated the room, sprang from this crazy problem. If the accusations could be muffled by the objections of the state's attorneys general, whose job it was to deny everything, it could very well be that the only reality that mattered, what was real for the United States, was what the judge heard and understood, never mind Willowbrook. After all, the judge was a layperson, with all the cultural biases of any citizen looking at Willowbrook through words and arguments. If an understanding of the issues and the dynamics of the institution did not accompany the images of hopelessness and grotesqueness of so many of the residents, he could easily say, "But what can be done when such widespread injury exists?"

The court was being asked to intervene in an utterly scandalous situation; its potential resolution was so challenging as to intimidate any public servant, even the court itself. In fact, the first question forced by the state was whether or not the federal court even had a right to hear the case. According to the state's attorney general, this case should be handled in its own state courts. The federal government had no right to interfere in internal state matters. Jurisdiction over the case was at stake. If the federal court were to back out and send the case to exhaust state remedies first, the situation could be tied up for two more years without resolution in the governor's juridical system. If the judge decided this was, in fact, a constitutional question that required federal intervention, relief would become the next profound dilemma. Just to deal with the staff shortage and the disastrous public health deficiencies would cost millions of dollars for renovation and reorganization. To what end! Willowbrook would still be a secret factory of dehumanization and violence. If Willowbrook were to be cleaned up somehow or other, would individual suits then have to be filed at each of the other institutions in New York not covered by this suit?

In addition to all this, the governor had presidential ambitions and strong ties to the White House, not to mention unlimited financial investment in a status quo that was almost entirely of his own making. With a family holding that approximated twice what the Federal Reserve System contained, New York's Rockefeller was not a man to cross lightly.

All these things hung over the lawyers, the parents, all of us—all the people in Willowbrook and all the other institutions in the land—as the hearing opened that pretty day in December. What would be said? What was going to happen? If we failed here, resolution of the problem around the nation would be deeply hurt. New York was the very epicenter of the historical justification for institutionalizing people. Nowhere were there so many people stacked away, unwanted. Any crack here would be felt everywhere. Willowbrook was more than a test case on the issues. Similar issues were already on the books in the few but powerfully conducted cases in Partlow State School in Alabama and Belchertown State School in Massachusetts. This was a test of power. Did the system as it existed offer any mechanism for ordinary people to defend themselves against privilege and power? Whose interpretation of institutions would be legitimized, the rulers or the ruled?

It was almost as if the federal court were on trial more than the state of New York. A drama was being played here that reflected other dramas elsewhere. These other dramas concerned the controversial nature of some recent court decisions and the court's role on behalf of the government versus mass protests and struggles for other human and political rights. The very act of turning to the court system was itself an indictment that the government had turned away from its theoretical origins. Mediation between the government and the public reflected the breakdown of the contract for shared power and accountability between the electorate and its representatives everywhere. For those in Willowbrook, the breach had always been complete. No ballot box had ever been seen within those stained walls. The institutional systems were islands of disenfranchisement, the debris of democracy, just so much refuse and wreckage outside of town.

My beloved mentor, Gunnar Dybwad, Mental Retardation Consultant to the World Health Organization and founding Director of the National Association of Retarded Citizens, had toured Willowbrook with me, Doctor Koch and the Lawyers, having earlier visited to give a lecture to the community family members in Staten Island, joined the peerless testimony team to bring his great wisdom and judgments of what he clearly saw to the historic Court trial.

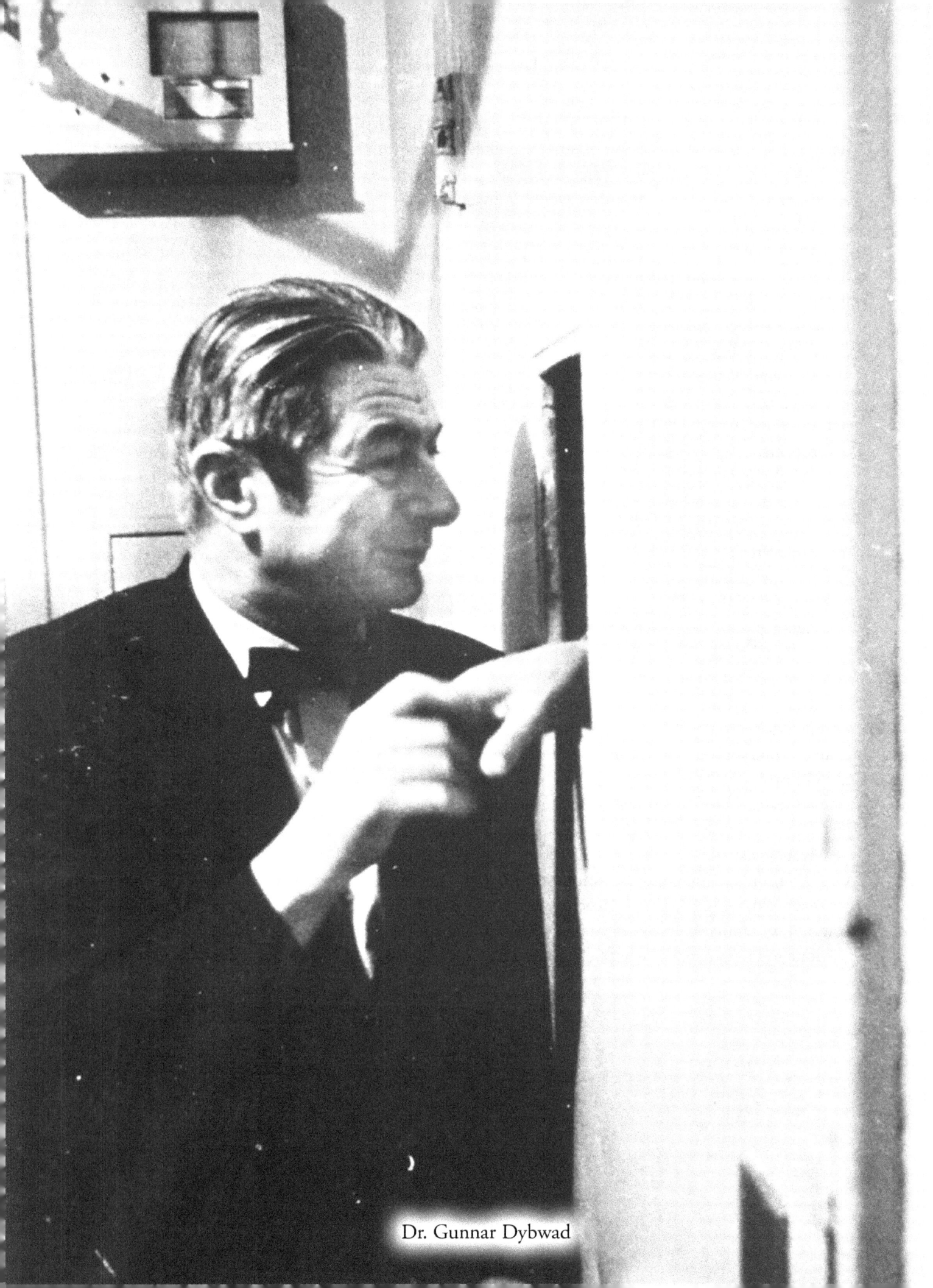

Dr. Gunnar Dybwad

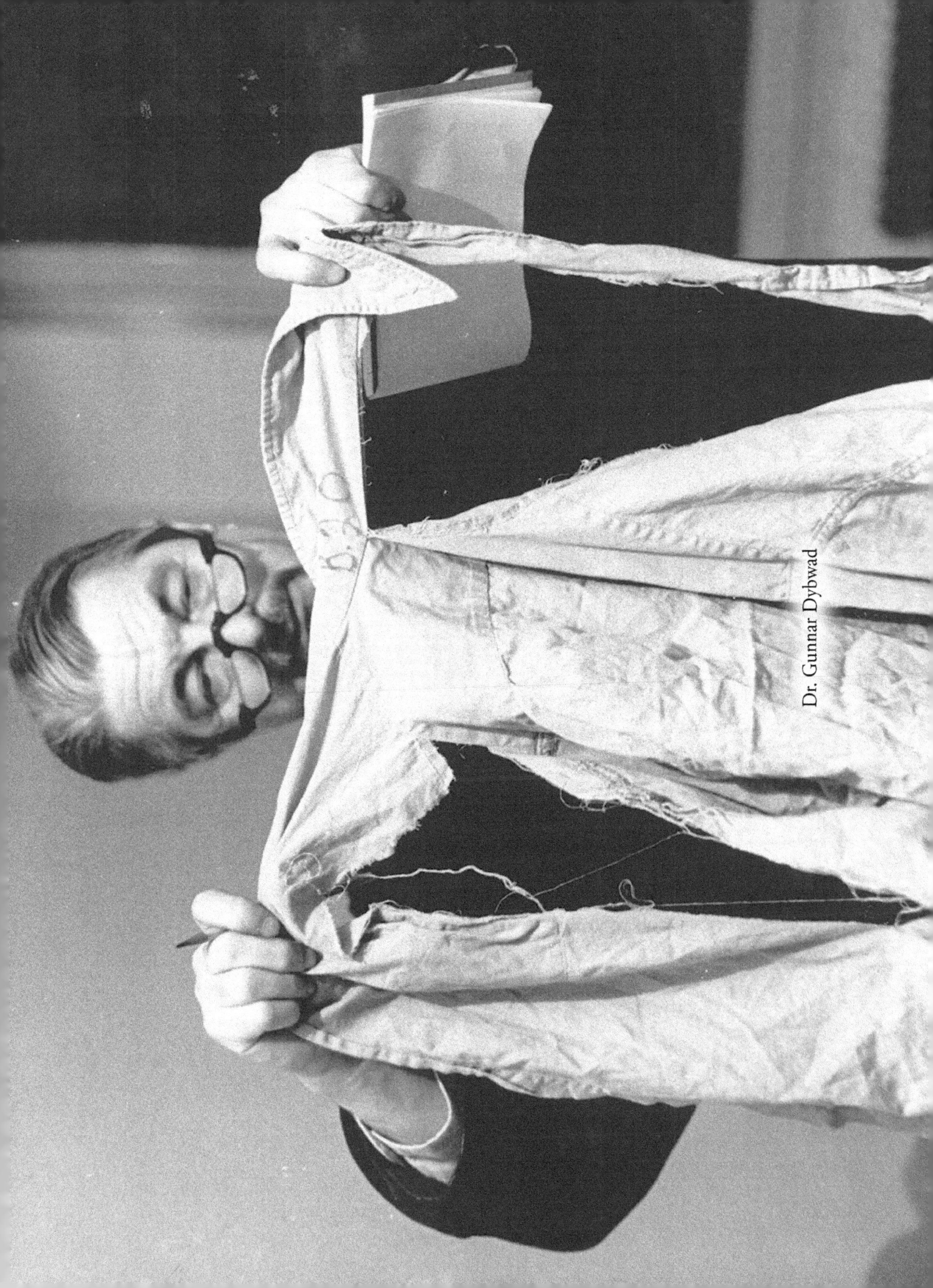

Dr. Gunnar Dybwad

The opening day of the hearing, the plaintiffs presented their case in hopes of obtaining a temporary injunctive order from the court that would command the state just to do something about the galloping and progressive deterioration in Willowbrook. Four parents took the stand and told stories of seeing their kin eaten up by the conditions. The stories of losses of speech, ability to walk, eyes, ears, teeth, weight, life were not extraordinary. It was the beginning of a human attempt to convince a man who held power over their destiny.

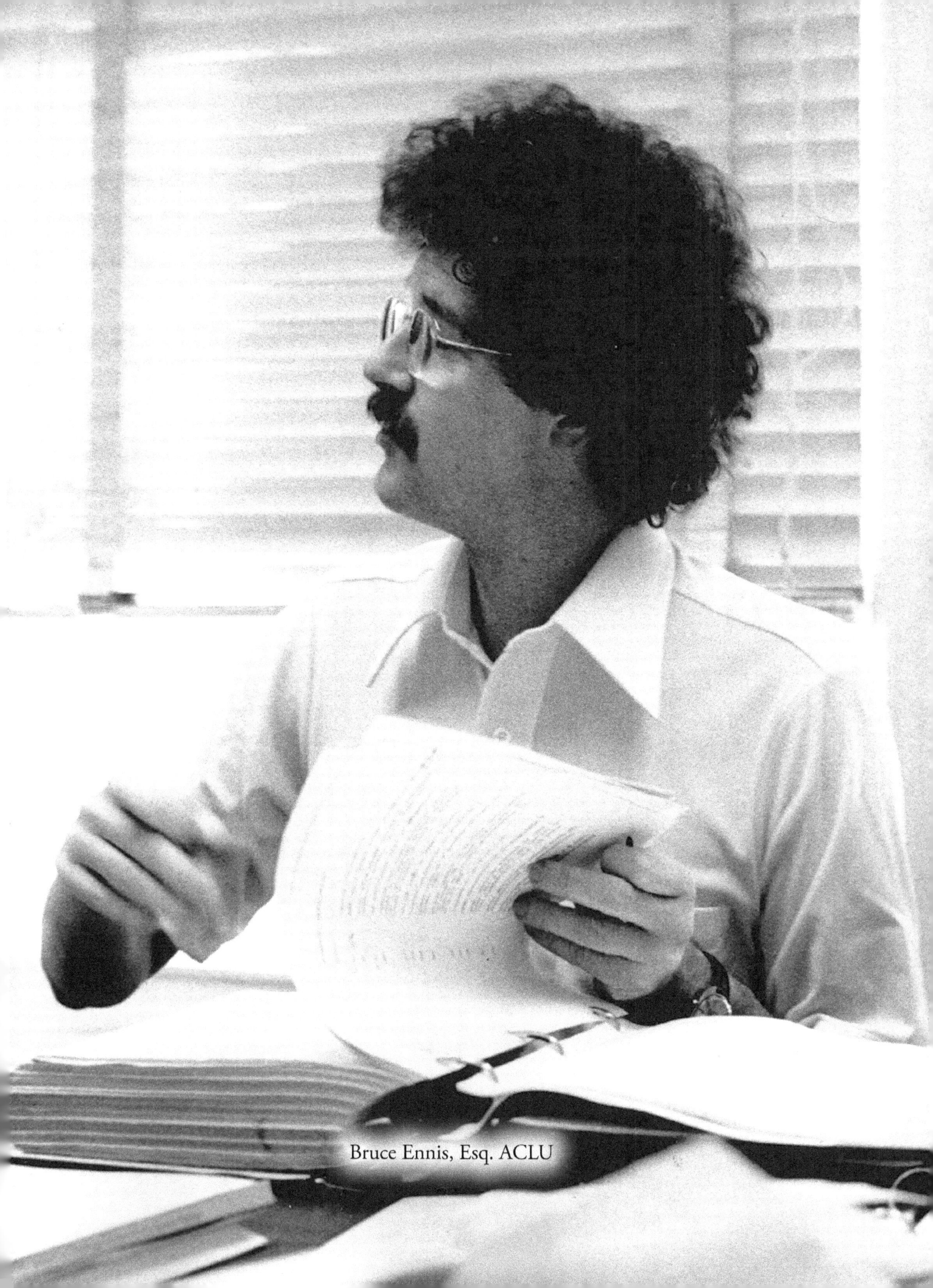

Bruce Ennis, Esq. ACLU

Only a few of us from the inside testified. It was critical that we testify, because we were the ones who could say that the conditions the judge was hearing about were not exceptional but were, in fact, terribly common and had long existed, becoming worse and worse over the very months since the lawsuit had been filed. Despite the departments being put on notice, given endless time to do something, the institution was continuing to decay.

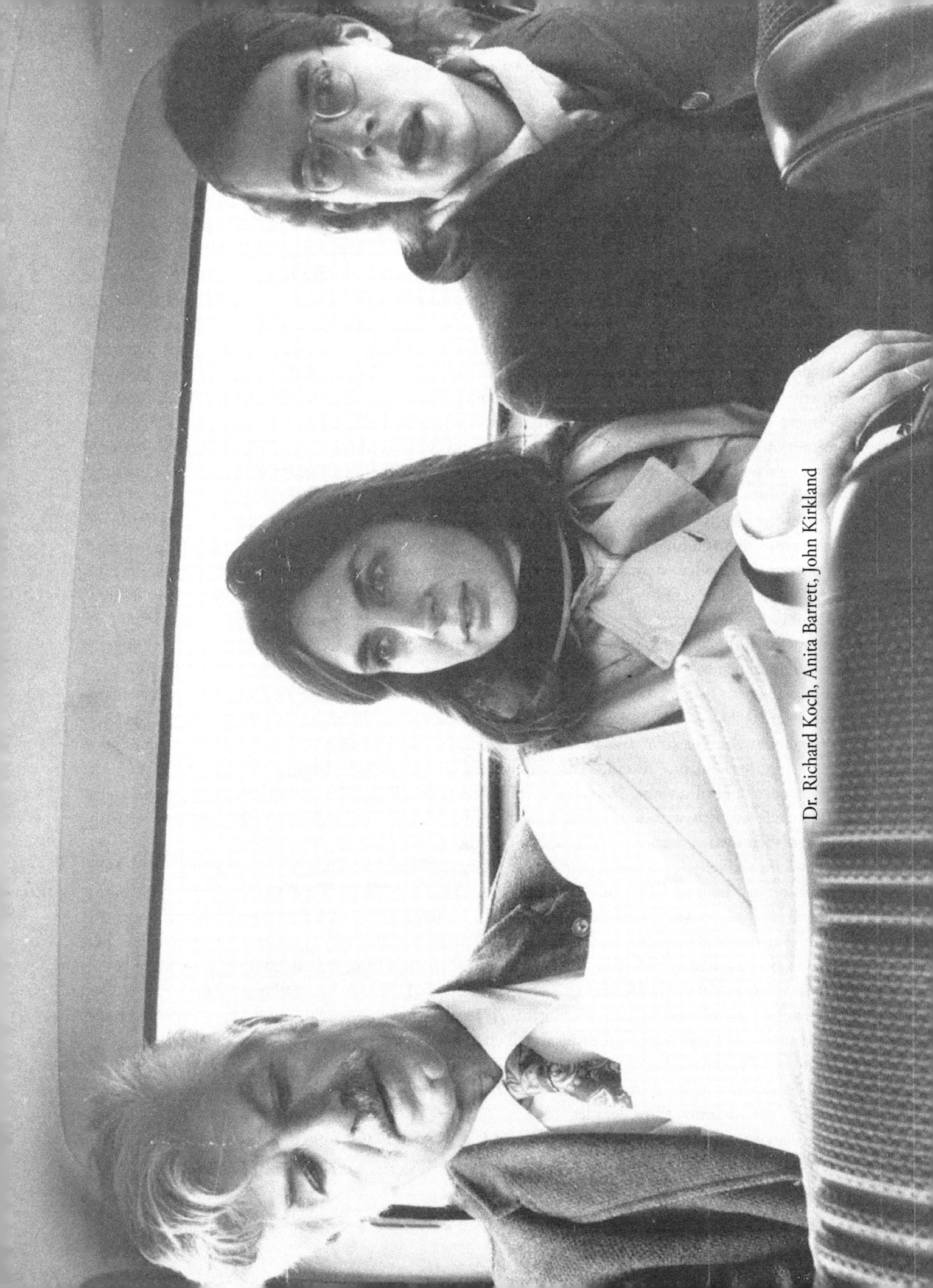

Dr. Richard Koch, Anita Barrett, John Kirkland

It was unbelievably hard to find coworkers willing and able to stand up against their employers. Ward attendants and nurses, especially, were very low in the order of things, and to stand up meant certain undeniable consequences. For those few employees who did speak out, there cannot be enough praise given: Inez Stevens, the nurse who worked in Buildings 22 and 23 with me; Nancy Begeley, the building supervisor on the afternoon shift in Building 23; Dr. Norman Rutnar, a new pediatrician who had come to Willowbrook as a result of the demand for the federal government to screen people to be placed back in the community; and Georgia Hayden, a nurse at Willowbrook for twenty years, had been responsible for the entire midnight shift. She had been blocked from an appropriate promotion because of her honesty and outspoken concern for workers and residents alike and because none of the top leadership of the institution was black, like her. Four courageous souls, out of the three thousand employees who knew the truth, understood the risks of putting others before themselves. They knew that antagonism would surely arise from their coworkers, who would see their standing up as exposing the rest who continued prostrate.

In every struggle, there are heroes. Often heroism is played out and passes quietly, unrecorded. But without these four, who are here recorded, the trial would have been carried on entirely by outsiders. What held up legal actions all around the state against the other institutions was precisely the critical fact that there was no voice of protest from the inside when the chips were down.

After the plaintiffs had presented their case, the leaders in their professions came to the stand to tell the court of their findings. Dr. James Clements, the incoming president of the American Association on Mental Deficiency (now renamed the American Association of Intellectual and Developmental Disability), the largest professional organization concerned with services to the persons with disabilities, and himself the director of a small institution in Georgia. He described vignettes of his visit to Willowbrook, "During the day, the children are kept in pens about 10 by 20 feet with no toys, equipment, water, or attendants in the pens. The floors were covered with urine and feces, and the children were lying on the floor banging their heads on the walls, spinning on their backs, or just staring at the ceiling. I saw many children trying to climb over the four-foot stone walls of the pens and being pushed back by the employees. The color TVs were mounted on the walls near each stone pen. The children did not seem to notice them, but the employees were sitting on beds outside the pens watching TVs."

Clements told of a young Roman Catholic priest, who had come to visit, pacing about in circles in the enclosed pens with four youngsters clutching his arms and legs, being dragged inadvertently through their own excrement. "Willowbrook is among the worst I have ever seen."

Patricia McNelly, director of nursing at Central Wisconsin Colony and Training School, an institution in Madison, Wisconsin, testified, "I don't see how they can call that kind of service in the medical building at Willowbrook a hospital. It's so medieval in there that their problems are really acute." Pat spoke of how none of the children she saw established eye contact for more than brief seconds. So devastating was their withdrawal and alienation from human contact. Dr. Phillip Roos, executive director of the National Association for Retarded Citizens, the national parent organization, testified that people with normal intelligence, if forced to live under the conditions at Willowbrook, would soon lose those human qualities we all cherish.

Intense preparation had gone into each witness's testimony so that the kernel of the experience could be rapidly depicted in the courtroom. Three days had initially been allotted for the hearing. Three days to describe three decades.

The lawyers for the plaintiffs were young people. Bruce Ennis was from the New York Civil Liberties Union and had constructed their case. For the previous three years, he had been immersed in the virgin area of mental hygiene law class action and the rights of the institutionalized. He was tall, elegant, and disciplined to the extreme in the technology of the law. He interrogated with deft certainty, like a neurosurgeon at work. His language was precise, concrete, balanced, every word like the wielding of a scalpel. Bob Feldt was the handsome bearded lawyer from the Staten Island office of the Legal Aid Society. He had spent months inside Willowbrook seeing, listening, learning, and thinking about the issues. He had been the impetus for the Aid Society's assignment of Anita Barret and John Kirkland, lawyers in the Civil Appeals Office in Manhattan. These three had fashioned the case that was filed alongside the ACLU case. Their presentation was rich with humanity and imagery. It raised the shabby obscurity of Willowbrook's dehumanization into metaphors and crystal-like examples that illuminated the reality. With the rangy, shaggy-haired representative from the National Legal Aid and Defenders Association, Stan Herr, they comprised the core of the legal team upon whose shoulders rested the task of defeating the New York attorney general's office and the Department of Mental Hygiene.

These young, beautiful people, nurtured in cleanliness and prestige from top law schools, and with very little personal to gain by establishing an alliance with the unwanted and the unglamorous, were locked into subsequent months and years of full-time involvement, on ordinary salaries, to translate the institution into the language of the law. They are heroes also. They each understood the toll of each day's delay. They felt, each at the center of his and her being, what was being risked and how vital every decision they made was to thousands of human beings at Willowbrook, in New York, and across the United States. They suffered with us, and it was not for money or charity or fame that they labored and remolded their lives to the needs of what was right. It was a purification that bound us together like a family. There was nothing we could not or did not ask of each other in the life's work at hand.

Drs. Grunberg, Ristic, and other members of the new Willowbrook administration were called to testify under the questioning of these lawyers. Grunberg admitted there was no plan to change the situation. He admitted things needed changing but said there were so many barriers—those workers, those residents, that lack of money, the public's disinterest. The department was doing the best it could in a bad situation. They would clean it up; just give them time. There was no abuse that was not punished, no negligence that was not remedied, no guilt at the department's door of wrongdoing. Ristic was interrogated by Bruce. It lasted four hours. Ristic denied that he had fled from Minnesota under fire. He denied that any real evidence existed that environmental deprivation led to injury, and he denied that Willowbrook represented a case of environmental deprivation. One staff person for every eighteen residents was safe although one for every ten persons was really needed, he said. When asked if he was familiar with national standards put forth by the professional community calling for one staff for every two to four residents to provide habilitation, Ristic scoffed. Ristic, backed by the department to stonewall the situation, slid about like a ball of mercury in order to escape containment. He was a man with another reality, another religion, whose devotion to preservation was consuming and total. There was nothing of substance to display. Shame, shame upon a Nuremberg clone for such a career.

Only five days passed in the courtroom, though the five-day hearings dragged on over four weeks, with time-out for a long Christmas recess. Through it all, the department promised change, in time. They had their plan, and besides, it was not the judge's business. This was an in-house affair. Those persons at Willowbrook were not being held against their will; they could leave if they wanted.

The hearing ended, and it was up to Orinn Judd to decide the fate of thousands. He had heard and seen all that there was time for him to hear and see. Again, like always, there was the waiting. The court had to sift the evidence, reflect on the legal matters, and decide what was right and possible, here in New York State.

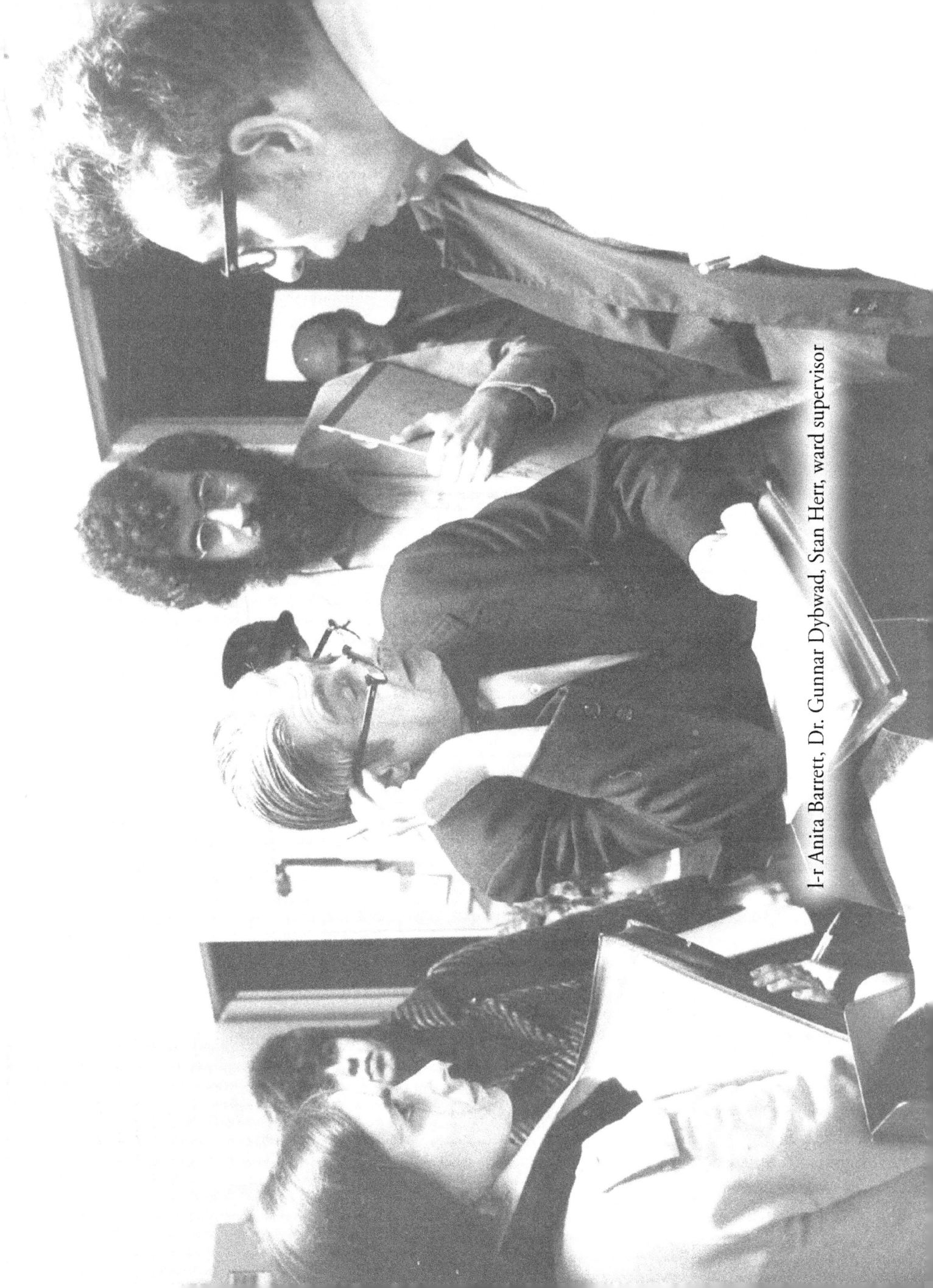

l-r Anita Barrett, Dr. Gunnar Dybwad, Stan Herr, ward supervisor

CHAPTER 23

The Toil of Transfiguration

IT IS COMMONLY HELD that events rightly are borne out as a result of action from the pinnacles of power. The court is such a pinnacle in the eyes of the people. It had the option to take nine months to bring the parents' Willowbrook emergency petition into a hearing. It had the option of drawing five days of testimony out into nearly four weeks. It had the option, too, to take as long as it wanted to deliberate on the indisputable facts. And every minute, life, crimes and death went on unchanged in the institutions.

Thinking that life is paced and given by the powerful is an error, and those in power turn every trick to produce that illusion. That is the magic of power. It must keep the people awed at its majesty and unassailability. If the people were those of Oz, where the green smoke and light belched a manipulated image of the great Wizard—a new popular awareness would occur. The truth of the matter is that the people, despite their confusion and isolation from one another and groping, are in constant political motion. This is, the motion that determines the course of events, which the powerful only certify and attempt to cloud and slow down to give the appearance of having immutable control. The greatest danger to those in power occurs when people spontaneously politically organize themselves to clearly challenge their relationship to an intolerable situation imposed by the system. Then rulers immediately react to change the arrangement of the system, to thwart the natural assemblage of people, and to allow themselves to interfere in the form or rules of the corrective game.

The struggle proceeded. The court had listened, but nothing was resolved. The period following the initial federal court hearing was an unbroken period of popular movement. Ever since late 1971, when Willowbrook's real struggle for change had begun, the contest had been played within this framework. The only force against the abuses in the institution was tied to the first real parent organization to accurately perceive the truth of the institution's situation.

All Willowbrook's residents were utterly held within the power of those people who administered the buildings that they lived in. For the parents, it had meant trying to put pressure on the central administration for this or that concession, an established authority that had minimized any petition for two decades, fostered only the most limited reforms and corrections, which were seen as singular and exceptions to the rule. Following upon the Building 76 affair, the parents of that building were encouraged to meet to discuss the common problems of that particular building. Dr. Mike Wilkins and his building's social worker Liz Lee had slowly encouraged the parents of Buildings 6 and 8, where they worked, to do the same. Their role was to assure parents of their unconditional support and willingness to be bound by parent policy direction and to provide all the facts and information about the most intimate details of the building, its operations, and experiences.

As these parent groups met regularly and grew, led by a vigorous small group at first, a new situation developed. The parents, seeing that the conditions that affected one of their sons and daughters were shared by all, began to demand changes that were wholly in order. Moreover, it became manifestly clear that the particular situation affecting one building was shared by all the buildings and was really a systemic fault within the institution, or even in the whole Department of Mental Hygiene.

The parents' demands for particular and personal favors and corrections gradually developed into a deeper understanding and led to fundamental demands for reform. The administration saw the spontaneous building organizations as an enormous threat, and moved tactically to end that development. Even the Benevolent Society's old-line leadership saw this development as threatening. Before, only a few parent leaders who were professional meeting goers attended. Membership now flourished with parents who wanted to take a concrete role in change at the building level. Action was demanded by more and more working-class families, who had little patience for the glibness and parliamentary dragging of the organization's board. Ensconced leadership everywhere was threatened with demands for change that they did not feel equal to effecting.

It was the militancy and strength of the Building 6 and 8 parents that finally resulted in Dr. Hammond's taking the step to rid himself of Mike and Liz. Invited to one of their regular meetings, Hammond was confronted by a group of parents who had sophisticated knowledge about the workings of the building and the administration beyond what even Hammond knew. Hammond blustered, floundering to regain his previously unquestioned authority. He was deflated and could not tolerate the assault on his personality, let alone the rejection of his unchallenged word. He saw Mike and Liz as the troublemakers and was blind to the fact that it was really the parents, whom he had patronized for years, who had come into their own and were exercising a power that had always been there but needed a little incubating.

This enormous struggle between the people and the power-playing authority continued right through the media exposés, the filing of the class action lawsuit, the hearings, and the waiting time that followed. A few weeks after the close of the hearings, a confrontation occurred with Ristic and was reported in the newspapers as an example of the new relations between the parents and the administration.

On one Sunday evening in February 1973, the parents' group from one of the buildings, irate at seeing the lack of laundry, the understaffed kitchen, and the many broken windows in the building, walked as a group to the stately backwoods mansion where Ristic now lived. Such weekend times were the only ones when parents could visit and meet comfortably at Willowbrook. The parent leader said, "We went over to his house like ladies and gentlemen, staff and parents, but he refused to see us on a Sunday." Dr. Ristic later left his house and went over to the building in question, and another confrontation took place. Somehow or other, the parents had obtained the help of a policeman. This so confounded Ristic that he said, "That's it. I've had it with you. If you called the police, that's it."

In retrospect, it is a comical scenario. Diminutive Ristic always strove to maintain a suave and detached air. When trapped by the parents, he began hopping around, gesticulating and pouring out angry, petulant resentment and expletives, surrounded in the gloom by real people who had a new sense of their rights and purpose. An administrator who pretends to know all and who does all to keep away from accountability cannot afford to be seen as fallible by those who are kept humbled. The people had drawn blood with their persistence. The wheel of leadership was about to take another turn. It was clear that Ristic was used up and that his days would be sharply reduced. His personal ambition to remain the master of this domain would not be realized.

All this was only too clear to the Department of Mental Hygiene. It was desperate to find a stable counterstrategy that would allow the storm to pass so that they could go on doing what they were constituted to do. Throughout the waiting time after the hearings, and even before the confrontation with Ristic, the department's strategists had been working hard on such a solution. Two problems had to be dealt with simultaneously. They had to give the impression of reducing the size of Willowbrook, since that was blamed for most of the problems. (In truth, size is a mechanical consideration and could never be a problem by itself. Abuse can occur in a foster home, where one person can be violated.) The second, real consideration was political. The department had to address its incredible newly discovered vulnerability. A situation had arisen out of its carelessness and the growing watchfulness of the parents, and now a broken window or injury on a ward could directly result in the commissioner's being thrust into the public limelight.

The department had to do two things: (1) get distance, so they could resume their magical remoteness and image of power and authority from the people; and (2) figure out a way to break up the growing parent organization, so that the bureaucracy could resume calling the shots and setting the rules for grievances. That was and is the continuous basic strategy of any elite minority for controlling the lives or fortunes of a majority. It was instinctive and took no genius to move in that direction. And it takes no more than a little experience to learn to anticipate the strategies of the bureaucracy and their leaders in self-preservation against the public.

As a first step in tackling its problems, the state, through its appointed citizen leaders on the Governor's Developmental Disabilities Council, put forward an auspicious plan agreeing that Willowbrook was just too big and needed to be broken down. Willowbrook served all five boroughs of New York City. The obvious answer, in its way progressive for the people in the long run, was to break Willowbrook up into five units corresponding with each of the five New York boroughs and ship all the out-of-city people back to where they came from or to some other remote place. Just get them out of Willowbrook! From a positive standpoint, the demand that local communities begin to look at and provide an answer to service responsibilities that were going unmet was historically essential. On the other hand, the reason that this plan became central was because it would serve the bureaucracy's interests to cool out the situation. It came to be called "unitization."

The force of the possibility that the federal court might intervene in New York, plus all the daily publicity about the conditions in New York institutions, resulted in the governor grandly upping the budget for Willowbrook by five million dollars. This was interpreted as money to clean it up— that is, the court really shouldn't bother itself when munificence, dedication to public service, and accountability animated the spirit of state leadership so thoroughly. The headlines hit New York on January 29, two weeks after the December and January federal court hearings closed.

Then on February 7, Commissioner Miller admitted that "poor management, not lack of money" was the real problem. "The problems of Willowbrook are not now soluble by a vast infusion of money.

The next phase is to change the whole massive, layered administrative situation at Willowbrook." This was after already having either spent or allocated the "vast infusion" of the people's money. Also, it completely ignored the fact of the other identical New York State institutions. This interview, printed in the newspaper, was merely the administration's next diversionary step, and neatly illustrates how verbal shuffling and "blaming of the victim" can be effectively joined to cover up doing nothing. Dr. Miller claimed that the previous administration was "so overwhelmed by problems that they had forgotten how to get things done. There are real problems when you try to make changes in a situation where problems were so deep, and added to the administrative issues is the difficult human problem of profound mental retardation."

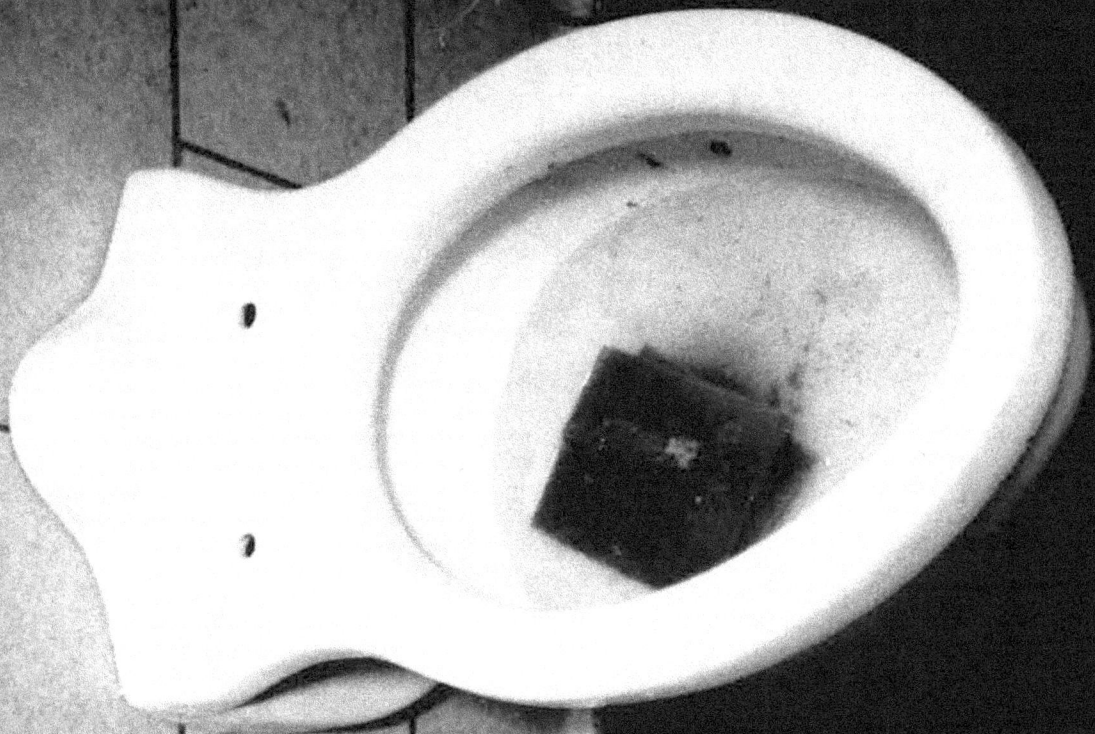

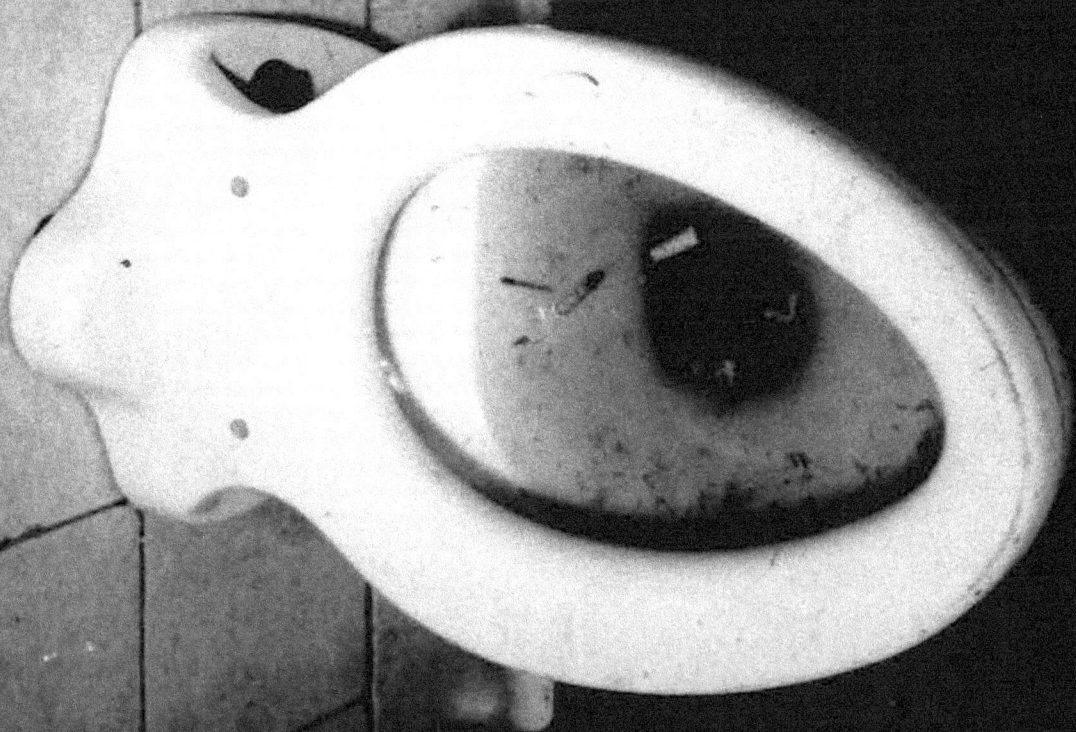

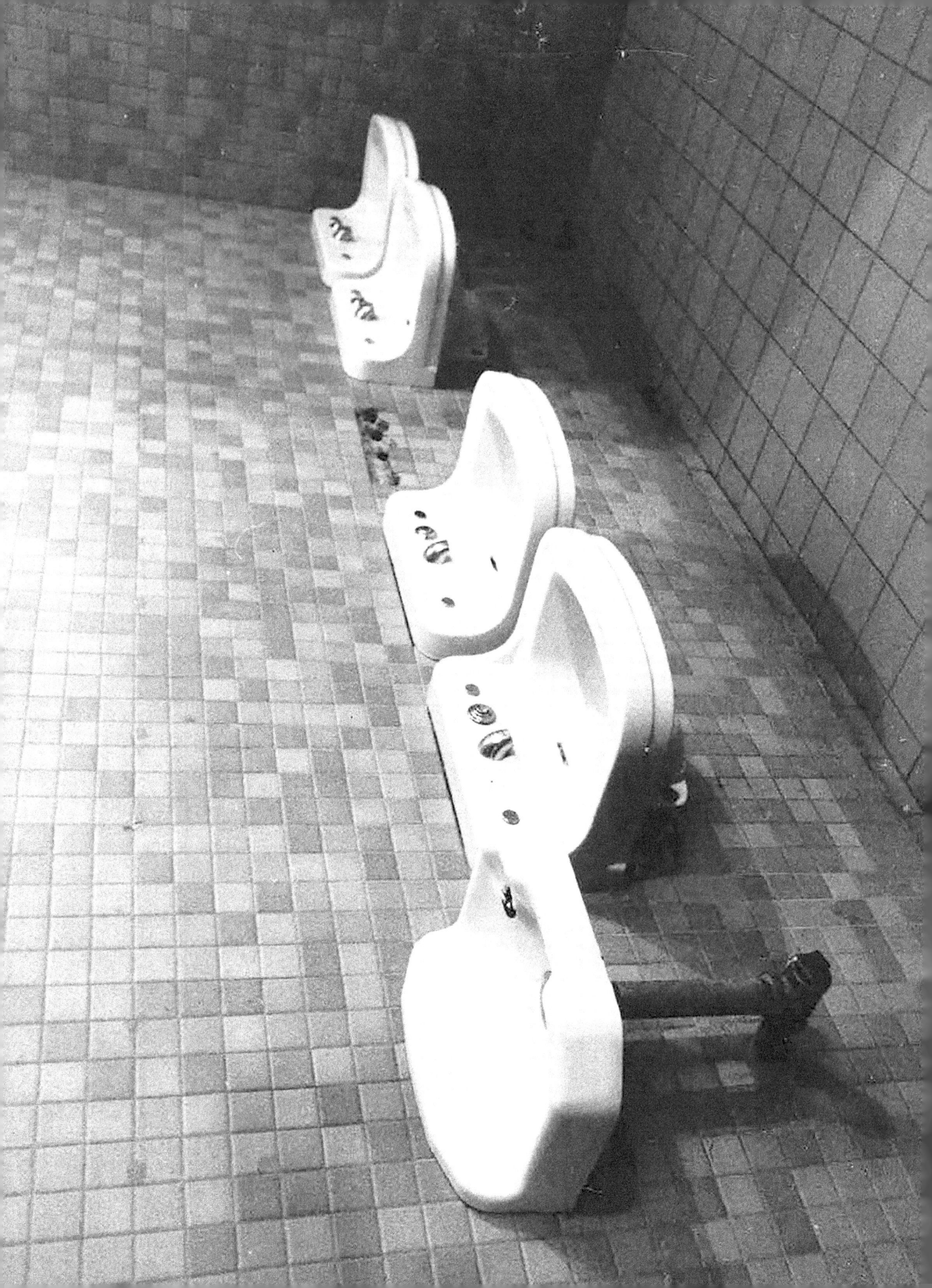

As a small cohort of residents were hurriedly farmed out of Willowbrook to depress the population, with no plan or purpose in the long run for the alteration of the quality of life of those powerless people, the next strategy of the department took hold: divide and conquer. It was under the central auspices of the Benevolent that the parents had marshaled and put together the strength of the new organizations that had begun to grow in ten different buildings. Now, could the Benevolent parents guard the conditions in Willowbrook and, at the same time, mobilize in the boroughs to do the same thing in four new institutions? A pressing need existed to organize in the five boroughs at a community level for all sorts of logistic and commonsense reasons. Further, the organization to act as change agent and watchdog should conform to the future service delivery system, which nobody could foresee. The planned and rushed dispersal of the residents to the other boroughs created tremendous challenges, problems, and questions.

The old Benevolent leaders opposed unitization, because they could not see the inevitability of it and because it was clear that they could be left alone again as soon as the parent "troublemakers" were decentralized and caught up in different boroughs, diverting them from the problems left behind at Willowbrook. The activist "troublemakers," on the other hand, were already challenging the old leadership of the Benevolent for power, and now, in 1973, they held seven of the twenty-one board memberships. Conflicting interests and opinions weighed do0077n the parents' organization. This turmoil within the Benevolent served the department well. The people would need time to sort out their differences and work out what to do. The department needed time too!

It was predictable that the sons and daughters of militant families would be moved away first to dissolve the core of courage and confidence as quickly as possible. Torturous decisions faced these parents when it came their turn to decide to have their kin moved closer to a newer facility, away from the overt violence and misery of Willowbrook. They recognized that this would demand that they drift away from the newfound community of struggle and comradeship that had deeply colored and given new meaning to their lives. Was it a bribe? Were they selling out for caring about their own lives? The old guilt and doubts flooded in, and a tension and uncertainty crept into even the best relations as these dramatic and touching decisions intruded. It was the end of a period of innocence and simplicity.

It was becoming manifestly clear than an enormous and complex social and civil rights struggle had begun, one that would lead into some unknown future. There were as many problems of personal values and logistics to deal with as there were outward problems. For some, the recognition of the depths of the struggle was frightening and signaled preparations for retreat. Perhaps everyone had to at least prepare for retreat as a serious contingency for surviving over the long run.

Some people felt so overwhelmed that they could not make sufficient plans for continuing on the offensive. They did not see that the struggle would ultimately be won if all the available social forces were effectively utilized. When delays were so painful, they could not see that time was what would be needed to begin to understand what the choices were and what was to be done. The growth of understanding and its internalization take a little time and effort. Nobody stands ready, alone, with answers to conditions and problems that afflicted their families. It is the hundreds and thousands that have the answers in their collective wisdom. One person, alone, can only act to catalyze, summarize, and to help separate progressive concrete options from things that had heretofore proved ineffective. It was three months after the hearings, and nearly thirteen months after the filing of the papers against the state. It had seemed like endless shuffling and waiting. But finally, the court was now ready.

The judge had made a personal visit to Willowbrook—walking through the buildings to see for himself what this Willowbrook smelled like and sounded like. Volumes and volumes of affidavits had been given by experts, who had examined every drop of the situation and unanimously condemned every aspect of the institution as revolting and unconscionable violation. The first order came. On April 10, 1973, a temporary injunction was issued. A ninety-page opinion was handed down directing the state to remedy the "inhumane and shocking conditions" at the Willowbrook State School.

Earlier, there had been an enlightened ruling in Alabama, in the *Wyatt v. Stickney* case over an identical monstrous institution, Partlow State School, where the federal court had expressed its position that appropriate individualized treatment is constitutionally guaranteed. Judge Judd in New York, however, sidestepped this point and based his judgment on the substance of the Eighth Amendment to the Constitution, which guarantees freedom from cruel and unusual punishment. It was a judgment of the most conservative theoretical pitch, for its thrust deferred the question of rightful habilitation services and dealt solely with a justification to stop the active destruction of people in the institution. In short, it bought time for the bureaucracy on that essential and already precedent issue. The real trial on that and all other issues was more than eighteen months in the future.

Here was an interim emergency order, thirteen months after the facts had been made known to the people of New York. It said that custodial care had a minimum floor and could not be construed to be bottomless. It could not dip into and affirm utterly atrocious negligence and barrenness. The Benevolent Society and the lawyers issued a summary of the thrust of the order, setting forth for the parents the timetable for resolution that lay ahead. The state had lost the first battle and had to bow to the intervention of the federal court, and its assumption of legal and policy jurisdiction, at least for Willowbrook, on paper. They would not wriggle free from the jaws of the trap that had clamped shut on one arm of the governor's institutional and political empire.

CHAPTER 24

The Decision of the United States

THE SUIT WAS FILED on March 17, 1972, in the United States District Court for the Eastern District of New York by the Mental Health Law Project, the New York Civil Liberties Union, and the NLADA National Law Office on behalf of the New York State Association for Retarded Children, two of its chapters, and parents of eight children who are residents of Willowbrook. A companion case, *Patricia Parisi et al. v. Rockefeller*, the parallel suit, was filed by the New York Legal Aid Society on behalf of parents of other children at Willowbrook. The ACLU and the Legal Aid suits, both of which sought class action status, were now consolidated.

On June 30, a motion for preliminary relief was filed, supported by depositions, massive affidavits from plaintiffs' expert witnesses, and numerous exhibits obtained through pretrial discovery. The motion was argued during several days of extensive testimony in December and January.

On April 10, 1973, the district court entered a wide-ranging decree granting plaintiffs most of the relief which they requested. This included a ban on the use of seclusion; a requirement of substantial additions to professional and nonprofessional staff by May 31; and a requirement that appropriate provision for medical attention to acutely ill residents be made. The order went so far as to require that the starting salary for physical therapists be raised in order to allow for effective recruitment. The conceptual basis for the court's decision does not rest on a right to habilitation but rather on a right to protection from harm rooted in the due process, equal protection, and cruel and unusual punishment clauses of the Constitution. The court in its opinion neglected the right to habilitation in its order for preliminary relief before hearing full legal argument or expert testimony concerning the right to habilitation.

Plaintiffs, New York Department of Mental Hygiene et al, therefore, moved for modification or clarification of the court's order of April 10, 1973. They argued that this ruling was premature since the April 10 order was one granting preliminary relief, and plaintiffs had not had the opportunity to present evidence on the constitutional issues.

The court issued a modification of the April 10 order on May 22, 1973, in which it reserved "final Judgment with respect to the plaintiffs' constitutional claims of equal protection and the right to treatment or habilitation, pending the receiving of further evidence, expert testimony, and legal argument relevant to those claims." In the same modification order, the court denied, without prejudice, plaintiffs' request to make the April 10 order applicable to all members of the plaintiffs' class who were residents at Willowbrook on March 17, 1973, at whatever public institutions they may presently reside. In addition, defendants were ordered to conduct a daily ward census of residents and direct care staff and to make a weekly report available to plaintiffs.

The United States Department of Justice was granted leave to appear as amicus curiae (friend of the court) and would participate in presenting evidence. The final trial was scheduled to last two weeks, the first week beginning October 1, 1974, and the second week beginning November 11, 1974. The trial would take place in the United States District Court, Eastern District of New York, 225 Cadman Plaza East, Brooklyn, New York. It began each day at 10:00 a.m. in the courtroom of Judge Orrin Judd, open to the public.

"Plaintiffs and amicus will present evidence that the mentally retarded can be habilitated, but that the environment that now exists at Willowbrook makes such habilitation difficult. Evidence will show that in order to protect residents from harm and deterioration, affirmative programming must be provided. Evidence will further show the advantages of community-based mental retardation facilities. Further, evidence will be presented on the right of the mentally retarded residents to receive education. Experts will testify for plaintiffs concerning the deficiencies at Willowbrook, the causes of these deficiencies, and recommendations to correct those deficiencies."

The state was genuinely stunned at the situation. But even when the bureaucracy is so paralyzed, it is deceptive to think it is now powerless. Even a flick of the beast's tail can crash and splinter the fragile container of the court's orders. It only takes time for the bureaucracy's brain to get its reflexes down through its gargantuan body. All messages take time in that body—even the message that it is exposed and mortally injured may take an interminable time. The people may even be fooled into thinking that they have not struck a mortal blow. And in the meantime, the beast will thrash and remain dangerous.

When a just blow has been struck at a bureaucracy, it requires scrutiny to correctly interpret that the blow has been properly aimed and indeed will become fatal. One must have the kind of confidence that rocketry experts have that their theory and mathematics and have set the proper trajectory, that their knowledge of the motions of the planets, the forces of the universe, that have a set character and are predictable, will lead the missile months or years hence to its ultimate target, even though the target is light-years in the distance and, at the moment of ignition, is nowhere to be seen. This kind of scientific clarity about social conditions is within the power of the people to master and use for their progress and social development.

A chronicle of events following the court order could fill a volume but would not really light our way to understanding the meaning of things. What must be understood is that even now the true target had not yet been reached. This target is not just the evil of institutions, nor the reform of the bureaucracy, nor even the plight of any group denoted by a social label as inferior. Such secondary targets absorb only a portion of the public attention and alter social conditions little in the end. The ultimate target is an intangible thing. It is this concept that inspired the expression within the court ruling. It is a promise dearest to all our hearts, a feeling about the quality of life among us in human society. It is the striving, despite all barriers and living trials, toward that condition of justice, of independence and self-confidence, the feeling of creativity and "lives of high spirits."

Such an aspiration may not be recognizable in the actions and efforts of the people as they strain, day after day, against the things that deny that promise. People may even deny that this is what drives them to take risks, to sacrifice, to act, day in and day out. It is a reflection of conditioning, of humility within people, which prevents them from expressing such "unrealistic," even embarrassing, aspirations. Lesser rationalizations are more common and acceptable. It is up to those who can unite these higher visions to the concrete efforts of the people's fitful social evolution and battles, to put in their proper place the lesser reasons. So that in the end, a sense of patience and confidence can be comfortably won by all of us, the great majority who are the society—we who create value from work, caring, mutual respect, and a hunger for the best.

The state, commanded to "clean up" Willowbrook, persisted in its interpretation of the problem—size, money, unsatisfactory workers, ungenerous public, questionable management at fault. The state was devoid of any higher value; devoid of recognition of the wonderful challenge to change, to embrace a new service paradigm, to turn to the public for energy and partnerships; and devoid of an appreciation of the true role of developmental science to serve the people. The state was doomed to fail at every scheme it constructed that dodged the need for radical change.

From time to time, New York City newspaper headlines told the story in its simplicity: "State asks delay in Willowbrook hiring" (May 15); "Court gives state week on Willowbrook hiring" (May 17); "U.S. takes action on Willowbrook (May 24); "Willowbrook acts on hiring" (May 26).

Ultimately, despite FBI monitoring of the wards and the mandate to have one staff person on duty during all the working hours for every nine residents, the administration was unable to comply. A raft of people were promoted into new administrative positions, with no change other than to break up the image of unchangeability within the institutions. Nevertheless, this led to the improved power of the workers, through their local CSEA, to defend against arbitrary demands on their thin numbers by people who shunned real caring themselves.

Miodrag Ristic's fruitless grasp was to hold the institution intact. So, it came to pass that with the state's effort to decentralize Willowbrook and efforts to create the proper numbers of staff-to-resident ratios and dissolve the parent organization, Ristic became a liability to the very bureaucracy that had sought his egomaniacal complicity in the first place. He was removed in midyear, after bitter internal struggles, only to be replaced by a temporary bureaucrat brought in from another institution in New York, and that bureaucrat was then replaced by another recruited from Illinois by the new governor Hugh Carey, who, in 1974, replaced the old corrupt Rockefeller dynasty.

Four institution directors revolved over three years. It no longer was important to the bureaucracy who it was or what qualifications were needed to head up the scandal-ridden warehouse where death and disease continued to prevail. It was the spasms of the dying state beast beginning to recognize the impossibility of its plight but without the adaptive capacity to do anything other than what it had been created to do, run a concentration camp riddled with immorality, out of the view of the public.

CHAPTER 25

Photos: Injuries

AFTER THREE YEARS INSIDE the bleak, hopeless buildings of Willowbrook, nothing made me sicker than the jolt of having to face a new injury. Something in me changed over the time I spent there. My tolerance for facing the ceaseless flow of gashes, burns, fractures, and massive bruises eroded and finally gave way. This occurred in direct relation to my growing understanding of why these injuries happened. And as I was pitched deeper into the bowels of the warehouse, from infant service to teenagers to adults, the magnitude of violence multiplied tenfold.

I remember vividly preparing myself in medical school for horrible things that a health worker must see and correct. I persuaded myself, over time and by gentle conditioning, that there was nothing too mutilated or offensive to approach rationally to see as a complex disruption of parts—blood vessels, nerves, skin, organs, tendons—each with a precise name and place. What is working, what is destroyed? Where does this or that part belong? Reassemble, connect, and mold the injured back together. What I did not, or could not prepare for, what drove me to wild rage, disgust, and even panic, was being helpless to stem the tide of injuries when the source was so tangible, so preventable, so inevitable, so clear. More than anything that tripped my fury and frustration was the incredible attitude of the institution and all its workers toward injuries.

Nothing more exemplified this attitude than the wry, mechanical tone of voice of the supervising nurse over the telephone when I was on night duty. "Dr. Bronston? There's a laceration in Building 22, one in Building 8, a burn in Building 20, and two temps [people with fever] in Building 12." That was all, a synopsis of four or five hours of the consequences of life for the hostages. Just as simple, cool, and matter-of-fact as saying, "There's a cloud in the sky," "The time is six o'clock," "I spilled a glass of water," "The phone is ringing."

Never, never could I understand that attitude—just telling me that somewhere among the stone structures, lying somewhere on a steel bed, there in a treatment room tied in a sheet was a person torn, violated, washed in agony, an innocent somewhere there within those 340 acres of grass, trees, and stately brick buildings. "A laceration in 27." That was all. No urgency, no anguish. God, what working there has done to my coworkers!

216

I so clearly understood why the injuries occurred. When you crowd life together and turn up the flame of boredom, confinement, hopelessness, deprivation, disdain, cruelty, there will be injuries, and injuries, and injuries; it can only be one way. Bites, tears, rents, avulsions, cuts, flesh so fragile, so scarred, so ready to yield to a blow from a hand, a shoe, a chair, a key, a stone wall, stone floor. No contest. These things I understood. To end them would require the demolition of the system of warehousing and dehumanization.

It was the detachment, the collaboration, the expectation, and acceptance of this carnage by the workers and staff of the institution that shattered me. Maybe they were too innocent themselves. Maybe they thought the injuries were a given, a river with an origin beyond eyesight, with a delta unimaginable. Maybe the confinement to one building where eight or ten injuries a day occurred seemed tolerable. I, on the other hand, had to see it all in five or ten buildings—scores, hundreds, thousands of crimes of negligence, dehumanization, institutionalization.

There is no defense against such an onslaught unless one has packed away or amputated one's humanity and sanity. Toward the end, after the lawsuits, after the TV exposés, after the memos, the meetings—it became too much. The announcement of an injury to me over and over and there was no defense. It was all over. I was a volcano. I cried. I cursed over the phone. I cursed in the buildings. I began to fantasize how to confront the director and the commissioner and do to them what they were doing to the thousands of their victims, their public hostages, for whom they received thousands of dollars each per year. Only the destruction of the jailors, only the razing of their murderous violent institutions could stop the river of suffering, blood, and ravaged souls.

I could not go on any longer on the inside. I somehow got a two-year paid educational leave to go away to Syracuse University. I was through. I fled to friends in Canada, then California, like an exhausted, deeply depressed, half-drowned man pulled from the floodwaters. I sought comfort, normalcy, humanity. There are limits to what each of us can continuously endure, regardless of support and understanding.

As you look at next agonizing evidence, understand that the flooding river of injuries still flows in the nation's segregated, congregated institutions everywhere.

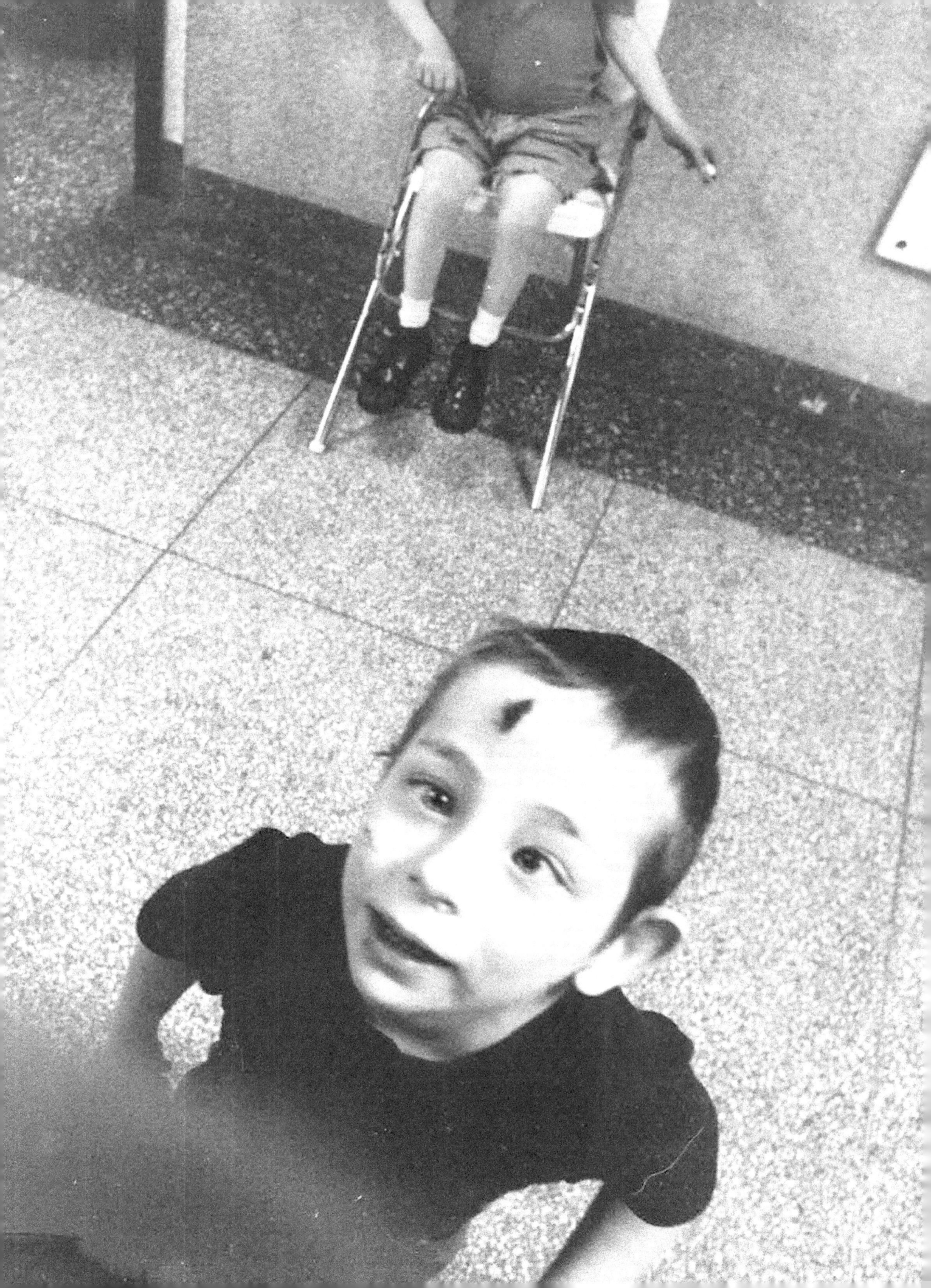

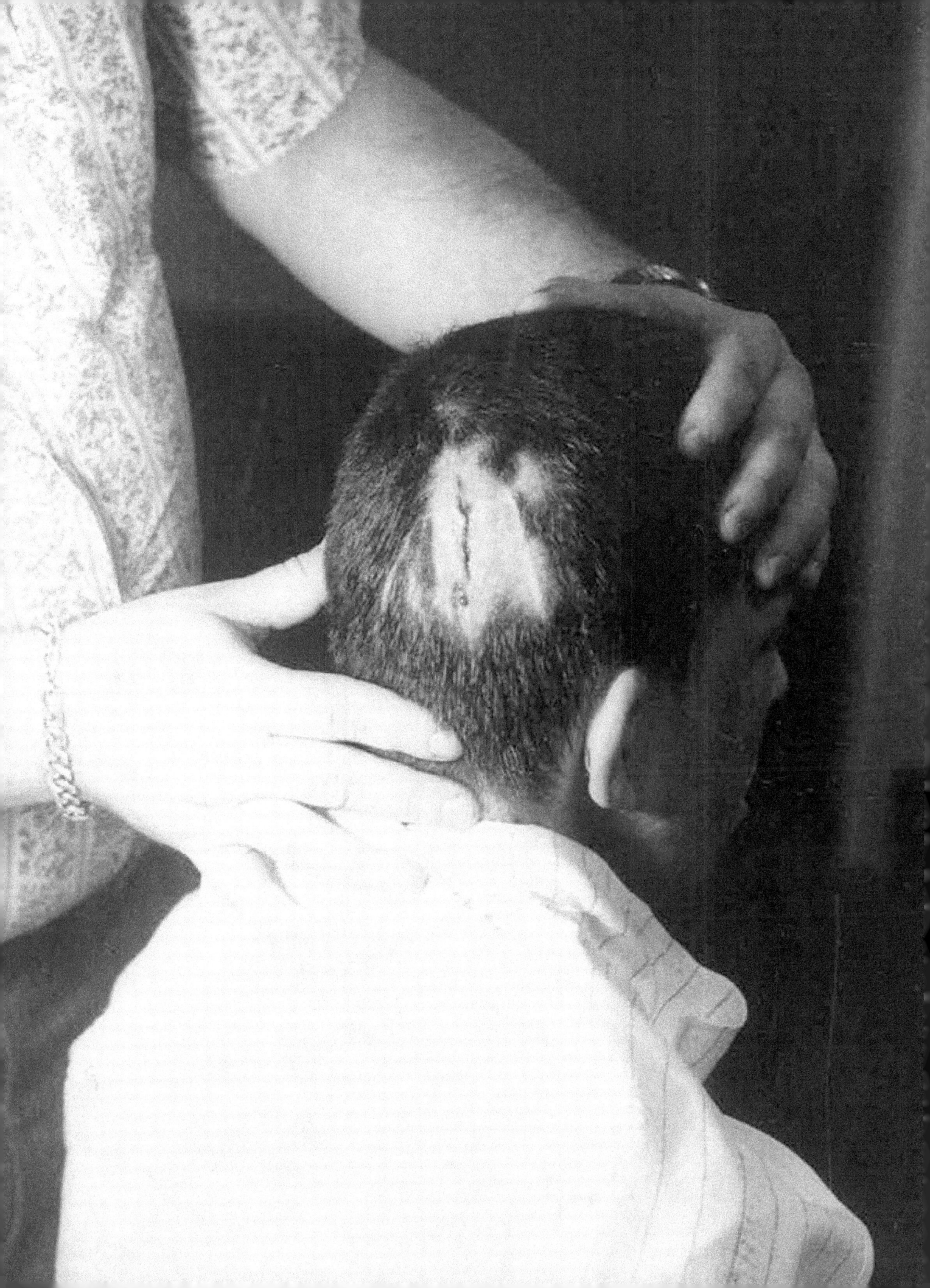

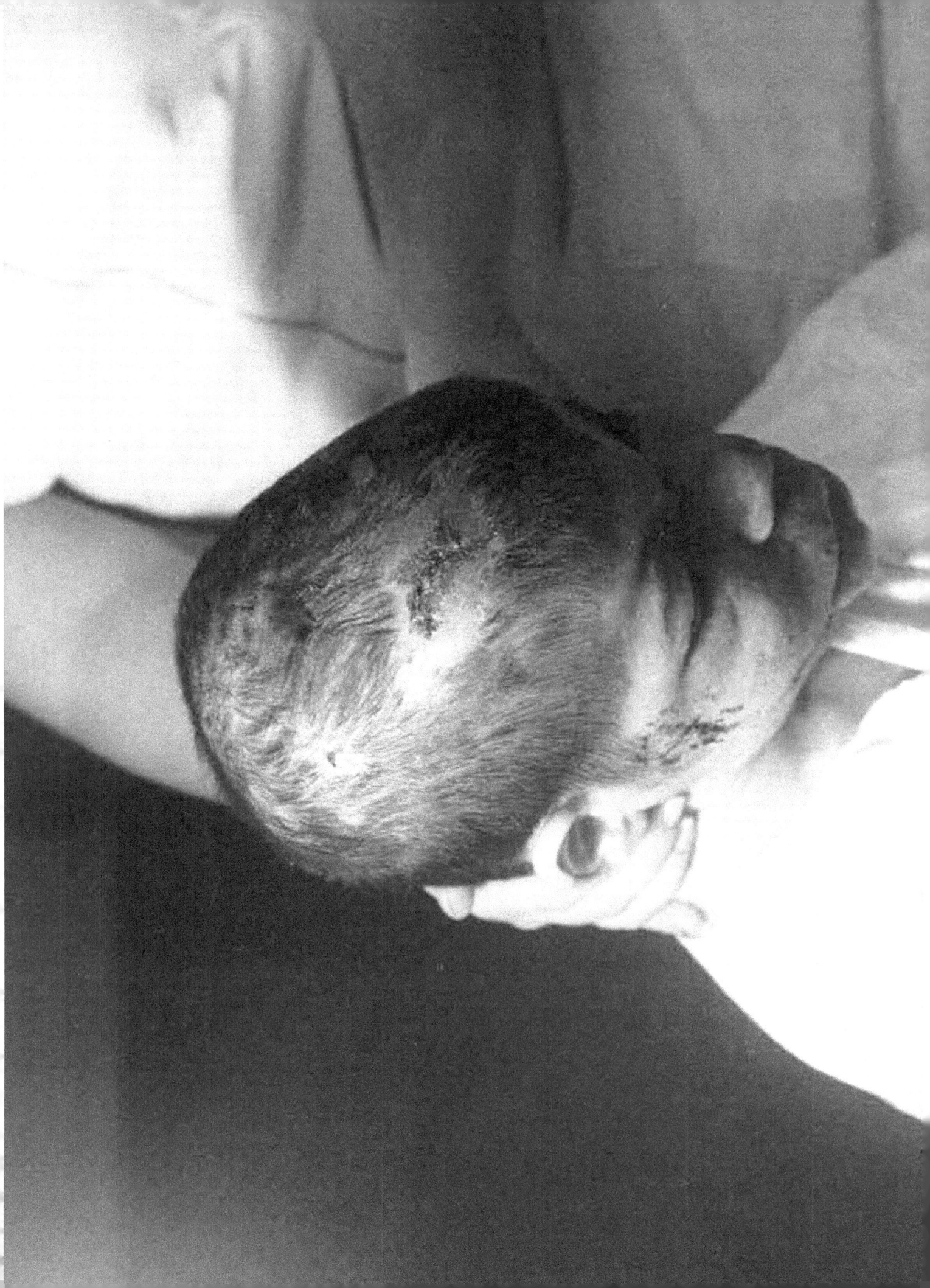

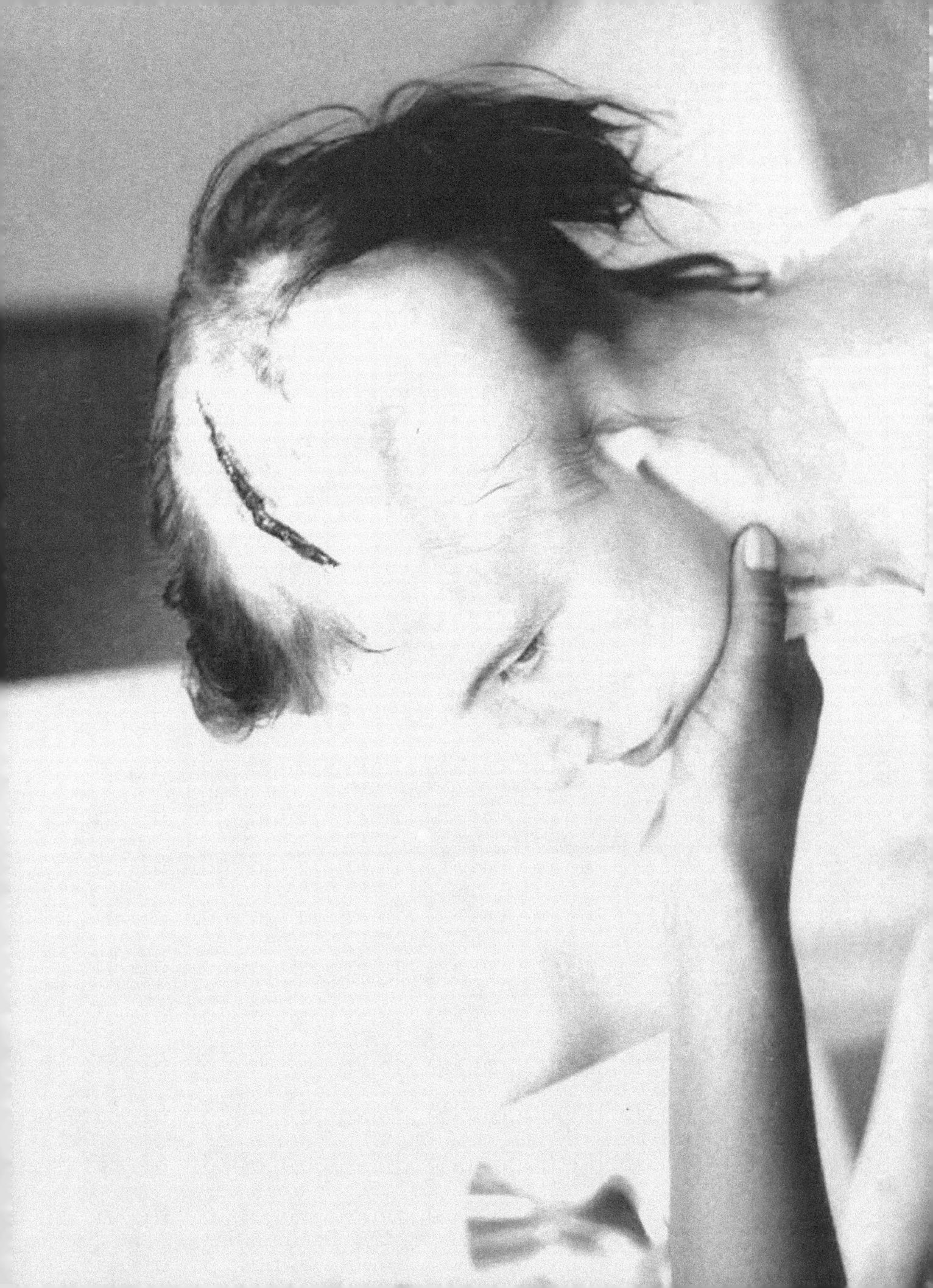

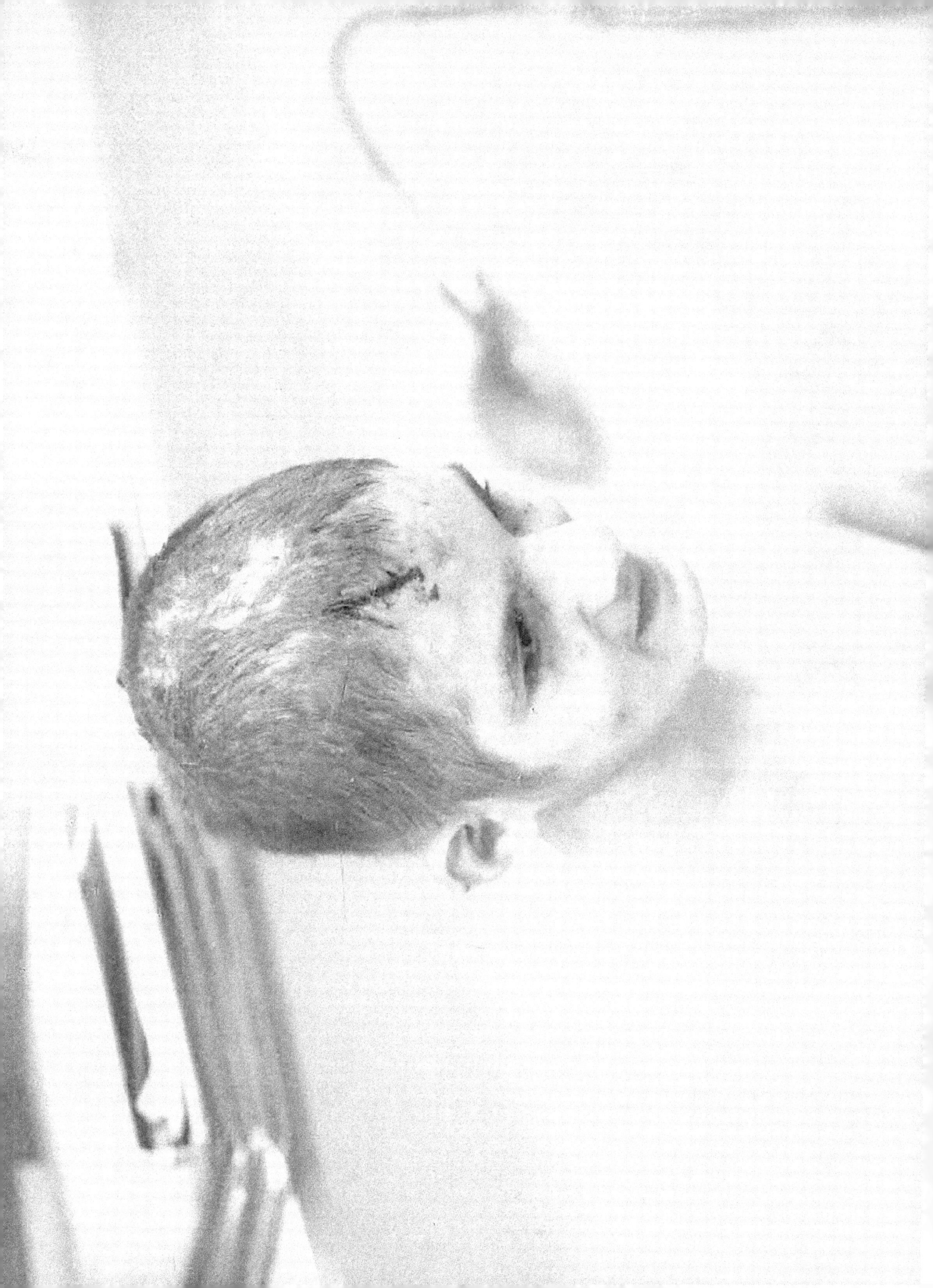

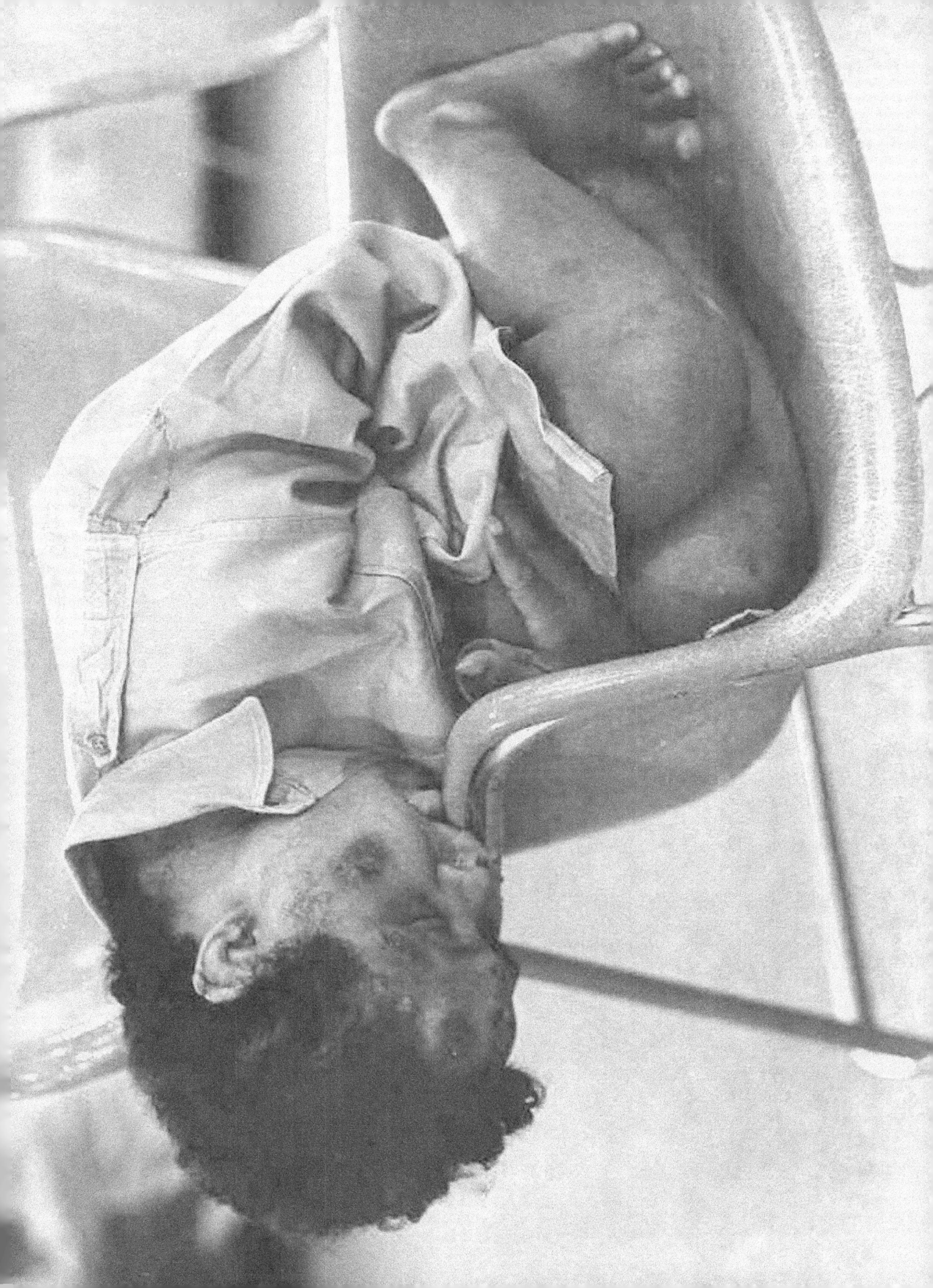

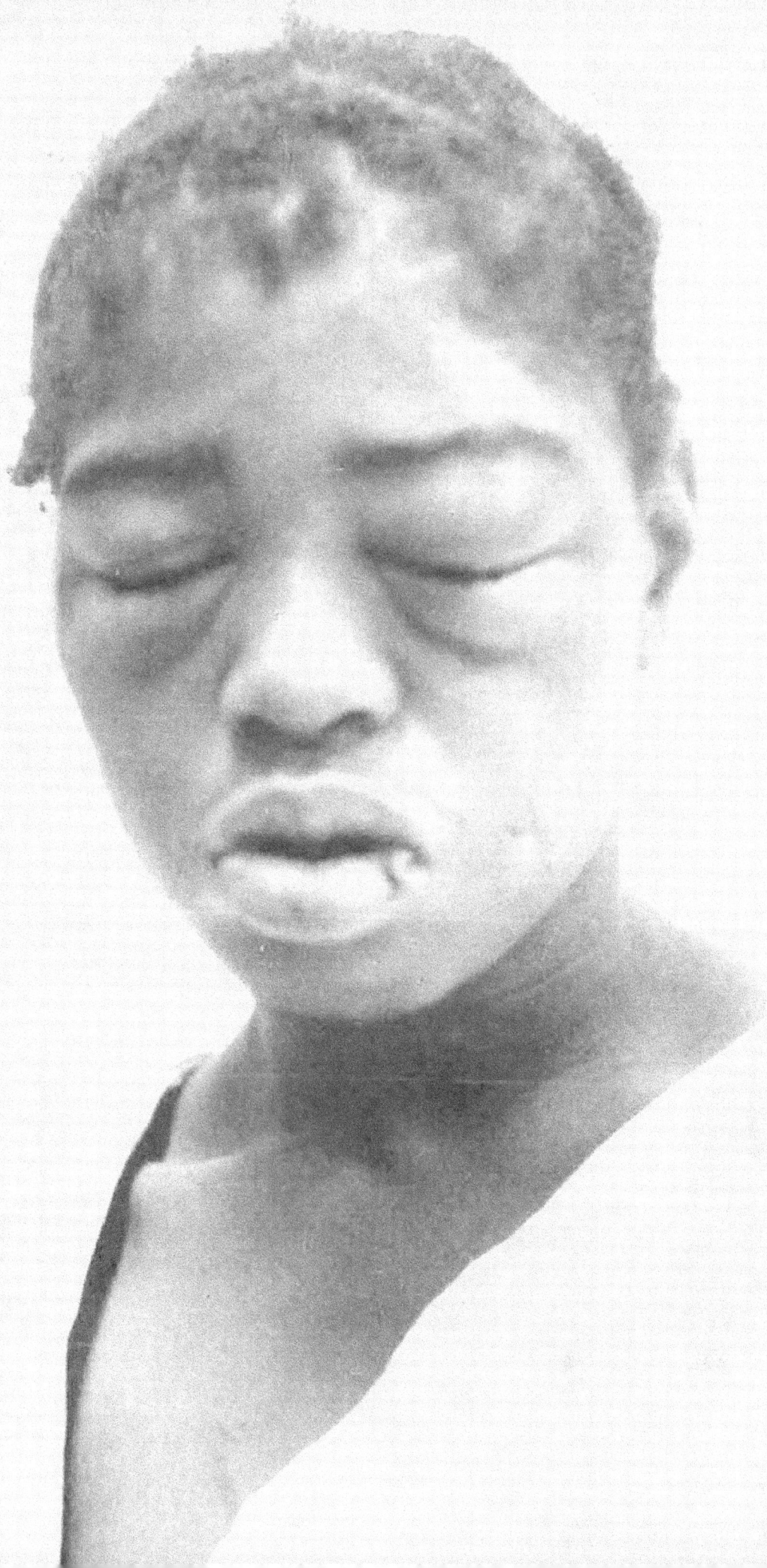

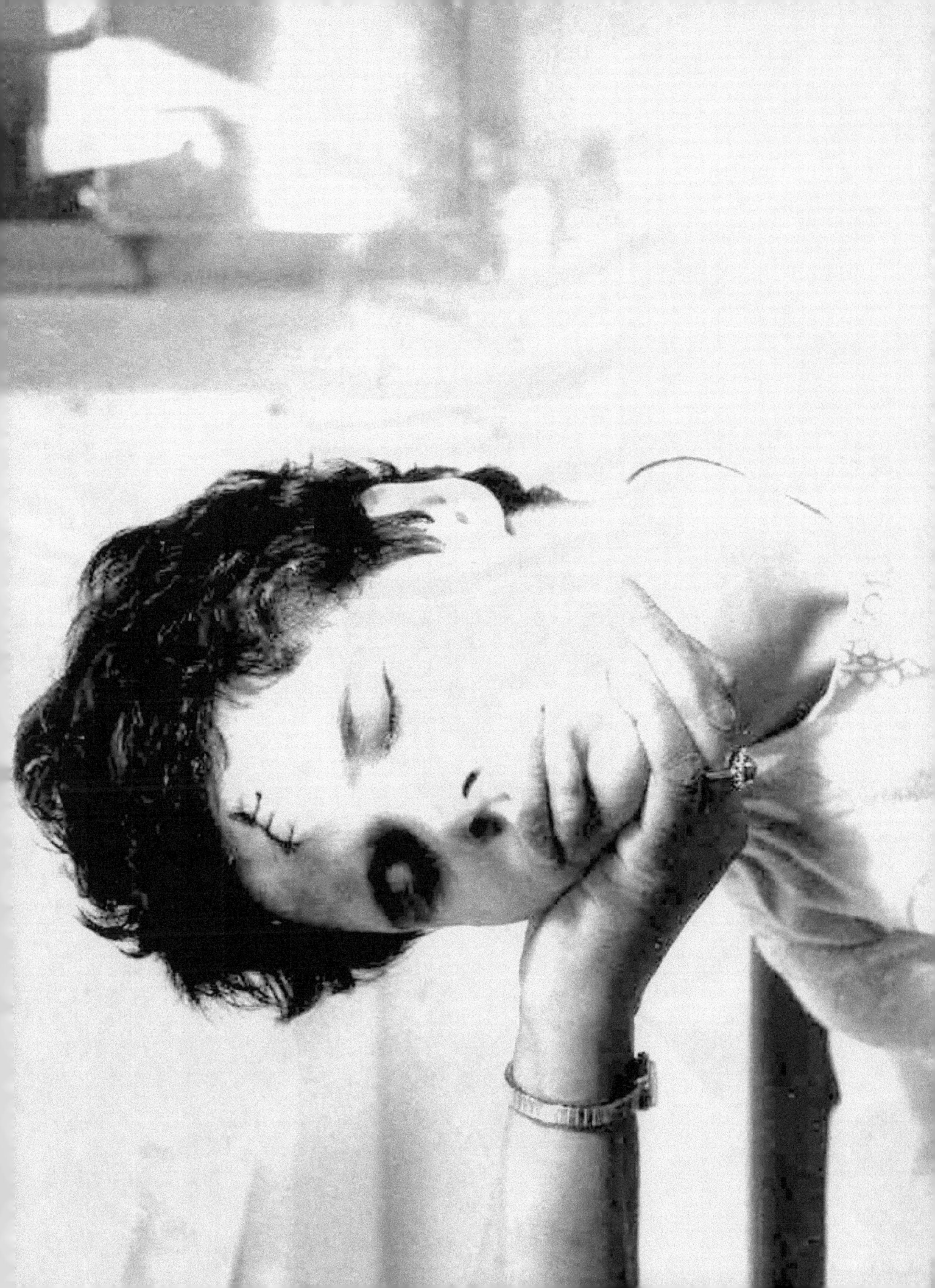

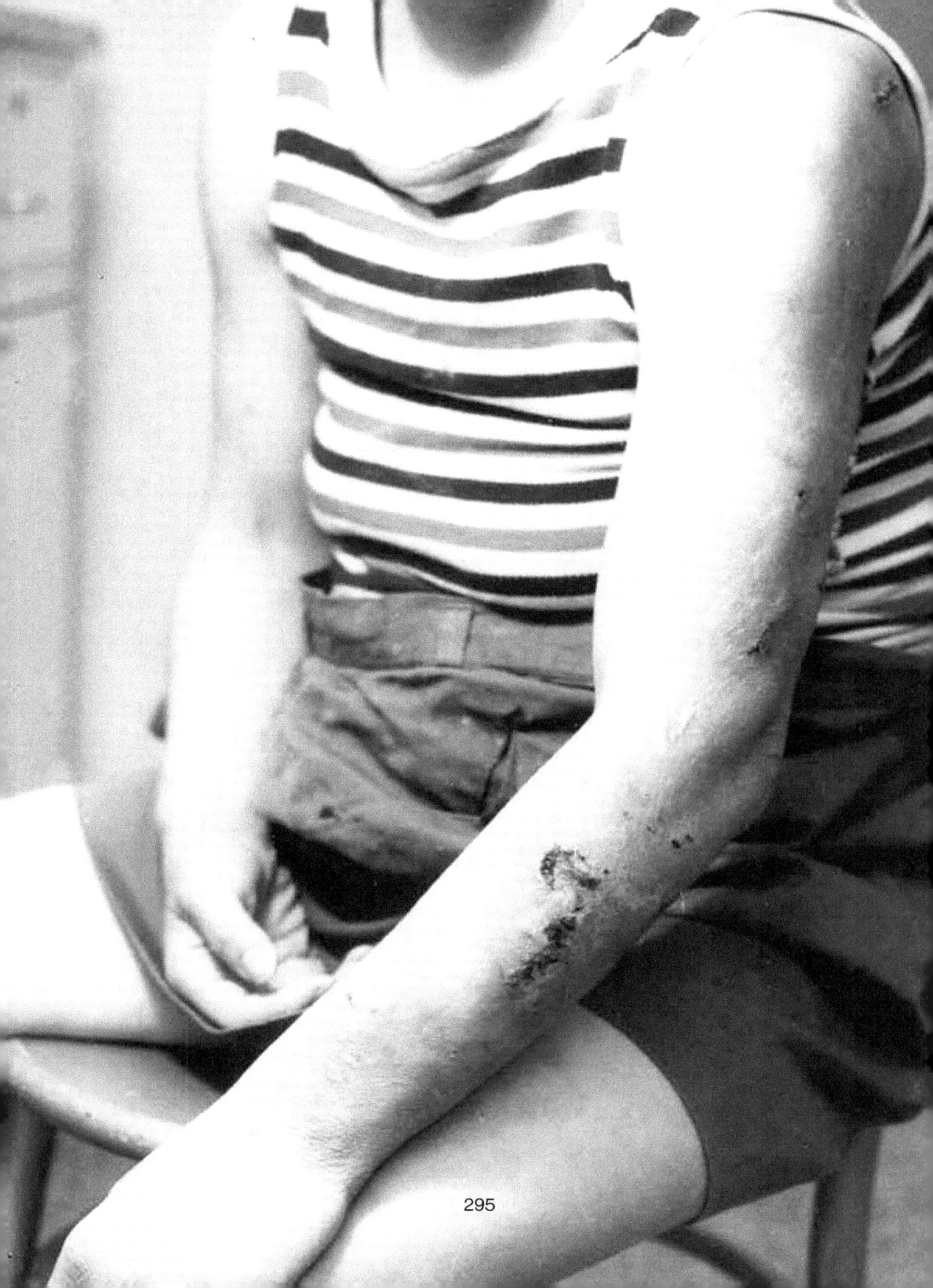

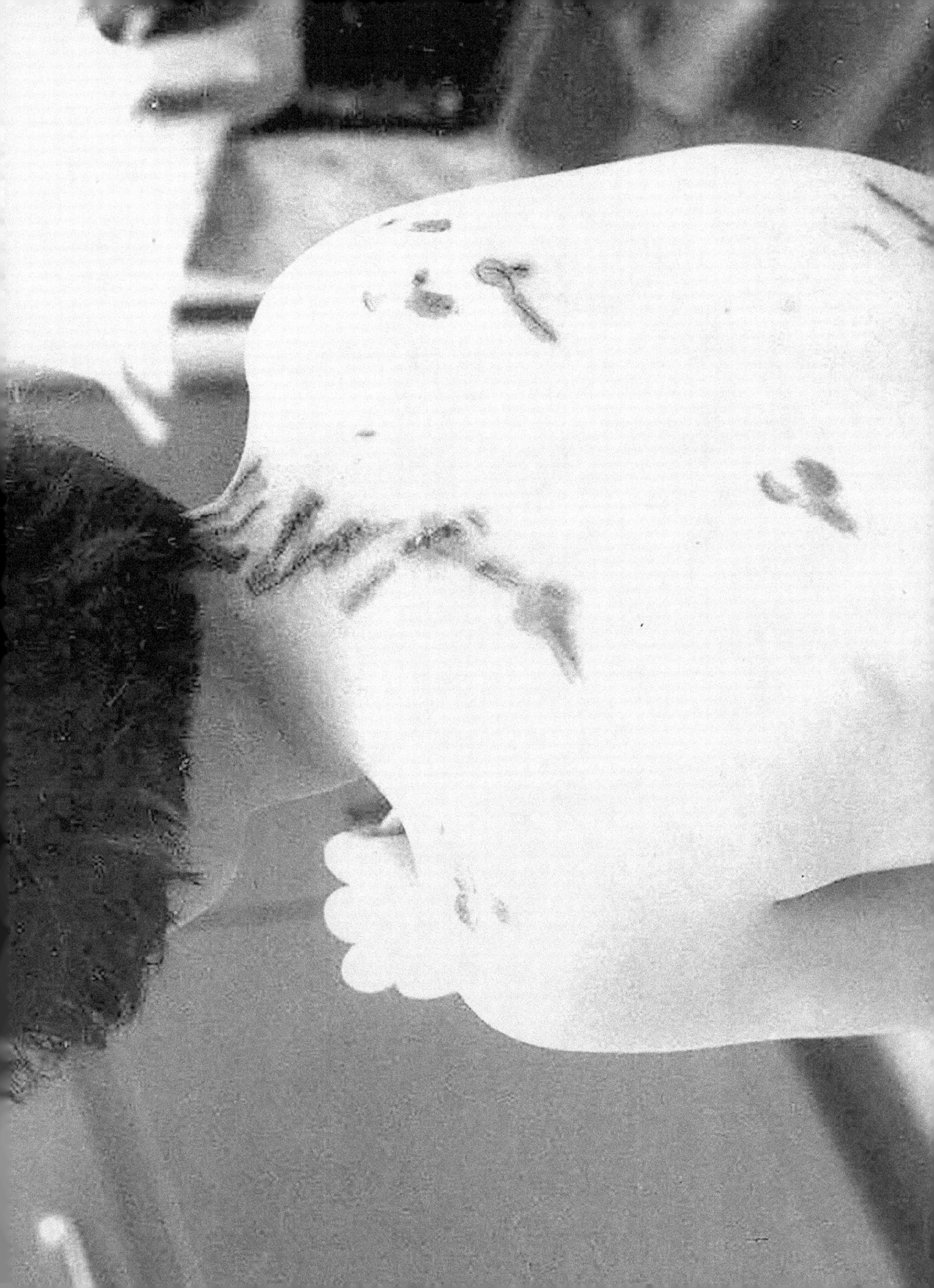

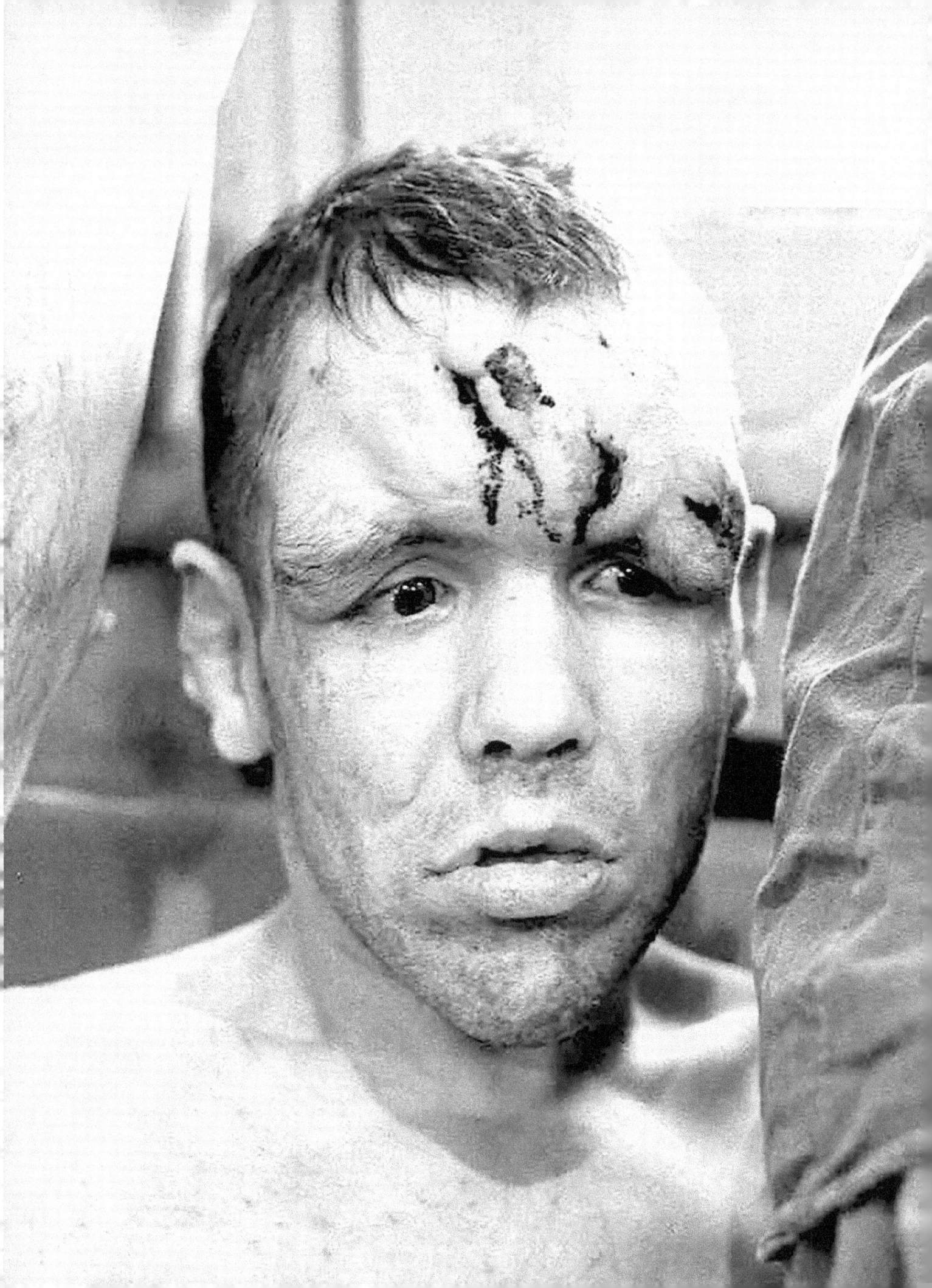

PART II

PUBLIC RANSOM

CHAPTER 26

Ransom

ONCE AGAIN, WE WERE waiting for the courts to act. It would be a year and a half from the time of the hearing injunction to the beginning of the real trial. During that time, intense activity went on in the department; all of it led nowhere. Few of us understood the deep and abiding strength of the institutional system and the reasons for it. Few of us fully understood that victory in the courts and judgments for change would not mean victory and change for the victims, the hostages of Willowbrook.

The staying power of the total institutions is intense and complex. It is essential to understand the basis of this staying power, or Willowbrook and all other institutions will live on just as they are, forever. The material center of the institution is expressed in the title of this book *Public Hostages: Public Ransom*. The ransom is literally the billions of public tax dollars flowing into the nation's institutional system on behalf of the tens and hundreds of thousands of unfortunates incarcerated therein. An analysis of how money is obtained and spent by the public bureaucracies is more than any other information a help to illuminate the true essence of the institution. Here is the sacrosanct and firm reality of what things are all about. Shorn of rhetoric, promises, plans, and publicity. It is the cold decisions measured in dollars and cents that tell the story. Institutions are immensely profitable for the state bureaucracy and private industries. They constitute the multibillion-dollar national industry that is tied to the center of the state and national economy at many points. Expansion of the institutional system is as inevitable and necessary as it is to any other major profitable enterprise in the economy. When the institution no longer expands and reaps benefits for the private and public sector, it will be junked and reinvented in more pernicious and aggrandizing forms if we fail to understand and turn public policy into the individual, home, and family direction.

The 1975–1976 public budget for the New York State Department of Mental Hygiene was $1.03 billion. The inflation change to 2020 dollars is a multiple by 376.5 %, today's amount would be $3.88 billion.

Of that year's budget, $878 million ($3.3 billion–2020) went to the direct costs of running the department's offices, institutions, and research programs. One hundred million dollars ($376 million–2020) of this is in "local assistance" funds. That means it goes back into the state's counties and municipalities in the form of state aid for local mental hygiene programming. The remaining $54 million was the department's "Capital Construction Budget" for the year, and was used for new buildings and renovations and repairs in the existing structures.

This billion-plus dollars of taxpayers' money means that in 1975, New Yorkers each paid an average of $57.33, or $229.32 ($86,000–2020) for a family of four just to keep the department and its programs going for one year at maintenance levels (*Albany Times Union*, May 4, 1975). That amount was two and one-half times what it costs per capita in all other states in the seventies.

The department had essentially two major thrusts: mental health and mental retardation, including children's services. Here, we are concerned with tracking down the share that went to mental retardation and children's service—$351 million ($1.3 billion–2020), a little over one-third of the budget. This money was utilized in 44 facilities that year, 25 of which were separate institutions; the balance were units associated with mental institutions where children or persons labeled retarded were housed. Of this budget amount, approximately $300 million was allocated to salaries and $50 million went to "non-personal expenses." That included supplies, materials, travel, contractual services, and equipment. The "Executive Management Budget" alone was nearly $17.1 ($64.4 million–2020) million dollars; this for the people in the central office of the department whose job it is to oversee and run the system. None of these people live or work at any of the institutions where citizens are housed, live, and die.

The top commissioner and deputy commissioners' salaries each exceeded $45,000.[2] The commissioner's salary was $51,150 ($244,000; 2020), not counting the massive benefits associated with that job. The public relations officer for the department, Harold Wolf, received over $33,700.[3]

Also in 1975–'76, for the first time, nearly $17 million was set aside in the budget to meet the cost of lawsuits leveled against the department for the abuses it would be found guilty of committing (Department of Mental Hygiene '75–'76 Budget). It is of vital importance not only to log the absolute costs of the system derived from public taxes and fees, but also to look at the growth rate of the system over time.

When I began work in 1970, the total budget for the department was $600 million, with the mental retardation portion at $200 million. The department's increase between 1971 and 1972 was $30 million; 1972 and 1973, $40 million; 1973 and 1974, $120 million; 1974 and 1975, $80 million; and 1975 and 1976, $180 million. If this growth rate continues even at its lowest level, this means a doubling of the budget each six years, with inflation further ballooning the growth.[4]

When I began work at Willowbrook in April of 1970, its budget was $20 million. The total census of the institution was 5,600 persons. By 1976, with the advent of the lawsuit, the budget had soared to a staggering $60 million plus ($287 million, 2020), even with the lowered population of only 3,200 people.

By comparison, the entire 1974 state budget of Nebraska came to about the same amount for all state-supported services. We will discuss the implications of this comparison later.

---

[2]   The annual adopted New York State Budget Acts of 1970 through 1976.

[3]   Ibid.

[4]   Ibid.

The expenditure of more than $60 million per year for the dearth of services and warehousing for 3,200 persons is clearly outrageous even in 1975 dollars. Equally outrageous was the department's attempt to account for this flow of money in relation to the human services it was not providing. For example, the cost per "patient day" allocated by federal standards for Willowbrook as an "intermediate care facility" was $21 per day. Multiplying the $21 times the 3,200 people, times 365 days in the year yields a figure of $24.5 million—just over one-third of the allocated budget. The challenge to locate where the unaccounted for $35.5 million went leads into the most incredible morass of spongy explanations and questionable endeavors defined as "fixed overhead." None of it accrued directly to the people who are supposed to be served.

In terms of New York's institutional growth, there had been a major expansion in the number of New York institutions every ten years over the prior twenty years without a single community-based residential home statewide! Seventeen brand-new institutions had been built between 1963 and 1975, at an average cost of $26 million ($124 million, 2020) each. The cost per bed for construction nationally ranges between $30,000 and $100,000, but the 540 beds in the 4 newest institutions in New York (Elmira, Capital District, South Bend, and Hutchings) average a per-bed cost of $214,818 ($1.03 million, 2020). The department projected that these institutions were mainly "outpatient service centers," planned to serve 6,800 people. This presumably justifies the incredibly high cost of the 540 beds for inpatient service.

The department did not grow to this size overnight. The course of its growth is the course of its capitalization. Here, in the most unlikely area of the rejects of society, there is an industry that involves the biggest banks and financiers in the world. Once its growth was underway, its geometric expansion occurred almost effortlessly. The critical point is that at no time was the department aimed at transitional services, where persons with special needs pass through a system of services based on personal relations and skill development, and on to more meaningful lives in open society. The department was always construction-industry financed that was aimed at the simple goal of investing to make long-term profits that led to the establishment of a vast sphere of political influence and patronage. These are the realities that can be traced in conjunction with the leaps forward in the budget. The little monies that actually trickled into the lives of those citizens in the institutions represent an insignificant benefit when compared with the dramatic profits accrued by the leaders of the construction industry and their friends in big banking finance.

The New York Department of Mental Hygiene was actually organized and founded in 1927, replacing the function of the State Hospital Commission and the State Commission for Mental Defectives. During the period until 1960, building derived from mostly federal or local sources. This allowed for very slow and limited facility development and residential services. In 1960, when Governor Rockefeller came to power, a statewide structure called the Housing Finance Agency was created. The HFA increased the ability of all state departments to expand greatly. Its role was that of a financial intermediary to obtain money from the investment communities through the sale of notes and bonds that would go to "eligible borrowers," and to monitor the repayment of these loans back to the private sector. Moreover, since it was a quasi-governmental agency, it was authorized to market tax-exempt bonds for the state, which meant that financial investors who bought the bonds would not have to pay taxes on the interest they got back when the bonds matured. Under the guiding hand of the governor, the legislature authorized the Housing Finance Agency to incur on indebtedness amounting to $1.05 billion ($3.95 billion–2020) after its founding for just the Department of Mental Hygiene alone. A master plan for financing was thus well underway.

In 1963, the Department of Mental Hygiene created its own corporate structure called the Facilities Development Corporation (originally the Mental Hygiene Facilities Development Corporation). This was the counterpart within the department of the HFA. Several years prior to the creation of this structure, the HFA had borrowed $350 million through a mental hygiene bond issue. When the Facilities Development Corporation was created, it assumed responsibility for this loan and launched into borrowing more money for construction. By March 1974, it had expended $683 million ($2.57 billion–2020) for construction.

The Facilities Development Corporation became a giant in its own right, created to plan and finance development of construction not only for the Department of Mental Hygiene but also the state's drug-abuse system, the Corrections Department, and the Department of Social Services. It made agreements with the HFA for raising the money it needs from the private sector.

When the department, through its Facilities Development Corporation, decides it wants to build a number of places and refurbish an additional number of its institutional jurisdiction, it puts together a proposal for a block of money with all the projects set forth. The HFA then prepares a written public prospectus listing all of these proposed projects and turns around to Wall Street, offering all the big banks and financial houses the opportunity to bid on the making of the loan on which the proposed construction bloc depends. This is a process in which the private sector agencies compete among one another to loan money to the state. Whoever will make the loan at the lowest interest gets the bid. In exchange for the money, it then gets the state-issued HFA bonds to sell to private investors as blue-chip, low-risk, tax-exempt securities. The HFA receives the money, deducts its fees for services, and gives the balance to the Facilities Development Corporation, which then goes about using the money to build its new projects. The bonds, just like mortgages on these construction projects, must be paid off by each of the construction projects in the aggregate proposal.

The repayment period ranges between 20 and 30 years, again just like home mortgages. The repayments to the private banks that hold the bonds are made semi-annually and include the principal plus interest on the loan. Despite the relatively low interest or debt service on these bonds, the cost of paying back the borrowed money is nearly equal to the principal sum borrowed. Therefore, when the bond issue is $103 million, as was the case for one sold in 1975, the ultimate repayment will be $200 million. So, for the four institutions built since 1963, the cost of nearly $215,000 per bed is factually more than $400,000 ($1.5 million–2020) per bed. This is the actual burden that falls on the public. The dynamics and rationale of this repayment make the blow especially cruel.

If a construction project such as the Capital District institution costs $37 million within a bond issue of about $103 million,[5] then that "institution" must make its own mortgage payment (a total of over $60 million) into the Facilities Development Corporation payoff. Where does it get this revenue? It gets it from the repayment on keeping its beds filled: Medicare, Medicaid, Social Security, insurance payments, and out-of-pocket fees levied for the persons residing in the institution. Not only does the state pay the institution a per-resident fee, but also, families may also pay fees based on

5   This is the policy of the State of New York in repaying building bond costs.

income. It is out of this total repayment that the institution pays off its gigantic mortgage over two to three decades. The structure itself thus becomes self-supporting. Each time such an institution is built, the public is locked into decades of indebtedness in order to buy out the mortgage.

This is the "ransom" that the taxpayers must pay for the institution residents, but it buys no freedom for most of them. All that is accomplished is that the residents continue to have a building in which to be held hostage, as long as sufficient money is available to pay off the mortgage so that a payment default does not occur. In its annual report, the HFA seeks to entice investors by its very claim of secure investments: "It (HFA) has a solid 13-year fiscal history of prompt payment of all debt service (interest) charges. All obligations are retired on a self-liquidating basis out of the revenue derived from the facilities which the HFA finances…The acid test of the soundness of the Agency's operations are the continued acceptance of its obligations under all market conditions." Not a single default, not a single institution closure.

If the institutional system was to be abandoned ideologically and any facility evacuated, the HFA would be saddled with the problem of absorbing the financial loss. It would have to pay off the multimillion-dollar outstanding mortgages and interest—buy out the debt. Such a default would send a shock wave throughout the HFA's unblemished record of "fiscal responsibility." This would immediately increase the "risk" to the private investment community in loaning money to the HFA, with a concomitant increase in the interest rates to the HFA in borrowing money, and an ultimate increase in the cost to the public. It is absolutely not in the financial interest of the system to do away with residential beds in these gigantic capital adventures. Any decision about institutionalizing or deinstitutionalizing people ultimately deals with the cardinal principle of "financial responsibility." That is to say, profits come first, and nobody, nobody, is going to expropriate and annul the hundreds of millions of dollars of investments plowed into the private sector banks and say, "The deal's off, we've made a terrible mistake." And since the bankers do not attend the department's human services meetings concerned with social policy, the key decision makers are invariably absent.

The private sector banks were always the other side of the Rockefeller public-empire coin. In the 1972 bond issue, which amounted to $148 million ($557 million–2020), Chase Manhattan and First National City Bank were two of the nine financial houses that bought the bonds. Both are Rockefeller family possessions. Additional partners in the purchase and sale included Kidder, Peabody and Company; their mother agency Lehman Brothers; the Morgan Guarantee Trust Company of New York; W. H. Morton and Company; Goldman and Sachs and Company; and the Salomon Brothers Company. The 1975 bond issue was covered by First National City Bank and Morgan Guarantee Trust. These two instances represent the general situation.

It is frighteningly clear where social policy in our society is made. It is equally clear how prostituted the so-called leaders of science are to the exigencies of their patrons and employers. Any scientific policy that might threaten the financial system must absolutely be rejected.

New facilities are being financed and built all the time. Then, as of November 1974, there were 34,700 "hostages" in 23 psychiatric centers and 24,000 hostages in the 30 public mental retardation warehouses waiting. This preceded the massive private industry development of nursing and assisted living facilities, since referred to as *long-term care* services, fueled by the initiation of Title 19 Medicaid financing that birthed the US out-of-home funding policy.

By 1975, the HFA boasted having borrowed a total principal of $35 billion ($1.32 billion–2020) since its creation in 1960. This means that the public repayment for the vast holdings of that agency was nearly double that amount. This indebtedness includes New York construction bonds for mental hygiene, state universities, hospitals and nursing homes, general and nonprofit housing, urban rentals, health facilities, community MH and HR projects, and youth facilities. All these construction operations are "mediated" by the HFA. As of 1975, only $200 million had been repaid on the principal of $5 billion. One may comfortably live with the debts to build housing, schools, and hospitals, but those structures are for independent people who have a great deal to say about where and how they live, who have access to the political process. For the persons in state-operated nursing homes, correction facilities, and mental-hygiene settings, there are no choices. Their continuation in such segregated and barren settings is based on the premise that these unfortunate inhabitants will unlikely return to open society, so significant is their deviancy.

This is the beginning. This is where the public insult begins. In the flow of much of our public resources, year by year, the most extraordinary abuses grow and flourish. Ideally, a decision maker in the government is elected by a constituency because of his or her responsiveness. If this elected official is committed to continuing in power, he or she has a considerable and natural interest in satisfying this constituency. One of the major elements in any political campaign is the need for money to run that campaign. Key money comes mostly from the rich. Nevertheless, it is the general public that votes, and they must be continuously wooed. Nothing sways people like the ability to provide life-sustaining jobs and supports in a community, public works. A significant portion of the service bureaucracy's budget is discretionary. That is, the governor has considerable influence over policy and allocation of that part of this budget not bound to civil service personnel salaries. The geometric expansion of institutions and the concurrent need to hire a lot of people to staff then becomes an immensely potent mechanism for transferring favors to entire communities.

Contracts running into the tens and hundreds of millions of dollars become channels for affecting the maintenance of influence and power. At the highest level, where personal favors and appointments can be affected for top jobs, the word *patronage* is entirely appropriate. For example, a decision was made to build a $22-million[6] 550-bed institution in a small, barely populated county in upstate New York called Broome. There is only one reason for building it in Broome—to exercise the discretionary power of the governor and grease the political machine. The governor's personal lawyer happened to have had a law firm in Broome County and was involved in closing the deal with the state for a massive fee. Then, the contract is awarded to a company whose leadership is coincident with the then county Republican Party leadership—all this a scant two years before a difficult election was to be held. It takes only the slightest research to uncover the multitude of hidden links that have resulted in millions of public dollars flowing into the private and personal coffers of the state's business elite.

New construction is the largest share of the pie at any given time, but the same conditions operate in all areas. For every contract let out, there is an opportunity for a favor, notwithstanding a bidding process. The annual budget for drugs alone was $8 million.[7] Here is the payoff to the companies

---

[6] The HFA bond issue that year

[7] See Budget Act line item year after year in mental hygiene numbers.

that make Thorazine, Mellaril, Valium, Haldol, barbiturates, Prolixine, and the other behavior and epilepsy control drugs. Then there are the lucrative contracts for laundry, trucking, food, hardware supplies, and the like, for in a system that is wholly centralized, everybody must submit to the central office's menu of the day, all over the state of New York.

Besides the contracts with payoffs inherent though not always totally apparent, there are purchase agreements that blatantly avoid state purchasing regulations and competitive bidding requirements. And all this to further ensure that favors are awarded to those who will support, and help to perpetuate, the elitist system that preys on so many and profits so few. An excellent example of this rip-off as it occurred at Willowbrook was revealed by the state comptroller's office and reported in a local newspaper. There was ample evidence that efforts were not made to obtain the most reasonable prices in accordance with state regulations on Willowbrook State School purchases.

Orders were split to avoid competitive bidding requirements, the bidders' list was inadequate, and in general, there was an open circumvention of the applicable purchasing rules. The auditors singled out the Empire Sales Co., which made sales of $44,000 to the school for fiscal 1971 without benefit of a single contract. Large numbers of purchase orders to this contractor were written for amounts just under $300 or just under $500. The quantities ordered usually were odd amounts because an increase of one unit would have increased the dollar amount to over the limit, and would have altered the regulations controlling the purchase. The audit said, "Of nine clothing contracts that were awarded to other than the lowest bidder, seven were awarded to Empire." The auditors called the proposals for these orders "vague or overly restrictive" in order to ensure that only a certain bidder would qualify (*Staten Island Advance*, September 24, 1973).

The bids or arrangements for all these materials and non-personnel services are made by somebody, somewhere in the bureaucracy. That person, invisibly, makes a decision for a million dollars' worth of this or that. That is the nature of institutions, as opposed to life in open society where people make personal economic choices about their purchases and the quality of their everyday lives. The risk of corruption and personal glorification is miniscule in our lives in comparison to that of the dealers in institutions.

The 1975–'76 budgets in Willowbrook earmarked $17 million ($68 million, 2020) for non-personnel expenses, a full four times that for any other state institution for people labeled retarded. Under the heavy scrutiny of the court and families, this may now represent a more appropriate expenditure for food, clothes, laundry, and supplies, but it also creates an enormous opportunity for money to be spent to gain more influence and further entrench the virtues of the institution in the eyes and pockets of large business that relies on such substantial contracts for success.

Returning to the issue of "small" construction, millions of dollars in contracts continually flow out, year after year, over and above the monies for building new institutions. For the 20 to 40 projects combined for each bond issue, money is continually pumped all around the state through the various institutions in order to keep things cooking with "friends." A new gymnasium, $815,000; renovation in Building 58, $2,725,000; alterations and improvements for modernization of laundry Building 37, $1,660,000; patient therapy center, $620,000; bakery building and distribution center for Upstate, $8,750,000; air-conditioning, toilet repairs, fire protection sprinklers; annex here, modernize there. It goes on without end. Millions and millions of dollars flow, like a mortal hemorrhage of the people's money, into what has become known as the largest dehumanizing warehouse system ever constructed.

Ed Goldman, then Pennsylvania's commissioner of Mental Retardation, presents a dramatic synthesis of the cost of fixing up our old institutions: "If we decided not to repair any institution if the cost for the repair exceeded 60 percent of the cost of new construction, then three out of four institutions would be out of business. Even if we did modernize the old places and brought the equally barren new ones up to individualized standards, half the bed space would be lost in the process. And there is no place to house the displaced persons in that event, as no provisions have been made even to that ignominious end. This is the dilemma of the institutional system."

There is yet another dimension of the situation which must be fitted into our examination of the "ransom." Given such an enormous empire, such a staggering take, the New York Department of Mental Hygiene—the system—is in a position to share its wealth here and there to ensure the orderly continuation of its expansion and profits. The first claimant in New York that might naturally have challenged the expansion of the state's empire was the parents' organization, the New York Association for Retarded Children, originally created to advocate for services and to defend the rights and needs of their sons and daughters.

Historically the family organizations began by rallying a few young parents back in the forties and fifties to develop among themselves the service needed for support and protection of their developmentally delayed children. As these enterprises became more organized and well-known, the families began to get a little money from grants and charity appeals and even to win some public support to continue their work. The rub is that at no time has there ever been a real commitment to require the public sector address this need fully on an informed and rightful basis.

This noncommittal attitude had many valid bases and objective realities at the beginning. New York parents did not identify with the institutions until they had to place their sons and daughters in them. The basic preoccupation with meeting their own needs, coupled with a sense of the remoteness of the state, allowed a parochialism to prevail. As the parent structures grew, they hired professionals to do the work for them and expanded their operations. This was not done on the basis of intentional planning, but was concretely tied to the evolution of their own families' needs. Thus, from children's programs, as the patients aged, they needed vocational programs, then residential and guardianship services. Initially, the parent organizations innocently and ignorantly drifted into the business of providing a parallel system of services that the state escaped. This token grant dependency comprised special schools, day care, adult activity and vocational settings, transportation, and residential and recreation services. With great pride, community families compared their evolving agencies and services with the impersonal and gloomy public services and institutional systems.

The state took good advantage of the underdevelopment of the parent organizations and increased its token payoff to keep the parents occupied with their "high-quality" projects. Gradually, the parents became more and more indebted and dependent on the state's benevolence. It is not difficult to see how such a patronizing relation could capture the parent organization leaders in a trap where all power to dissent, all militancy and advocacy were sapped. In fact, parents were lulled into thinking that they were providing leadership and exercising influence when the state would enlist their help to lobby for more and more money for the state programs—that is, institutional construction and expansion—in order for the parents' organizations to qualify for their comparative pittance grants from the state.

The sadness is that the many parent leaders are in so deep that like old alcoholics or long-time gamblers, they no longer can admit to their dependency habit. This is the deep conflict of interest and lack of real power that they have encumbered upon themselves. They delude themselves that they are potent, that they have the ability to persuade or influence the state. They have been brought into line with the state financial strategy and taught in the most deliberate way how to play the game of token rewards. This is the deep sickness that pervades much of the leadership of the parent and voluntary service, nonprofit structures.

They cannot bring themselves to realize that not only must they build a truly organized and educated base, but also that from this base they can deliver an ethical, political blow against injustice and token co-optation. At this moment, they do not even fully understand what true change is. In New York State, the greatest sellout occurred under the very nose of a parent structure that boasted of its greatness and tradition of leadership. The venerated leader and founder of the New York State Association for Retarded Children, Joseph Weingold, accepted a token $8 to 14 million for the association's institution, and sat by while the state built its own empire at 500 times the magnitude. More tragic yet, the ironfisted Weingold became the counsel to the Joint Legislative Committee on Mental and Physical Handicaps, thoroughly drowned in the sense of his own importance and ruling his organization by sheer prestige and handmade control. The New York State ARC became the handmaiden to the crime of believing that telethons, pity imagery, charity—all the old hat-in-hand rubrics—could replace the entire share of the state's bounty that was rightfully theirs. And who else in the state would stand up for the families' needs if the ARC did not?

They could not even summon the ability to organize the poor, black, and Puerto Rican families and neighborhoods, whose communities had the greatest special service needs and whose force would have given the ARC real power. All of these errors led the state ARC to become just another possession of the bureaucracy's empire, a self-inflated, prattling puppet, fed scraps from the groaning table of the state's tax and financing wealth.

So, it was and in large part still is in New York, and so it is in other states as well. To a greater or lesser extent, most of the established parent structures have had to live with state strategies, forcing them to be the natural providers of last resort and focus most of their attention on survival, having yielded or been suffocated under feelings of impotence, ostracism, or undeserved pride in their own private little charity based empires—at a desperate political and social cost. They have gotten a kickback from the ransom, complicit in the maintenance of the public hostages who are their own kin.

CHAPTER 27

The Deep Alternative

CAN THE SITUATION BE so monotonous and bleak? Is there no break in the backwardness? In this tumultuous period of challenge that burgeoned against many state's institutional dependence and abuse, financing strategies varied widely. Not all states financed out-of-home placements and construction in the same way as New York; some states had not seized on the opportunity to do what the New York financial community did. The pressures on all the states to do something about the wretched conditions in all their institutions in their jurisdictions sparked a massive commitment of funding to modernize, provide new earthquake and other safety standards and rudimentary cleaning of their outdated warehouse systems.

Texas

At the time, a significant example can be seen in the situation in Texas, where there were 12 institutions for persons labeled retarded, with 13,127 residents. Texas's Department of Mental Health and Mental Retardation is constituted similarly to that of New York. A simple chart shows the trend clearly:

	1974	1977
Total budget for mental health and MR	$174.4 million	$303.6 million
Budget for Denton State School	$7.2 million	$15.6 million
Budget for Austin State School	$8.2 million	$15.3 million

I have selected the Austin and Denton state schools because a class action suit similar to the Willowbrook suit had been filed against these institutions. It is striking that the growth rate in Texas of the institutional budgets were nearly double over a four-year period—an even sharper growth rate than in New York. Furthermore, of the twelve Texas state schools, two were built and began filling beds in 1973–'74.

And yet at the height of the struggle, there was hope for another way. A way that would offer an avenue toward an increasingly mainstream existence for those persons who differ from the mythical "norm." Approaches were beginning to allow them to exist as valued and useful people. Such alternatives would rely totally on existing living arrangements for people with special needs in the community, rather than in specially built facilities. Such community living arrangements would be identical in appearance, size, and feeling to the homes where ordinary folks live. Such a system would emphasize the vital importance of having skilled and devoted people working to serve the entire range of client needs, in leased or rented settings in every neighborhood.

This kind of model staff and facilities continuum, established for the individual-and family-sized integrated group, a true community-based status-and identity-enhancing service system is virtually still nonexistent. Such an ideal experience would develop a total range of family and service worker care mounted on the foundation of a developmental philosophy that does not rely a congregate out-of-home or institutional system for properly serving even the most in-need person. This eventuality would require states to close their monolithic institutions and plow resources into home and community development, or not have any segregated institutional system to begin with. Neither of these circumstances currently exists following the June 22, 1999, landmark federal class action ruling in *Olmstead v. United States* that established community service standards for detailed care and services to people with developmental disabilities as a dedicated national policy. It is interesting to look at examples where large-scale community-based programs were begun in synch with growing public awareness, political action, and enlightened professional leadership.

Pennsylvania

In Pennsylvania, even in the early seventies, a special section of the Office of Mental Retardation (which basically ran an enormous institutional system) was formed to create a model of comprehensive community living arrangement and services. Legislation in 1972 established, earmarked, and protected money specifically for homelike living services with local county fiscal responsibility rather than 100 percent state funding. As of mid-1975, the community living arrangement system was serving 1,438 clients, with 285 apartments and 124 homes that were supported by state or local money. Around 750 people had passed through the community living arrangements. Of this matriculated group, 445 had learned to live independently; 138 were living in their natural homes with support; 31 were in foster homes; and 112 required more restrictive services and have been put in nursing homes. The total number served was 2,188 people. The budget for the community living arrangement program in 1974–'75 was $11.32 million ($42.6 million–2020), and for 1975–'76, $13.5 million ($50.8 million–2020).

The community living arrangement program was only one component in Pennsylvania's experimental comprehensive service system. Pennsylvania also budgeted $36.8 million[8] for all other community programs, including preschool, recreational, social, and vocational resources. For the 11 institutions in the state and 7 "mental retardation units" in state hospitals, housing 12,000 people, the state's share of costs amounted to $105.4 million. Thus, of the total $153.5 million dollars ($576 million–2020) expended in 1974–'75 for services to people with intellectual disabilities, and in spite of an extensive and evolving residential continuum, two-thirds of all monies was still tightly tied to an equally vigorous and expanding warehouse system.

---

8   Pennsylvania 1974–1975 annual adopted budget act and personal communication from Ed Goldman, Pennsylvania State MR Commissioner.

Canada

Though the comparative costs forty years ago are ridiculously unreal, it is keenly interesting to examine what the rare thinking and budgeting progress was unfolding in North America to further show the contrasts in costs of institutions and community services, looking at Canada's pre-national health entitlement program for persons with mental retardation, prepared by Alan Roehrer, then executive director of Canada's National Institute of Mental Retardation.

There were some 25,000 mentally retarded people in Canadian institutions. The cost of maintaining them is at least $100 million yearly ($376.5 million–2020). The number is increasing. According to federal data, during the last ten years, the number of patients on the books in "mental institutions" in Canada decreased by 41 percent while for institutions for the persons with intellectual disabilities, it has increased by 40 percent. The only way to reverse the trend for people with special needs is to do what was done for the people labeled mentally ill—increase availability and utilization of individualized community resources.

A key 1971 report to the Ontario government issued within the context that Canada's heath care system had shifted to its universal rightful Medicare for all coverage begun in Saskatchewan, July 1962 states, "If a mentally retarded person is institutionalized for life, and if we assume a life expectancy of only fifty years, the expense to the government at $20.00 a day (without allowance for increase) would be $365,000 [$1.37 million–2020]. Realistically, one can plan on spending $500,000 [$1.88 million–2020] for each resident who is to stay in an institution for life." Capital cost at $30,000 a bed is not included.

"Present planning (in Ontario) calls for 1,800 additional beds. To provide these 1,800 beds along traditional patterns, capital construction would be approximately $50,000,000. Over the next fifty years, without any allowance for capital cost for maintenance of the buildings, it will take $900,000,000 [$3.38 billion–2020] in 2020) to maintain only 1,800 persons in an institutional way of life which has been almost universally condemned." In the case of two institutions in Ontario, "The delay between the planning and the finished structure was such that the thinking behind them was obsolete before construction was finished."

The clearly obsolete figures in the Ontario government's policy focus of March 1973 showed that gross cost of maintenance per person per year in a community residence with counselors was about half the cost of institutional care. Additional "community" services such as a sheltered workshop and personal allowance bring the total to something under two-thirds of the $20 a day cited by the report and reinforced by the Ontario government statistics on institutional costs $6,760–$10,642* per person per year.

The cost of apartment living, with minimal supervision and counseling, is less than $1,000.00 a year. The average cost of maintaining a resident in the Manitoba Hospital School is $12.00 per day. The 60 residents in the 5 small community residences throughout the province cost $35.50 a day each (2020).

As Canada slowly emerged into their national health care, universal coverage system, the Canadian association for the Ontario-based *Mentally Retarded Association Canadienne pour les Deficients Mentaux*, at least half of the people in institutions should not be there. Many could support themselves, given a period of work training and rehabilitation counseling. A few people have been moved to an "approved boarding home" in the community. If they can obtain and keep work, they are eventually "released" and become tax-paying citizens. The incidence of institutionalized people who eventually learn to support themselves is small (about 30 in Ontario's largest institution), partly because institutions are purposefully located away from urban centers with opportunities for work training and community living experiences, partly because they are traditionally custodial facilities and there are few training programs.

The Vocational and Rehabilitation Research Institute in Calgary was founded with the object of training people with disabilities to the stage where they can function independently and keep out of the Canadian institutions. Since 1969, more than 200 of the 889 trainees placed at the institute have become self-sustaining members of the community. One hundred eighteen are in supervised community accommodation. In Toronto, 30 percent of the trainees at the Foster Training Centre go into regular employment. In 1965–'66, the Federal Department of Labour reported, "Cost of support before rehabilitation of 272 people with mental retardation—$207,626 [$7.66 million–2020]. Earnings after rehabilitation—$380,010 [$14.3 million–2020]."

The cost of keeping 20 people in an institution for 60 years is $9 million ($33.84 million–2020). If the special individualized help they need was available in the community, we estimate the cost could be reduced by more than 60 percent. Nobody can predict how many babies diagnosed with suspected intellectual disabilities could grow up to be tax-paying citizens if they had the right kind of special training during their first eighteen years of life. Research findings to date suggest that infants with retarded development, can make remarkable progress toward independence and socialization—expectations, skilled help and a positive environment are the keys.

Evidence from the two major experimental vocational and rehabilitation centers for persons with retardation is that about 25 percent of trainees "graduate" to regular employment after one or two years' training. None of these trainees has had the benefit of early childhood stimulation or new knowledge in special education. It seems fair to predict that the success rate will accelerate greatly if the right groundwork is done in preschool and school years.

Once these "graduates" join the workforce, most become virtually self-supporting. Any special help they need in legal and business dealings is offset by the taxes they pay on earnings and purchase. What of people with intellectual disabilities who can never become self-supporting? Less than 1 in 50 need continual nursing care. Supervised living accommodation and a sheltered work situation are all the support most require. The kind of accommodation and the extent of supervision varies with the individual, but in all cases, it costs profoundly less than maintenance in a large institution.

According to figures based on Ontario government estimates, costs vary in other provinces because of regional wage disparities, differences in housing, and other living costs. The ratio remains constant—$9 million ($33.88 million–2020) to keep people shut away, or $3 million ($1.13 million–2020) to help them thrive integrated with us as fellow citizens in the community.

Nebraska

Jumping back to the United States, by far the most complex and creative situation began and existed in Nebraska. As clear-cut as the dominating institutional versus the community-service model is in states like New York and Pennsylvania, the situation is diametrically the opposite in Nebraska. There the community budget was actually larger than the institution budget. For the first time in the United States, we catch a glimpse of the possibilities of the not-too-distant alternative future. A résumé of some of the facts provides the greatest paradigm shift that all animated progressive advocates now use in their calculus.

The state of Nebraska had the most advanced demonstration of a near-ideal community system in its time. It was not only structurally ideal, but also, more importantly, it was ideologically developed by the work of Wolf Wolfensberger, PhD, where an amazing service staff averaged under thirty years old. Dr. Wolfensberger constructed the comprehensive vision of approaching human service delivery from a place of enlightened common sense and unparalleled scrutiny of normal society to confer high social value on all its members. His dynamic model service forms were not seen as enduring and permanent. Rather, they were created as transitional steps toward the full individual integration of all the state's citizens with special needs into open society. They include individual-enhancing supports as well as safeguards against abuse and rigorous research and data gathering with true social integrative outcomes. Furthermore, Nebraska had but a single large institution, Beatrice State Home.

The total budget at Beatrice for 1975–'76 amounted to $11 million ($41.4 million–2020). That for a population of 1,039 people, plus about 1,000 employees. A construction campaign proposed to build cottages on the grounds of the institution at the rate of 3 per year until 18 were completed would cost the state $1 million cash[9] per year for four to six years. By comparison, the community budget for MR services for the entire state was then $17.4 million ($65.5 million–2020). The state provided developmental needs services for its six geopolitical regions by contracting with local agencies set up on a quasi-governmental basis.

The Eastern Nebraska Community Office of Retardation (ENCOR), Dr. Wolfensberger's initial idea, was established in 1968 through a cooperative agreement among the five most populous counties at the eastern border. Including Omaha, the five-county area had a population of 520,000 people, which was a little over one-third of the state's census. ENCOR began with a consolidated plan and the empowering legislation to serve all the citizens labeled retarded, to empty out Beatrice, and to demonstrate the primacy of values and beliefs in constructing human services. It was the conviction of the planners that costs would plummet down as service quality improved in the community, and that more consumer and community volunteers could be enlisted in developing real comprehensive human services that would work. Starting with $200,000[10] from a state and county grant, and a systematically worked-out approach, about 70 clients were initially served. Some of the staff for the services were even drawn from high schools, where students were given six weeks of training with the emphasis on "normalization" ideology about helping people without stigmatizing them. Each year, successful services expanded, and the growth zoomed. In 1970, the budget was about $950,000 in 1971, $1.7 million in 1972, $2.4 million in 1973, $3.5 million in 1974, $4 million in 1975, $5.8 million $21.83 million(2020).

The community services and service organizations were spread through the entire five counties, with the young brilliantly trained workers sharing in the everyday affairs of community life at the

---

9   See Nebraska Budget Act 1975–1986.

10   Personal communication with Wolf Wolfensberger.

markets, stores, schools, and hospitals used by everyone. Further, there were no three work shifts for staff but a full week's work and life shared in living settings with the people who were being served! Significant numbers of the special needs adults who came through the system now earn a living and pay taxes in their production training settings, which function as a part of regular industry. In Beatrice, there continued only subsidized inactivity, drugged dependency, and social control. The bulk of the clients in the community living system were taken from Beatrice with great care not to also transplant their institutional behaviors and culture into the community settings. The Beatrice population gradually declined by over one-half, though the budget for the institution continued to grow as usual.

As of 1976, ENCOR had established 114 service sites in their comprehensive system, with an emphasis on using those services in a transitional way—to move people from the dependence and segregation of the past into interdependence and integration in regular neighborhoods. A constant shifting went on as service sites were continuously scrutinized for their appropriateness. Some were phased out as the need and growing awareness of unnecessary stigma demanded changes. Among the service sites were 99 individual living units in 13 training residences or specialized group homes, with 6 to 8 individuals residing in each, unheard of in its time. The nature of the training varied according to the special needs and ages of the persons served. The most expensive unit was called the Developmental Maximation Unit, a typical home designed to intensely serve no more than 8 very young children with profound multiple developmental needs and 24-hour medical-care-required conditions. In addition, there were 81 persons in alternative living arrangements, which were generally more apartment-based settings than the training residences. Finally, there were 5 structured correctional apartments designed to serve people in trouble with the law. About 225 persons were being served within this residential continuum, at a cost of about $1.4 million[11], a figure on its face close to that of the institution's.

The rest of the ENCOR system included 5 vocational services, 7 workstation sites in regular industry, 5 developmental settings for school-age youngsters, 15 integrated preschools, 5 infant stimulation programs, motor development services, and 5 family counseling and service centers. A larger number of services had no walls at all; there were staff-intensive services in the home and community, directly focused on ensuring the success of the individuals being served. A total of about 1,400 individuals were being served. Thus, with the additional community services, only a small proportion were seen as needing any out-of-home residential programs.

And yet, in spite of the overwhelming humanitarian advantages of the community-based service system, the state of Nebraska continued to press its massive institution cottage-building campaign. The bureaucracy was fighting for its very life to hold on to Beatrice.

In a firsthand report from an ENCOR worker who made an extended visit to Beatrice in 1969, a few lines affirm the situation so familiar at Willowbrook:

"Through the double doors the group entered a world of yesterday, a world of tile walls, lined with benches, toilets without seats; no provision for toilet paper, no soap, a post mortem table for bathing; beds two feet apart with few pillows, no blankets... and that odor...you couldn't escape it. On three

---

[11]   Personal communication with Wolf Wolfensberger.

floors the sight was the same—men shackled to benches; men aimlessly wandering or rocking; men laced into straitjackets; television sets with no volume so the attendants could listen to the radio; men wandering in bare feet among puddles of urine; camisoled men being fed by fellow patients off steel trays with tablespoons so fast that the meal is vomited up almost as fast as it is swallowed; no pictures, no drapes, hospital white bedspreads; men with skin so dry and scaled it resembled snake skin; men who if lucky get bathed twice a week. It was in this building that on one floor of 81 patients, one attendant was on duty."

In March 1975, I received a letter from another worker in the Developmental Maximation Unit at ENCOR. A portion read:

"Since writing you last we got another girl, Susan B. All I can say is, chalk another one to Beatrice. Susan is almost 3 years old now. She had (and still does have) a 'severe seizure disorder' and. at 5 months. was institutionalized. Weight—18 pounds. She kept developing respiratory infections and became a "feeding problem" so they stuck a nasogastric tube down her and fed her Complete B. Only they just gave her 2 ounces every 4 hours. Bill, that child was starving to death. When she came to us a month and a half ago she weighed 18 pounds—the same weight she entered Beatrice at... about 2 years ago. I don't know what goes thru those people's heads! I get so angry and damned near maniacal when people tell me "Those are the kind we need institutions for. Extermination camps is a better word."

It was such conditions, coupled with the battle to establish the community-based system, that resulted in a class action suit against the state of Nebraska. This was the definitive precursor to the 1995 *Olmstead v. L. C.* suit filed on behalf of two institutionalized young women that had been in Georgia Regional Hospital for treatment that ultimately reached the US Supreme Court for the 1999 landmark-defining decision in the United States. Here in the Beatrice, filing the most decisive issue was yet to be adjudicated. Given two parallel systems able to care for people, the institutional system was alleged to impose restrictions that breach the constitutional guarantee of the right to equal access and due process. Thus, the suit maintained, Beatrice's very operation was to be judged unconstitutional. Given a choice, people have a right to community services. Here is not the less precise right-to-treatment issue, but a direct shot at the very essence of the institution's nature.

Under a flood of overt and covert pressures in Nebraska, possibly from other states as well, the decision was made to let up on the sharp issue and compromise by just making the state clean up its warehouse. The argument went that a decision would take time and certainly be appealed, meaning endless delays that would impose devastating suffering upon the residents and their families. The faction that supported obtaining a definitive ruling for a national as well as local precedent was suppressed, and instead, a consent proposal was submitted. But the state, in its encrusted position, rejected the compromise and threw it back into the face of the conciliators, thus setting the course for ultimate collision and a return to the federal court for a full hearing.

Here was even more evidence against retaining the institution. In one of the more rural regions in Nebraska, the Mid-Nebraska Mental Retardation Service served 22 counties and was spread over 15,000 square miles. The administrator of the service prepared a cost analysis for the state legislature, which was debating whether or not to build a new institution to serve the people. The plans were meticulously drawn up. They offered total services for 450 persons, in an institution modeled on the services available to people in the community. Costs for the building alone were estimated at $4.75

to $5.25 million ($19.76 million–2020), with $2.5 million ($9.41 million–2020) to run annually, with a continuous population of 450 persons. The identical community-based services would cost $1.5 to $1.7 million ($6.4 million–2020), with no new construction needed.

We need to understand the reasons why the state retains institutions at all, given such facts. In the face of a highly developed, publicly supported community system, with a lawsuit pending, with but a thousand people and one facility in operation, why does the state persist in holding off understanding this would bring us to the most important insights about the entrenched and hidden ground of the institution. We must have this knowledge in order to wage an effective war on the institutional system.

The institution claims it provides "total care" for its residents. Yet we know that the quality of life in the institution is at best stagnant, nonproductive, if not downright ravaged. The community system, on intentional, ideological grounds, assiduously avoids the provision of "total care" except for a very limited few, and even has expectations and services aimed at gradually moving their clients to live in the community in increasingly useful, productive, and valued roles. Conscious effort is exercised to protect clients from the stigma of "community institutionalization," and to guarantee a relationship within the natural flow of community and family life, in which each person can continue to develop and mature.

Again, the question, why does the state cling to the institution? Could it be that the politicians protect the highly paid bureaucrats out of a dedication to their needs, in the spirit of fraternal loyalty? Could it be that the state bureaucracy is so laden with rigidity that the idea of a fluid and changing community-based service system paralyzes the decision makers? Community services would be in the hands of younger people, people not subject to direct state control. The decision makers would have to surrender a service model based on authority and complexity, both of which make those beneath them more compliant.

In a tiny town like Beatrice, with a population of fifteen thousand, do a thousand families have no other means of survival than to be employed by the institution? Rather than tackle this fact of social life, does the state feel it is preferable to use the institutional setting regardless of its moral implications? Is the outspoken opposition by a few families against the "return to the community" for their relatives the real reason for perpetuation of the institution? Or is this an excuse for the state to cover up its true motives? Are the state decision makers aware of the tradition that they uphold? Do they find it impossible to close out a despicable past? Is there no end to this cancer? Must it metastasize and encumber us into the future? What policy prescription will allow our persons with special needs to become whole and contributing?"

Like a lingering cancer cell, the institution can, at any moment, regenerate to play its evil role. Surely when the institution is completely outlawed in Nebraska, it will be another strike at the very heart of the system that has humiliated so many Americans for so many scores of years. The question is no longer which is cheaper or better. For those who value open-society living and human integrity, these questions have been fully and adequately answered. For those who are held hostage by the Title 19 public ransom they generate, those questions are not even asked. No decision, no choice is available to them.

It is an informed public that must take measures to deal with this bondage. First, we must understand the diagnosis: The entire system of profiteering and privilege, built on deep societal prejudice against devalued people, is the corruption that tyrannizes us. The laws in our system legitimize and perpetuate exploitative financial relations, privatization of essential health and human services, and protect obligations to the financial corporate leaders as they go about their business. Only a systemic approach that creatively promotes universal human empowerment can challenge the impossible and perverse conditions that give rise to the multibillion-dollar traffic in an artificially generated domestic refugee population which plagues our society. As we will see, the true solution will be in establishing guaranteed health care as a right through expanded and improved Medicare for All.

CHAPTER 28

Janus

INSTITUTIONS, LIKE FESTERING OLD boils, still exist. But not just in New York State. They can be found everywhere in both the United States and Canada. I have now spent forty years away from Willowbrook. The forces and interests that kept Willowbrook alive and well for decades after its assignment to closure are the same forces that keep the institution system the land over alive and well. The challenges that are raised in opposition to dislodge those forces are, in the main, propelled by the same hopes everywhere. In 2015, the US Department of Justice was involved in federal lawsuits in forty-four states, Puerto Rico, and the District of Columbia regarding the integration mandate of Title II of the Americans with Disabilities Act. For an observer entangled in any one of these struggles, it is very easy to miss, to simply not know the magnitude of the national movement challenging the institutional, out-of-home placement system that is grounded in the national movement for universal health care as a right, expanded and improved Medicare for All, and the broad advocacy movements around special needs that exist.

While I was writing this autobiographical documentary, I received a document published by the President's Committee on Mental Retardation titled "A Compendium of Lawsuits Establishing the Legal Rights of Mentally Retarded Citizens." This study, commissioned in 1974 by the Council for Exceptional Children and published in 1975 by the Government Printing Office, reviews the breadth of social litigation filed against such abuses on behalf of people with special needs. At the time of that report, eighty-three major class action cases existed, spread through thirty-eight states and the District of Columbia, the oldest of them dating back no earlier than 1971. The cases were classified under nine categories: (1) right to equal educational opportunity; (2) right to be free from inappropriate educational classification, labeling, and placement; (3) right to community services and treatment in the least restrictive environment; (4) right to be free from peonage and involuntary servitude; (5) right to be free from restrictive zoning ordinances; (6) right to free access to buildings and transportation systems; (7) right to be free from unconstitutional commitment practices; (8) right to procreate; and (9) right to equal access to adequate medical services. Each of these calls for the recognition that people with special needs are in fact being daily deprived of those rudimentary needs, pleasures, and relations to which we all have become accustomed and expect in ordinary living. The articulation of guarantees of these basic human rights has been one level of the embrace of justice.

In these cases, rights must be intimately depicted in relation to the actual conditions, both real and theoretical, where citizens who have been devalued are forced to live. So complicated are the habits, traditions, rules, regulations, and laws within our society, so deep-seated are the prejudices that animate and provide the brick and mortar of our human services that the job of exposing the abuses that exist as accepted practice requires sharp persistence. Ultimately, it is the many—ordinary people—who discover and live out the drama of transforming our society. But who can fathom the implications of such technical reasoning? Who knows of this mass of litigation? Distressingly, only the few. The technicians, the professionals, the experts forge ahead by means of their mobility, privileges, and power from the rest of society.

The progressive lawyers and their agencies have their hands full just doing what most other lawyers are unwilling or unable to do for devalued people. They labor under advocate and family demands to be organizers, day-to-day translators, and popularizers of the meaning and implications of their work. Without a two-way bond between courageous professionals and plaintiff institutionalized constituencies who are socially valorized or crushed on the alliances made, a justice gap opens and grows wider. This gap continues to widen as the established and invested stakeholders and structures that feed off the institutions regain their composure and seize the initiative to define the issues and impose their traditional violations. States cynically delay, distract, deny, and hide truth, confining their negotiations with the lawyers, not the plaintiffs or public.

Even if these negotiations result in injunctions for relief of the plaintiffs, ever more brutal problems are uncovered. Court decisions must be enforced. Each apparent advance holds out a promise. Each lulls the general public into thinking that because a decision becomes imposed policy or the law of the land, that law will be given the material support and the public involvement for getting rid of the offending situation. What actually happens, however, is that these human rights pronouncements from the bench—when and if they do arrive—may commit a community or consumer organization to the full-time monitoring job of seeing to it that a reform is carried through. All the while these scarce and thinly spread advocacy groups do not have the membership strength or even the organizational inclination to do something that public authority should and must be doing.

It is a problem of the first magnitude. If there is nobody else to mind the child when you have to battle to get that child into a good classroom, what do you do? Withdrawing from one responsibility may injure the other, and there may be no right choice. This circumstance tends to inhibit the volunteer organizations from demanding reform in the first place. They realize they will be saddled with the responsibility of making sure things are carried out, instead of being left to the task of building a social or political structure that will ultimately do away with the need for such reform in the first place. All the early considerations and problems were present in the Willowbrook trial. As the political and legal situation ripened and evolved around the class action trial, more and more people were gripped in a dilemma that they felt was of their own making.

Meanwhile the bureaucracy, unencumbered by the ethical preoccupations of right or wrong, progressive or regressive, just sat it out. Unless people expend enormous personal energy to discover and protest the grievous conditions in the institution, these conditions continue unabated, court orders and laws notwithstanding. A thousand ready excuses are available if such a subterfuge is discovered.

"Oh, we didn't know… Well, we needed more time, we were going to do that…You are mistaken in your accusation. What you see is not green, it is yellow, isn't that so, Commissioner? I don't see any problem …You are not the expert …We're not responsible for that, they are."The evasions are endless.

Ordinary people begin to think they have lost their wits when confronted with such insanity and vulgarity. Activists, whether they be parents or professionals, come home every night after such tilt and feel they are going mad. In the realm of values that affect so much, with no agreed-upon standards since the faux political and professional leadership are often complicit in the deception, where does one gather the confidence and assurance to take a stalwart position? This duality the parents had to grapple with between the rational work of the law and court system indicting the brutal and confounding realities versus the intentional irrationality of the institutional bureaucracy is the 'apparent no win' conflictual experience, symbolized by Janus, the opposing two faced Roman deity. In our degradation as a culture with such relativism rampant, benefiting only those in power, who is to say a spade is a spade? That is why, despite the potential burden of a legal judgment, people may turn to the courts as a temporary means of sorting out the madness in human services. Sometimes it helps. Certainly, it does in the matter of definitions and words. For this reason, we may have to accept, for the time being, the disadvantage of dependence on the elitism and the mystery of judgments, laws, and lawyers. The work of actually bringing about change, however, continues to reside with the many, not the few.

Lawsuits, complaints, and court records are available online at disability justice. tpt.org.

As of 2013, in a "State of the States" report by David Braddock,[12] there were fourteen states without state-operated institutions for people with intellectual and developmental disabilities. The fourteen states include the District of Columbia, New Hampshire, Vermont, Rhode Island, Alaska, New Mexico, West Virginia, Hawaii, Maine, Indiana, Michigan, Oregon, Minnesota, and Alabama.

---

[12] Communication with Dr. Colleen Wieck, executive director, Minnesota Governor's Council on Developmental Disabilities.

CHAPTER 29

Guilty and the Aftermath

IN MID-1974, WILLOWBROOK STILL awaited the approaching trial that would give its residents a judgment for relief. I had been gone from Willowbrook, barring two visits, for more than a year. On one of my returns with Mike Wilkins, we thoroughly looked at many buildings including our own old building's records. This was a time when the $50-million budget had been in effect and census was purportedly down to 3,500 persons. There was essentially no real change. Most telling was the tone of voice and the manner of the many workers and building supervisors with whom we spoke. There was the tinge of whining that we recognized immediately, as if the respondent were trying to say, "Please don't blame me for this. I would not have it this way, but you have to understand how things are here. I've got this job, and for better or worse, I've got to do what I'm told. You just can't do certain things, but it'll get better." People were still on the floor. A few pieces of broken-down furniture, placed there in a pitiful attempt to mask the true and indelible import of those stone rooms of despair. Humanity still writhing, for it was expected to writhe. They were there in the first place because they were "they," not "us."

The lawyers were battling behind the scenes preparing for the trial. The defendants' predictable behavior of deny, delay, divert, deceive, and defy the federal court prevailed. The state put incredible pressure on the federal court to squash the plaintiff's case. It took full advantage of the judge's refusal to address the central issue about which the case really revolved—that is, was there a constitutional right for people with special needs to be served in such a way as to maximize their potential, and to base these services on community living standards?

Instead, the issue was doggedly confined to the Eighth Amendment's right to freedom from cruel and unusual punishment. This narrow focus, this keyhole to squeeze through, threatened the thrust of the whole case. How could questions about community services be admitted that could expose, in comparison, the violence and backwardness of the institution? The lawyers were terribly worried. They felt that Judge Judd was simply too overwhelmed by the magnitude of the problem and the political and economic demand that would fall upon the state if the ruling went beyond the abuse question. Nevertheless, Bruce Ennis, Anita Barret, John Kirkland, a new lawyer Chris Hansen, and Mike Thaler, the lawyer from the United States Justice Department who had entered the case as an amicus on the side of the plaintiffs, forged forward. They marshaled a mountain of expert testimony, data, photographs, and analysis that spilled well over the boundaries of Willowbrook. Now with residents having been stashed all over New York in similar old institutions and similar new ones, the experts had to look at scores of facilities in pursuit of the interests of the class bringing suit.

For the public in New York, the issue had appeared closed for more than a year. Publicity about the 1973 emergency ruling had been thorough, and the department, under the deft public relations management of Mr. Wolfe, continued to bend every effort to carry its campaign to depict itself as a paragon of compliance, virtue, progress, and humanity. But nothing had changed. Only to people directly involved with the lawsuit, to families who suffered the continuation of the insults to their intelligence and the injuries to their kin was the full truth known. The FBI continued to monitor and turn in reports of failure to meet the "cleanup" order that had been issued so long ago. A new feature was added to the whole debacle. Governor Rockefeller had stepped out of the picture and was pursuing more serious policy matters concerning future challenges to his financial world. The lieutenant governor, Malcolm Wilson, had assumed the governorship. An electoral challenge by the Democrats loomed as a sure thing against the colorless politician who sat on New York's throne. Everything in the state was at a standstill. The bureaucracy, paralyzed under normal circumstances, was simply nonfunctional and hung like dead weight on anything requiring a decision. These circumstances prevailed when the final trial hearing opened on October 1, 1974. It was two and one-half years after the case had been originally filed, seventeen months after the emergency order had been handed down. One hundred million dollars[13] had been budgeted and spent at Willowbrook, and nearly twenty times that much had been used statewide. Nothing had changed except the ransom had gone up and off the charts.

I attended two days of the trial to listen and help wherever I could. I had moved to Syracuse, New York, and was carrying on my studies and my teaching trips from the university's Division of Special Education. I had been assigned there by the Department of Mental Hygiene, at my request for an "educational leave" to keep me out of their hair. During the sixteen days of the trial, the lawyers again were able to forge a powerful and compact concentration of testimony, as they had in the 1972 hearing. They outdid themselves in honing the testimony of the professional and scientific leaders down to the most precise and telling evidence. Fifty witnesses and three thousand pages of court testimony were recorded.

Linda Glenn, the executive director of the Eastern Nebraska Office of Retardation (ENCOR), had been with the case since its inception. She testified after seeing Willowbrook again and visiting numerous sites around New York City. Referring to the children she saw at a facility on Wards Island, Linda testified that though she hated to say it, she thought they would be better off back at Willowbrook. So complete was the isolation and lack of any semblance of an environment to raise any child.

There was no break in the theme of the testimony; Willowbrook was absolutely unsalvageable in any form. It had to be closed. The very attempt to provide an education within the structure was sure to "miseducate." There was no conceivable way that any person in the institution could be

---

13   New York State Budget Act approved for 1974–1975.

shaped to develop any fraction of his or her actual potential. This miseducation could only be seen as violence—an abuse. Thus, the greatest teachers, physicians, parent organizers, nurses, researchers, system designers, administrators squeezed their enormous and prestigious bulk through the keyhole for the Orrin Judd trial. As they squeezed, the keyhole soon became a window, then a door, and finally there was no doubt the whole ugly terrible nightmare of the thing lay split open.

The deficiency in programs; the excessive use of drugs; the half-million dollars in clothes that never reached the residents; the food shortages; the collapse of all efforts to solve the laundry crisis within and without the institutions; the high absenteeism of staff; the incompetency of the new administration and all their underlings; the abuse of technology, such as behavior modification pedagogy, being used to conform people to the most inane if not inhuman conditions; the paper programs that were primitive or not in operation and that could not have any value upon those they were intended to emancipate; the grossly inappropriate setting of the entire place, coupled with its history, marking every person who entered those pastoral grounds with a stigma that simply stained their entire lives. All these realities were sounded and shown again. It all boiled down to the absence of any clean-cut philosophy, goals, or objectives that could be measured in familiar human and ethical terms.

The experts came, one after the other, to explain in detail that things didn't have to be that way. That there were, in fact, myriad approaches to solving these seemingly unsolvable problems. That we lived in the twentieth century, not the nineteenth. One did not have to see the challenge of serving such citizens as a futile burden. It could be a joyous opportunity to enrich, in profound ways, the lives of everyone involved. In fact, doing the job right would cost the taxpayers less than half what it was now costing. The key was to see each person as an individual and to tailor individual services to that person in open settings where the very pressure of the congregation of differentness did not render the situation logistically unthinkable.

The role of parents was carefully set forth to the court, especially in planning for the future of their sons and daughters. Parents had a major responsibility to shape these futures, to provide insights, to address specific problems and objectives based on family priorities, to participate in the implementation of any and all programs, and to evaluate and monitor the results. No stone was left unturned or unexamined in all the possible implications of any decision. The court hearing came to a close, and again the familiar curtain of waiting descended.

This time, the lawyers took the initiative. They had gotten immense encouragement from the resolution, after four years, of the Partlow case in Alabama. The case had been appealed from the federal district court ruling of Judge Frank Johnson, and had been sitting before the Fifth Circuit Court, which had to decide the constitutionality of a judgment. The delay was unprecedented. Finally, with another full-blown right-to-treatment order won in Cambridge, Minnesota, against the institutions from which Ristic had come, the circuit court ruling affirmed the "right to treatment."

The lawyers for the Willowbrook plaintiffs, with the help of the parents and their experts, compiled a seventy-page order to be submitted to the judge and hoped it would be adopted as the court's judgment. It became apparent that Judge Judd preferred that all parties could arrive at an agreement among themselves that would establish a "consent decree" rather than require a judgment. The delay pending the consent negotiations again extended the wait.

As had been predicted, Rockefeller's placeholder, Wilson, was defeated by the Democratic contender, Hugh Carey. During the lame-duck period from November 1974 until January 1975, as is always the case when an election causes a reorganization, the bureaucracy was impossible to get anybody in the DMH to negotiate anything. Any decision had to wait until the new administration assumed control and could "study the matter." Again, one had to feel sure that the missile had struck home, for it was damned hard to read the signs.

On April 21, 1975, a news release was sent out:

FOR RELEASE: 11 a.m. Monday, April 21, 1975

NEW YORK, APRIL 21, 1975—The New York Civil Liberties Union, The Legal Aid Society, and the Mental Health Law Project today announced that the parties to a federal law suit involving Willowbrook Developmental Center had reached agreement upon the terms of a consent judgment that would, if approved by the court, resolve the lawsuit. The agreement established detailed standards to guarantee the constitutional rights of the more than 5,000 mentally retarded persons who were all residents of Willowbrook in March, 1972, when the lawsuit was filed. This became known as the Willowbrook Class.

Governor Carey announced that Attorney General Louis Lefkowitz had approved this course of action, and that attorneys for plaintiffs and defendants would promptly be filing a motion asking Federal Judge Orrin G. Judd of the United States District Court for the Eastern District of New York to approve the consent judgment. A hearing would be held on the motion in the near future. After the hearing, Judge Judd would decide whether to approve the agreement and embody it in the form of a consent judgment. Key points mandated in the landmark agreement included:

• Reduce Willowbrook to 250 beds within six years— to serve only people requiring institutional care from Staten Island.

• Establish within a 12 month period, 200 new community placements in hostels, halfway houses, group homes, sheltered workshops, and day care training programs to meet the needs of residents who will be transferred there.

• Request the State Legislature to provide at least $2,000,000* for financing, leasing, and operating the 200 new community placements.

• Request the Legislature to provide additional funds to develop and operate community facilities and programs annually for the next five years. ($5,000,000*)

• Develop an individual plan of care, education, and training for each of Willowbrook's 3,000 remaining residents to prepare them for life in the community.

• No resident shall be transferred from Willowbrook unless the Director determines that the new placement will offer better service and opportunity.

The consent decree sets on-duty ratios of direct care staff to residents of one to four during waking hours for the majority of the residents (children, multi-handicapped, and residents requiring intensive psychiatric care). At the time the suits were filed, the ratio of staff to residents was 1–40 and 1–60 in same wards. It also required an overall ratio of one clinical staff member for every three residents. At least one-third of the clinical staff must be at the professional level. Implementation of the ratios must be accomplished within 13 months.

The decree absolutely forbids seclusion, corporal punishment, degradation, medical experimentation, and the routine use of restraints.

It sets as the primary goal of Willowbrook the preparation of each resident with regard for individual disabilities and capabilities for development and life in the community at large. To this end, the decree mandated individual plans for the education, therapy, care, and development of each resident.

Further provisions in the decree required:

- Six scheduled hours of program activity each weekday for all residents.
- Educational programs for residents including provision for the specialized needs of the blind, deaf, and multi-handicapped.
- Well-balanced and nutritionally adequate diets.
- Dental services for all.
- No more than eight residents can live or sleep in a unit.
- A minimum of two hours of daily recreational activities—indoors and out—and availability of toys, books, and other materials.
- Eyeglasses, hearing aids, wheelchairs, and other adaptive equipment where needed.
- Adequate and appropriate clothing.
- Physicians on duty 24 hours daily for emergency cases.
- A contract with one or more accredited hospitals for acute medical care.
- A full scale immunization program for all residents within three months.
- Compensation for voluntary labor in accordance with applicable minimum wage laws.
- Correction of health and safety hazards including covering radiators and steam pipes to protect residents from injury, repairing broken windows, and removing cockroaches, and other insects and vermin.

The procedures must be accomplished within 13 months.

An extremely important feature of the consent agreement involved the creation of three boards:

- A seven-member Review Panel with primary responsibility for overseeing the implementation of standards and procedures mandated in the Consent Decree.
- A seven-member Consumer Advisory Board comprised of parents and relatives of residents, community leaders, residents, and former residents to evaluate alleged dehumanizing practices and violations of individual and legal rights.
- A seven-member Professional Advisory Board giving advice on all professional programs and plans, budget requests, and objectives; investigating alleged violations; and assisting in recruitment and training of staff.
- The terms of the Consent Decree applied only to the 5,209 persons who were the Willowbrook Class residents when the suits were filed. Thus, the agreement directly applied not only to current Willowbrook residents but also to those residents who had been transferred to other state institutions for the mentally retarded.

On April 22, a meeting was held in Manhattan, and all the principals signed the agreement. The suit was over for the moment. The state had been found guilty on all counts. It had been forced in some small measure to begin the process of making amends for its crimes at Willowbrook. It had taken a little over three years, an unimaginable expense of time and effort by the country's top leadership in the field of human services, the top lawyers, the most extraordinary group of mothers, fathers, sisters, brothers, and friends of the hostages in Willowbrook.

On the heels of the incredible victory began another episode that had yet to be played out. The order had to be converted into reality. Though the judge and the federal court retained jurisdiction, the composition and efficacy of the review panel referred to in the press release was at the heart of the matter. This extra-departmental body had unparalleled potential power from specific authority given it by the court. It virtually was to set aside the primacy of the New York State Department of Mental Hygiene bureaucracy in decision-making for the first time in all these months. Real power was vested in this body, the majority of whose members were to be agreed upon by the plaintiffs.

The dinosaur was far from dead. It is only Willowbrook that has been challenged to some extent, while new lucrative construction for more Willowbrooks proceeded everywhere in New York and around the United States. The war was far from over. It was but a momentary plateau from which we could survey the long struggle ahead.

What can we see in the aftermath? The implications for the states are mixed. The thought of closing the institutions is in a way secretly appealing to state governors and the rich. Thousands of civil servants would be dumped out of work, relieving the states of an enormous financial burden. But closing the institutions also poses an inconceivable shock to the system that far outweighs the potential monetary benefit. Even where action has been taken to close institutions, the states have usually taken the easy way out, dumping the institution residents precipitously into the community without preparation. Notwithstanding the outcomes of subsequent class action suits in various states where the courts finally created standards for community settings that required statewide, system-wide training and sometimes required reaccreditation of facilities, measures have not been taken to provide the kind of community resources that would help people to develop "lives of high spirit and creativity." Almost universally, the states seemed either uncommitted to a total responsible plan or incapable of devising one. Pressed by the massive front of multistate litigation, it is predictable that the targeted states would be perpetually in noncompliance and begrudgingly shift their monoliths to neighborhood warehousing as the population ages.

Most vulnerable and sensitive to the situation were the families who had already adjusted to the institution as a solution. They had accepted it as a preferable alternative to no help at all, or in distrust of the state's commitment to community services—in fear of betrayal. As decades passed, the public sees the precarious conditions on the streets of America for people who may not have all the abilities to fiercely compete for enfranchised status, personal life space, and essential care. To these families, the institution, the Title 19 Medicaid-funded network of profitable nursing and assisted living "homes" is a culturally familiar symbol and concrete guarantee of security.

As the institutional path now forked to establish community-integrated and inclusive life, a wrenching breach occurred among the parent groups. There were those who clung, without pause to reflect, to the secure image promised by the institution. There were others, the "community parents", who would rather put their kin to death than allow them to be absorbed by the monstrosity of the institution. And yet these are people who have a common claim. They breathe a common air of oppression. So terrifying is this division, so irrational is its expression that it is almost impossible to reconcile the bitterness that we saw escalate among these struggling and sincere families. On this discontent and confusion the beast thrives, for it can beguile, stall, and slither backward to try to stem the hemorrhage that it is experiencing. It may appear to become stronger than ever. Its assailants have become locked in combat with each other over the possession of the carcass, one to use it as a shelter, the other as a museum to remind us of the lessons learned in another time—Dachau, Bergen-Belsen, Auschwitz.

The tragic breach among the parents is well illustrated by excerpts from a letter written by the mother of a child with Down syndrome I received. She describes her experience at a parent meeting where she attempted to oppose support of institutions and speak out for the community living concept.

March 17

Dear Bill,

Well, I hardly know where to begin describing the fiasco of my first confrontation, When the meeting began, the head woman made it clear that this was an organization only for parents whose children resided in state schools. (The newspapers did not specify that). As her speech continued, she sounded very middle-of-the-road and nonbelligerent, stating they did not oppose community services for those who could utilize then, but their own children could not, so they were a special interest group for this area. At this point I almost changed my mind about speaking up in favor of community services, but my husband encouraged me to speak up. And I thought of all the people I had committed myself to including and most of all, you and my daughter.

When they finally opened the floor to discussion, a woman stood up in the audience and spouted off about the "normalization conference" earlier this year and was everyone "aware" that "they" are preparing to close down institutions and throw your children in the street where they would live in group homes with alcoholics, derelicts, drug addicts, rapists? And they want to do away with diagnostic labels! Then one very calm person explained the Association for Retarded Citizens' middle-of-the-road policy in not wanting state school's budget cut but merely wanting to request additional funds for community services. He also said he wasn't aware of any group homes such as she described.

Then another father got up and parroted the middle-of-the-road thing & then said, "Yes, institutions used to be very bad. Many times our child was abused. But in the last few years this has changed due to this parents group making changes in the system. Now, we're very grateful to the administration for allowing us to see our children."

God, I nearly died when I heard that!

I couldn't contain myself any longer and got up. I started out by saying I didn't realize they were a closed group—the newspaper hadn't pointed that out—and I was concerned about the same points that were publicly stated and the fact that the public would also easily get the impression that their group represented all retarded people. Woman #1 said it was stated twice in each article that membership was limited only to state school parents. I said it wasn't, and continued I talked about the successful alternatives that exist in Nebraska & Pennsylvania.

At this point, the president of the group cut me off by saying, "Oh, you just think Nebraska's program is so successful. What you don't hear is that ENCOR's death rate is 25% higher." (She didn't say higher than what!!) A friend was so angry she blurted out, "Lady, where are your statistics to prove that?" The president said she didn't have them with her and at this time said we were not here to debate issues and could see no reason for me to continue. I turned to the audience and said, "I am a parent and think I have a right to say what I feel. May I please be allowed to continue." I got a round of applause. So I continued. Then I finally mentioned "normalization" all hell broke loose over that word. There was noise & shuffling around and talking and people got up to get coffee. But I just talked louder.

Finally one of the women who had spoken earlier got up and walked over to me and interrupted, saying, "The meeting is temporarily adjourned for refreshments and you are out of order!!" I never had a chance to continue and say all the uniting words I planned to in the end.

One woman from the audience came up to me and said, "I can't believe they did that to you. They are horrible and uncivilized." Then another woman got up and tried to smooth ruffled feathers and get back on the damned middle-of-the-road track again, at my expense. She said, "We just can't have this arguing like we've seen tonight. We need to pull together. Just contact your legislator and let him know what you're in favor of." She went on and basically said what I was trying to get across, but instead of saying one word to support me, she made me sound like the troublemaker!

We decided to leave after that. I couldn't listen to any more of that shit. On the way out, a couple of older parents came up to pity me, saying they knew how I felt—that they had all fought when they were young, too, but they feel too old to fight anymore and have found a measure of security in having their child in the state school and they wouldn't have to worry about what happened to her after they were gone. One asked me about my child and I said, "She's 6 years old, Down's syndrome and rubella, classed as severely retarded, and lives at home." She said, "Oh, honey, she'd be so much happier in the state school with her own!" I said, "No ma'am!" She wouldn't! She's very happy right where she is. She is accepted in our community and family and I wouldn't think of having her live somewhere else!

No one else that was supposed to have been there in my support even came up and acknowledged knowing us, except these people. I held up okay till I got home and then it all came out. I didn't sleep much that night. My husband assured me that the rest of my compatriots were just too scared to speak to me or for me that night but that they would contact me the next day. Well, one did, I still haven't heard from the rest.

Well, I thought about it long and hard, but I'm not sorry I did what I did. It may not have accomplished all that I set out to, but my words did expose what a closed-minded, uncivilized, rude treacherous group they are.

I am most upset to discover that my "friends" would rather compromise their ideals than to budge from that damned middle-of-the-road approach!! And I don't know how all this will affect our future relations. If anything, I am stronger than ever convinced that I want to fight for my daughter's right to be a part of normal life (even with its risks) than to be subjugated in a place where I lose all say about what happens to her and where I would be forced to accept crumbs from a damned bureaucracy that might "allow me to see my child!"

What I hate so about this group is they are purposely spreading awful lies and making the most of issues by sensationalism to scare the shit out of all these old parents who only want a little peace in knowing their child will be cared for after they die! They are purposely playing on the emotions of these old people! It's despicable and I want to throw up!

Love,
Patricia

Almost nowhere is the clear analysis presented that would blast away the false dichotomy and unite the family voluntary organizations in a stronger union than ever. The families have yet to learn how to agree on issues and programs, and let the best outcomes determine where their effort is to be directed. In no way can even the most radical profession turn out the quarter-million institutionalized hostages overnight into the underdeveloped human service systems that exist everywhere. Every effort had to be bent to create successful models at local and regional levels as ground to assure the unbelieving. Policy and public investment had to drive the complex tasks, professional and volunteer resources committed to social development. Otherwise, there can be only catastrophe. In the conflict, the sad spin-off from the internal struggle of the parents is that the wounds of the beast heal, rather than a balanced plan devised to create the choice that would end the tyranny.

It is the thesis of this work, repeated over and over again, that there can be no such thing as good institutions. Their very nature stands against the virtues of humanity. They are a political creation predicated on values and assumptions that deny liberty, life, growth, and achievement. At any time, congregate segregated institutions can turn into centers for concentrated neglect and abuse. It is just not worth the effort to police them when we need to be about the business of building a new future. Betrayal is always close at hand.

Institutions in the United States could be closed down in ten years! Compromise adds decades more of backwardness for every year of timidity—now when the issues have been drawn so sharply, when the courts have lent their weight, when almost virgin conditions exist to launch the proper ideology. Where will the offensive spring from on the national level if the National Association for Retarded Citizens still feels the need to play ball with the perpetrators of public hostage relations and their sycophant promises of protection? The leadership feared losing touch and confidence among their membership and were still supplicants to the old order. The Association faced the challenge to marshal its progressive forces, win new friends, establish alliances with all groups demanding social change, recognize the profound political implications of it position in the country, cast aside its false respectability, and don modern armor. Without risk and boldness, there would be no gain. "It must dare to struggle and dare to win."

Burton Blatt in his beautiful book *Exodus from Pandemonium* sums up this modern reality:

> It is possible that this Movement will fail,
>
> That there will be no reformation of State Schools,
>
> It will fail, if we have miscalculated and struggled for
>
> reform, when, all the while
>
> The need was to Revolutionize.

CHAPTER 30

From Underdevelopment, the Agony of Change

THE ASSAULT ON THE institutional system that was launched by people indicting Willowbrook has been a constant around the nation. The expressions of outrage and protest have been a gut response on the part of grassroots parents and new generations of young professionals. The situation had looked so simple. Where there is evil, address it, name it, and it will be swept away—that is the American ethos. The movement gained its momentum and inspiration through this kind of idealism. A sense of purpose and righteousness ignited the struggle against conditions that had gone unchallenged for decades. The promises for help and a better life had come to be cruel deceptions. Persuasion, appeals, and petitions had failed, and the courts seemed to be the only recourse.

There was growing turmoil among those parents who could feel the dilemma of the responsibilities to be thrust on them by a legal judgment. Still, the courts symbolized for most a setting for the redress of grievance. It was a stage colored by the wish for justice and relief, by the conviction that change was but a judgment away. The institutions, invisible and unaccountable, would be brought to heel and forced to obey the law of the land. It was that simple. And the bigger and loftier the court, the belief held, the more legitimate, the less tainted with vested interests would be the judge. So, suits were raised from state to state to emancipate the thousands of people in state institutions. Trial after trial opened. Idealism blew like pollen on the wind from New York to Tennessee, Minnesota, Massachusetts, Texas, New Jersey, Indiana, Illinois, Kentucky, Alabama, Florida, Colorado, and the rest. Fernald, the first institution that had opened in Massachusetts in 1848, closed in 2014. Lanterman, the old Pacific State Hospital, closed at the end of December 2014 in California.

The thing that was not expected was the consistent intransigence of the institutional system. The lawsuits dragged on and on. Hearings were postponed. Delays plagued every legal action. But more disturbing than the delays were the complex changes that evolved in the parent community. All were struck with a new insight. It came from a revulsion at what they saw and the recognition of the sobering implications of the challenge against the institutions.

The numberless tendrils and roots that the institutional system had sent out, binding it to the very core of society, became apparent, and in the effort to change the beast, a new knowledge of society slowly spread among all of us. New breakthroughs poured into the ranks of the change agents. But this flood of new information and a more objective understanding of the tenacious roots of institutions in America led to confusion. We had initially bitten off more than could be swallowed. Now all state advocates were urged to move toward community. The evil we were culturally fighting was the commodification of people, people with disabilities, and the entire elder population. What unfolded was the realization, the practice that evil can be locked in a group home because there is no staff to take a person out or ensure a minimum of a private shower once weekly, where clothes and possessions are commonly stolen.

It may well be that this experience of initial shock is in store for all people who embark on a course of anti-institutional social action and change. The feeling of being overwhelmed is the unavoidable and predictable opposite side of idealism. Here, the greatest test of strength emerges. For those of us caught in this struggle, there was a truth about established forces in society that had to be recognized and accepted. Otherwise the enthusiastic expression of idealism would crumple, ultimately unraveling the wave of activism and movement that had spread so remarkably in New York.

It is well worth sketching this agony of change the context in which the public movement gradually found itself. It appears that unless we respect the feelings and experiences that had always threatened to slow down the militancy of the struggle, we may miss the most important lesson of this entire period as it relates to the present. In periods of confusion about who and what is the problem at hand, when it seems that everything may be lost, paradoxically, there exists the greatest opportunity for a leap forward to unify greater numbers of people.

The tumultuous period of the 1960s was when the anti-institutional protests, the acceleration of the disability rights movement evolved, a period when the civil rights movement, the Vietnam War, domestic economic depression, with its spiraling costs and savage cuts in public human services struck. The long history of warehousing devalued citizens and the immense cost and confidence invested in this monolithic service approach had resulted in the starkest underdevelopment of services in every community and neighborhood. Alternatives were not on the public agenda. A broad-based organized impetus for the evolution of noninstitutional New York models was still to be mounted. Thus, when the early call for service needs did make itself heard, private enterprise was the default sought to fill the need and, opportunistically, develop community services. The New York AHRC established ownership of group homes, real estate that erased the line between nonprofit and for-profit entities. The drama of the Geraldo Rivera ABC exposé led to the search in the nonprofit sector for expedited "homes" to be generated in distrust of the ponderous and corrupt state mental hygiene system.

The fact is that human services, properly provided on an individualized basis, are not very profitable, because such services are based on people's sharing skills and lives with one another. Yet, it was always profits that guided the building and maintenance of new kinds of institutions engineered by the always hungry private insurance industry and defense-oriented charity sector. When services were needed in the community, the "smaller" nursing home with its fifty to three hundred beds was almost universally the only response that proprietary and "nonprofit" agencies found remunerative. Giant corporate enclaves drawing on the massive flush of Medicaid dollars to states and locales saw the clear chances to fill their tanks. Despite the clear shortcomings to really change the fundamental quality of life for the people with disabilities who were housed in them, the times generated a growing river of society's elders and the victims of endless Mideast wars that matched and dwarfed the traditional cohort of those with developmental disabilities. The commercial conclusion was drawn that the value and need for such "small institutions" had to be seized with a fury.

In the wake of Robert Kennedy's visits in the 1960s and Geraldo Rivera's coverage of the conditions there in the early 1970s, in a meeting with key leaders of the Willowbrook panel, the advocacy leaders of the sister class action lawsuit at Pennhurst State School in Pennsylvania learned that between 1972 and 1977, nearly two thousand people had moved out of Willowbrook. However, none of the court's review panel officials knew where they had gone, or if they were "better off."

Under the aggressive research leadership of Jim Conroy, and Temple University, an intimate quality-of-life follow-along study was mounted. Every Pennhurst class action lawsuit member was personally visited with scientific quality-of-life measurement tools every year. Every next-of-kin family member or guardian was surveyed by mail and telephone every year. Conroy started the study with the hypothesis that people would be significantly worse off after leaving Pennhurst, because by 1978, that was known to have happened for Americans with mental illness who were deinstitutionalized from state psychiatric hospitals.[14]

The comparative findings were dramatically different. People who moved from Pennhurst into Pennsylvania's small group homes, with three or fewer people, were better off in almost every way the researchers were able to measure. Self-care skills and independence went up; challenging behavior went down. Services delivered went up, integrative experiences went far up, the opportunity to make choices about matters large and small went up, time occupied during daytime hours went sharply up, and satisfaction expressed by all the people able to communicate was dramatically higher. (About half of all the Pennhurst folks were unable to respond to interviews, whether verbal or by signs or pictures.)

In all the years of interviews with the people themselves, only a handful ever expressed a wish that they could return to Pennhurst. And after a few years, even those wishes changed. The oldest person at Pennhurst did not want to leave, but later he told interviewers, "These years [in the small community home] have been the happiest of my 90 years."

Most powerful among the outcomes were the changes in family attitudes. At the time the court ordered community placement, about 80 percent of families opposed the idea. Later, over 90 percent supported it. Of all the four hundred plus families interviewed in 1982, not one said their Pennhurst relative was "less happy" or "much less happy." These were among the most compelling findings of the entire study. Families saw the changes in daily life, and they were stunned. Hundreds of letters were written to the survey scientists at Temple, and many expressed the sentiment that they were very sorry they had worked so hard to keep their relative at the institution. They had no idea that life could be so good for their relative. At this time in history, no one knew that people could be so much better off after leaving an institution at such a cost savings. More kindness, more empathy, more quality of life—at less cost. It becomes objectively clear what was right, but the economic forces that built the institutional infrastructure was, and is, so strong. Most awful is the dependence of so many human care public unions with their workers concentrated in such remote areas where the big money located their largest institutional structures.

Among the Willowbrook class that were the first wave to be deinstitutionalized, anecdotes showed astounding parallel benefits in every category of behavioral and emotional improvement and success

---

14   Bassuk, E. L., and Gerson, S. [1978]. "Deinstitutionalization and Mental Health Services." Scientific American, 238, 46–53.

in the community. However, the underfunding and low social value of the emancipated population naturally resulted in continued segregation, low wage, and poor person staffed community "alternatives" that barely met the developmental needs of young adults. Initially, many families, though distrustful of the remote Albany, New York, state bureaucracy in the first place, became convinced that the institutions might again be their only salvation and that the "community alternatives" might, in fact, be a worse solution after all.

Still, forced to comply with growing pressures for deinstitutionalization, the public bureaucracies thrust into unprepared low-income communities the very members of society who for decades had been excluded and warehoused. As if cynically seeking a backlash, many departments of mental hygiene released thousands of mental patients into communities, with an incredible insensitivity to the cultural conditions in America's neighborhoods that led to exploding homelessness and rubbing raw the age-old attitudes and prejudices of society. Not the slightest meaningful preparation of the public was undertaken. Large numbers of people were put into areas where land was cheap or where zoning there provided considerable initial openness to accepting stigmatized population neighborhoods. Here, persons could be plowed into what soon became zoned ghettos of deviancy. The public backlash was fueled with predictable consequences of organized NIMBY neighborhood resistance. The mindless and rote actions of the bureaucracies were seen as assaults on property and community values, and were and are fought vigorously. Dumping, the general practice of piling people into communities without any preparation or material integrative supports, created its powerful opposite force. The real issues and beneficiaries were intentionally obscured.

Communities responded in deeply emotional ways. In a powerful monograph titled "Out of Their Beds and into the Streets," published by the American Federation of State, County, and Municipal Employees in 1975, Harry Santiestevan wrote:

> Twelve years after the initiation of community mental health centers, only 500 of a planned 2,000 had been built. In 1972 there were only 10,609 beds in community mental health centers, compared with 360,578 in state and county psychiatric hospitals (these would include people in mental retardation facilities).
>
> The libertarian court decisions pushed mental health costs upwards from $6 per patient day during the mid-1950s to $20 today. The courts were handing down complex court orders that called for major improvements in institutional care. For financially pressed state governments, the easy way out of the cost squeeze was to cut hospital budgets and send the patients to private nursing homes eligible for federal (resources such as) Medicare, Medicaid, and Social Security payment.

In New York and California, the two states that pioneered "deinstitutionalization" of mental patients, hastily reversed their policies after a wave of nursing home scandals, violent crimes, and protests from communities forced to accept ex-inmates.

The general credibility collapse of elected and appointed officials throughout the nation did not begin with the likes of Watergate. In almost every state, scandals had been characteristic of the crude and halting actions of departments of mental hygiene. In almost monolithic monotony, bureaucracies had fostered warehousing, cloistered systems, and human abuse that would burst every so often with a newspaper exposé or other such exhibition of the untrustworthiness of the public service sector.

Accompanying this phenomenon was the consistent bureaucratic and professional defensiveness that rarely, if ever, admitted to failures or to its increasing lack of touch with the public. It preferred a safe retreat behind "expertise" and authority, a retreat leading inevitably to cover-up of the scandals.

An equal battleground has historically been rivalry between the mental hygiene profession paradigm and the educational and developmental professions over who should or should not be responsible for the budget and services to the population labelled as "mentally retarded." Traditionally, the mental health profession, with its heavy jurisdiction over the word "mental," its medical approach, and its long-established institutional history, claimed ownership over the definition and medical management of the chronic, "incurable" condition peculiar to "the retarded." Since the money and prestige that are involved are no mere trifle, the rivalry still continues as fiercely as ever, with the general society and the people who need services caught in the middle of the professional turf fight.

The fallout of this jurisdictional struggle for control is earmarked by the constant top-down shuffling of service forms and structures within the competing bureaucracies themselves. A new commissioner, a new department reorganization, or some other such paper change keep things looking fluid and frustratingly inaccessible to the public. In fact, the whole situation is bankrupt from Band-Aid reforms with no fundamental recognition of the root causes of the social and management challenges.

Following on this interprofessional competition, the consumer community and especially the parents who rely on and trust the medical and educational professions are constantly realigning and splintering in relation to a new label or new condition "discovery" made within the scientific community. Terms such as "brain injury," "autism," "developmental disability," "intellectual disability," "PTSD," and "drug dependency" result in the change of jurisdiction—power and money—within the bureaucracies and professions. Parent charity and advocacy defense organizations consequently must also group and regroup. As the institutional system loses its heretofore unquestioned reliability and monopoly, so the parents' organizations, previously rallied about the institutions, become splintered and insecure.

The pragmatic unity that had generally prevailed in a simpler time has been shattered. Simultaneously, organized human service workers, institutional workers, and teachers in the community have been made to feel insecure by the uncertainty of jobs, the attack on their living standards, the differential in wages between public and private, state and local workers, the unwillingness of the public power structure to meaningfully assume basic responsibility for human service development, and the trend toward decentralization and community control. In their vulnerability, human service workers tend to be easily manipulated by many union misleaders. These public-employee union bureaucrats use the narrowest and most selfish economic concerns to pit their members against the developments that challenge the backwardness of traditional institutions. At the same time, the fragile alliance between the union leaders and the political power structure are increasingly threatened as new democratic militant leadership arises among the rank and file. The need to keep the workers under control and to keep them turned against consumers of service as well as against their natural allies in the community grows more desperate every day for the old-line union bureaucrats.

The controversy over integration and mainstreaming is just one of the issues that has rattled teachers against community family demands. The introduction of an additional youngster into an already overcrowded and impossible classroom situation, especially when that child needs individual attention, is more than most teachers can bear. To top off the whole mess, the need for mediation in this confusion has caused the system to produce the concept of "advocacy," which is a new branch of work for people to monitor and watchdog abuses. All too often, these advocacy positions are sponsored from within the bureaucracy itself in an attempt to capture this responsibility for its own employees, over whom it maintains power and control. These are but a few of the phenomena that boil and confront us.

Some clear forecasts of our gains and losses can be made and are rooted in the conditions that surround us. We can use these forecasts not only to prepare us for the temporary losses that we must inevitably suffer, but also to help us plan objectively toward the gains that are possible to win.

If we render down all the many varied value systems operating in most of the world in this new century, there are two basic and divergent roads that divide people. On the one hand is the ideological system that presumes all people are equally valuable, share a common destiny, and therefore deserve respect. This view holds that each person is basically more alike than different. All human beings develop and grow from experience, from environmental and social conditions to which they are subjected. Differences in people are a function of material reality, not a mystical specialness within a person, culture, or race. Differences among people are a cause for celebration and a source of social enrichment. A gain is any event that strengthens the integration and public value of all citizens, no matter what their degree of dependency on society.

On the other hand, the ideology exists that presumes that basic superiority, enhanced through competition, creates deserved privilege. There are some who win and some who lose. That is the way of all things. Individuals are more different than alike. If you are too different, you are less valued, stigmatized, less deserving, and fall lower on the ladder of success (or survival) than the rest.

One loss that can be forecast is that due to unprecedented wealth consolidation among fewer and fewer of the rich, fewer resources will be available for human and social services in general. Thus, a service funding shrinkage is likely toward the more traditional and impersonal services solutions. What is familiar and has worked in the past will be reflexively reforged. Within this frame, there will be a greater and greater search for individual relief, rather than people openly recognizing the need for society-wide solutions to the pressing problems of our lives.

There will be more bureaucratic shifts to avoid root changes in human services. The bureaucracy will continue to be deregulated and grow out of control, rather than be dismantled. Many actual services will suffer the cuts and constrictions of declining budgets. Segregation will increase, as will depersonalization and dehumanization— despite lip service and even laws to the opposite. We see the established order creating mechanisms to legitimize class and ethnic differences, segregation and labeling policies with ever more elegant rationalizations and brutal structures. An ultimate case in point is the growing medicalizing of age and warehousing of older people, excused by the equating of being old with a bankable commodity.

Another painful reality will be the continued weakening and corrupting of advocacy and voluntary associations, saddled with dwindling resources as people increasingly ignore charity appeals because of the tightening of the earnings at home.

Looming ahead most ominously are the increasing cloaked pressures for killing off the unwanted. Euthanasia and extermination pressures will mount as surely they did in Germany before the Second World War. These will come under the guise of humanity, dignity, and democracy, and they will fall first upon the neck of people with disabilities and the aged. The ground has already been laid for such contrived atrocities, from years of medical and social labeling, burdensome cost of care to the oligarchy, changing public perceptions about the social status and integrity of such folks, and having a major tradition of segregating such people and interpreting them as "less than you or I" in every subtle turn of phrase and reference.

The two major groups of special needs Americans owe their survival to the professionals and to the taxpayers, each looking for their own special way out of these responsibilities.

We now exist in a world of frightening demagoguery, economic insecurity, rising unemployment and underemployment, inflation, recession—and of privileged special interests that increasingly command the nation's wealth. This creates a paradox: The call to not forget the lowly, to help out, to give "them" the right to a life carries the taint of second-class citizenship. These slogans, sooner rather than later, will backfire and easily be recruited to fuel familiar euthanasia appeals and efforts unless a paradigm shift to advance human rights is inspiringly asserted.

It can also be certainly forecast that there will be continued reliance on and expansion of private enterprise in human services, as is monumentally enshrined in the Affordable Care Act (Obamacare) where the public sector continues to reject its responsibility for serving people in need through studied propaganda against expanded and improved Medicare for All as the most obvious solution to universal rightful health care. The bought-and-paid-for Congress majority will continue its obedient role of pouring public money into all more than a thousand huge private insurance coffers as ransom, $787-billion subsidy to the private insurance industry in Obamacare.

There will be an unabated surge in the construction and expansion of large and small segregated institutions, which is unavoidable, in the short run, because of the momentum of the Medicaid-fueled machinery that has been established to that end and the unwillingness on the part of the public or private sector to halt this market and family extortion as we all age.

This tendency is best exemplified in the four newer New York psychiatric centers—Capitol District, Elmira, Hutchings, and South Beach. "These institutions are committed to the maximum use of outpatient treatment methods and minimization of hospitalization."

This statement is absolute insanity. Here stand four of the largest construction projects that were undertaken in the Department of Mental Hygiene, all built within five years after the Willowbrook case was filed. Capitol District cost $37 million ($176.7 million, 2020); Hutchings, $26 million ($ 124.2 million, 2020); Elmira, $20 million ($95.5 million, 2020); and South Beach, $32 million ($152.85 million, 2020). These four symbols of the past were built to house inpatients, yet as the pressures upon the department grew, the rhetoric changed. These examples of gross public waste must now be interpreted and sold as "outpatient" centers.

The crushing public cost, waste, charlatanism, and scandals intrinsic to large state and "nonprofit" institutional empires will continue to be exposed. This must lead to their transformation and their ultimate dismantling. The taxpaying public cannot long sustain the costs imposed by a facade and claims that are not able to show health benefits but instead inexcusable drops in all globally based indicators of health and well-being—longevity, maternal and infant death and morbidity, and chronic disease incidences. Institutional culture and psychiatry in particular doggedly hold to rationales and service approaches that are totally opposite to all social norms and expectations at unaffordable costs.

There will be a slow but accelerating application of public health prevention and screening technology as it becomes manifestly evident that more than half of the conditions that disable our fellow citizens can be prevented and solved. A life of institutional care now costs us nearly $6.6 million. Early intervention of many disabling conditions with screening and helping intervention may cost $33,000. Home care and direct family subsidies must develop more broadly once "long-term care" Medicaid policies are replaced and humanized. Nationally there has been an embargo on providing direct subsidy and support to the parents of a child or adult with special needs. Out-of-home placement has been required before assistance is available that is only slowly being replaced by state "waivers" to allow money directed to the home. The demand to support the family, home, and neighborhood is the most creative and functional way these natural realities will grow stronger.

Without system-wide imposed drug company reform, we will see more and more self-serving and profit-driven research. The conflation of public university research ending in private pharmaceutical cartel patent hands is everywhere evident in the staggering essential drug prices and redundant repackaged products. For the better part of the twentieth century, elite professional organizations like the American Medical Association and the American Dental Association, through significant leadership wealth, greed, and conflicts of interest, support the worst and most backward public policies rather than taking a true leadership position to assure universal health for all and by not making contemporary science and technology popular, understandable, and affordable to the public. The more obscure and secretive the healing science can be made, the more it maintains the mystique, privilege, and ease of commercial exploitation by the professional class. This is at the expense of quality, universal, and accountable open-source research that relies on an informed and competent population for direction, priorities, and benefits.

Our contemporary experience is that extremely well-funded political demagoguery will reign and significantly block the chances for enlightened democratic leadership. This robs the public of truly unifying public policy and the volunteer and grassroots memberships of their ability to organize around their own creative power. Misleadership means opting for short-term and self-interest rather than long-term gains, excusing conflicts of interest. It means mishandling disputes among people with common interests because of entrenched male chauvinism, class and racist biases. It means a piecemeal and competitive approach to problem-solving. These backward tendencies are always hinged to profits, personal fears of exposure, failure, loss, or isolation.

Culturally, a potent underlying cause of our system cruelty is our manipulated practice of blaming the victim—the poor, black and brown, undocumented, addicted, unproductive, homeless, mentally ill, illiterate, aged, and on and on. Our language conveniently allows us to define the problem, via a label or some such device, as an intrinsic defect in the individual. We seldom hear that society cannot creatively make a meaningful place for persons who are genuinely different in the way they think or function. In our modern obsession with the convenient, the comfortable, the plastic, the easy, the magical way, we ignore a basic reality: all growth is slow, risky, and more likely to fail than succeed at first. Our mistrust of the concept and realities of development and our cultural reliance on experts, superstars, and spectacles plague us all. Somehow, we must shed these corrosive fallbacks, or we are in danger of being forever alienated from our collective social class power and destiny as human beings.

We can count on a number of things that will be chalked up as positive gains in human services. The overwhelming digital technological revolution in the means of production that is connecting us in infinite ways to share, learn, understand, influence, and access all human experience has changed all society that will continue beyond our imaginations. There is now a relentless expansion and sophistication of public understanding and activism for human rights, especially among our youth. The demand is growing for individualized services delivered ever closer to every home and neighborhood for all people. No longer is it necessary to require that people travel great distances to the population centers in order to have their health, education, or social service needs met, even those that are esoteric and have specialized needs. As the genius of the Internet continues to expand even into the most remote and rural parts of society, access to information and one another, within seconds, becomes asymptotic. With it will grow a local reidentification with the kinds of unusual people who formerly have been sent away to get help and been lost to society.

Last, and most important, there will be the advent of national right to tax-based, guaranteed, quality health-care services for every American resident in concert with the rest of the developed world. This pending system will universalize expanded and improved Medicare for All, what is referred to as single-payer health care. Of every great social problem we face, health care, as a right, is the only solution that is already fully funded for all US residents now as the United States pays fully twice as much as any other country in the world. Eliminating all the private insurance middlemen, radically simplifying the current administration nightmare, and forcing genuine negotiations for price reductions for all hospital services and drugs will free up hundreds of billions of dollars that will ensure comprehensive health care for all and have a profound impact on our grassroots democracy. People will have to democratically own, plan, decentralize, and reorganize existing and new medical resources and personnel to be available in every neighborhood, including the most geographically isolated or poor urban communities. Health services, like a public utility, require the public consolidation of all dollars for health, wellness, dental, social determinants, and lifetime care through a public single payer resulting to an expanded and improved Medicare with no out-of-pocket costs of any kind. The implementation of a national healthcare service, such as it exists in the developed world, is an inevitable step to end the rampaging annual inflationary cost and to truly take corporate profit and greed out of all health-care delivery. As education, fire and police, and highway maintenance is accepted as a tax-based right of all citizens, health care is even more fundamental to life and must be available in the highest quality for all people, regardless of any socioeconomic differences.

All of these things will evolve not because they are good ideas, but because of larger philosophical and economic forces that are as much at work in our society as those oppositional forces that have a stranglehold on the status quo. We are largely a society of individuals, poorly united together, to wield our democratic power. We are vulnerable to being manipulated by mass media, rampant consumerism in the hands of a small minority, and their funded apparatchiks who profit from and promote our fears, divisions, and secondary differences. If we are to achieve gains, we must find our essential collective power and compassion.

What appears to be an anchor inhibiting our social development must be turned into its opposite, a rocket to thrust us forward into the future. Seeing the dual aspect of all things is the agony of change.

CHAPTER 31

Continuo

IN 1974, NEW YORK State's new governor, Hugh Carey, was sworn into office. There was also a new commissioner of the Department of Mental Hygiene, Dr. Lawrence Kolb, respected but long loyal to the bureaucracy, holding both public and private sector full-time mental health positions for many years, and having received the highest recognition from the psychiatric profession—presidency of the American Psychiatric Association—assumed the post of power. What was the prognosis for reform? Surely, with new leadership and with campaign promises to clean up the institutional system, there would be a surge forward, a new spirit of responsiveness. Surely this new governor and this new commissioner had nothing to gain from being identified with the old way.

In January 1975, four people died at Rome State School. There was some question about the circumstances of four people dying in just one day. There was some concern that no licensed doctor was on duty to attend to the matter.

There were some questions about the contribution to the deaths by the over-crowded institution itself. Its ancient brick buildings were filled with 3,500 people, deposited there from all the state of New York without any adequate parent watch-dog mechanism to speak for the rights of those hostages. There were, in fact, a lot of questions.

A demand to investigate the matter was made of the governor, who agreed some questions existed. Dr. Kolb was instructed to carry out the investigation. On May 3, this effort began. Harold Wolfe, assistant commissioner for communications, called Dr. William Vorhees Jr., director of the newly formed regional office overseeing the DMH empire in upstate New York, where Rome is located. Interestingly, Dr. Vorhees had been first deputy director, an appointed job, under the Miller regime. The job was vacated, and Vorhees seemed to be out under the new appointment of Kolb as commissioner. Then lo and behold, here was Vorhees, one of the key architects of the institutional system, in a civil service slot, protected with an income for life from the vicissitudes of political change. According to a newspaper report in Syracuse, "Wolf said Vorhees had reviewed 'detailed information' given him by Cornelius Walsh, Director of the Rome 'Developmental Center' (renamed from State School during the trial), and ruled that there were no grounds for further investigation."

Walsh had confirmed the deaths of the four persons—a seventy-three-year-old woman who choked to death, a twenty-year-old woman and a ten-year-old boy with bronchial pneumonia, and a seventy-eight-year-old man with pulmonary congestion. "Based on the information provided him, Vorhees has ruled that there was nothing questionable about the deaths or the way they were handled." Thus, that evening, the same day that the investigation was to be launched, it was called off by the state.

It was decided to mount a citizens' investigation independent of the department with its new commissioner. The prestigious American Association on Mental Deficiency (AAMD) was the largest of the professional organizations in the United States and Canada interested in services and research for people labeled retarded. The association moved via its state chapter in New York to inform the governor of its concern. It established a blue-ribbon committee of physicians to have a look at the medical situation in Rome firsthand and provide a report to the governor and the professional community. The president of the Onondaga Association for Retarded Children and the Center on Human Policy, the political and advocacy arm of the Division of Special Education at Syracuse University, actively endorsed the investigation by the state AAMD.

Correspondence was sent to the governor indicating the fact that given the long history of cover-ups by the infamous old department, this issue was a political one. Only an accountable elected official should be in a position to respond and clear the road for the AAMD visit.

A letter from Dr. Kolb to the state AAMD chairman arrived, indicating that the governor had requested he reply concerning the deaths at Rome. "The deaths to which you refer were investigated, as are any deaths, but our investigation and that of the county coroner have shown that they were not part of a pattern or in any way suspicious. With that and a paragraph indicating to the AAMD that mechanisms already existed and were active in reviewing and evaluating the standards of care in the institution, Kolb believed that the "authorized accreditation procedure is the appropriate way to carry out the purposes you suggest."

Another correspondence was sent to the governor, indicating that a time had been set for the physician team to visit Rome. A request was made to have the records of all the persons that had died at Rome in the last twelve months available along with other public health data on the institution.

Again, a letter from the department came back indicating, in cordial language, that the right to privacy and confidentiality prohibited the department from allowing anybody to see those files without specific parental consent (and one could not find out the names of the deceased people because that would also be protected under the policy of the right to confidentiality by the department). "Come and look around but we cannot show you records or charts you understand."

CHAPTER 32

The Heart of the Matter

WILLOWBROOK, PER SE, EXISTS no longer. It has been all but "disappeared." Instead, a renovated college campus, the College of Staten Island, stands, where its students attend, largely oblivious of the human atrocities that occurred behind the new false interior walls and now linoleum-covered stone terrazzo floors that now are fully architecturally hidden. New doorways to enter and exit each of the pastoral campus buildings have changed the geometry everywhere. In the back of the huge old New York State property, behind a fifteen-foot fence, two disheveled one-story stone abandoned structures remain, unmarked and inaccessible, that were the Spastic Buildings 27 and 29. No one knows or asks about them. They are just nameless detritus for some reason spared conversion or demolition. Along the back winding street sit a dozen stately old, deteriorated two-story mansions with a few different-looking, drab adults standing about outdoors, some rocking with typical self-stimulating hand flapping and gestures, who have drifted outside their "living arrangements" that now have replaced the once elegant homes of the institution's director and selected executive Willowbrook staff. Only a few newly placed signs exist to commemorate what had been.

Cloistered, adjacent, behind a grove of high-manicured hedgerows is a glass and steel complex that is the multimillion-dollar Behavioral Research Center that held the vaccine and viral research work that used Willowbrook's children as its "test" subjects, administered by the top medical virologists in the world. At the time, these famed researchers benefited from unfettered lack of informed consent requirements, unethically using access to human subjects without safeguards and prohibitions when subjugation to being inoculated to crippling diseases was the ticket for their admission to Willowbrook. All, for me, an unspeakably sad, haunted, and unreal plantation of memories and ominous ongoing public ignorance.

Are there lessons, issues, actions that can be embraced and asserted today, in our overwhelmingly inchoate and complex lives? Life expectancy in the twentieth century has increased by nearly 30 years until it plateaued and began to decline in the last 3 years. Global politics has drastically changed from the Cold War through 9/11 triggering endless and secretive twenty-first-century Middle East wars and 137 million refugees worldwide. People, seemingly everywhere, blow themselves up or gun down innocents in an endless stream of daily desperation and slaughter that leaves us overwhelmed, striving for meaning and some path to ending this violence and shaping a just and sustainable peace. Climate change, linked to the fossil fuel industry and human use, plays its profound part on the ravaged world's stage. Planetary sustainability demands urgent action, wisdom, and vast political community, heretofore unthinkable. Questions of human rights and population growth boggle the machinery of civilized life. The epochal revolution in the "means of production," through the instantaneous and relentless invention of digital communications with its change in time and space, unimagined possibilities of social reorganization, and interconnectedness through human hands, engulfs us. Our US presidency, at this historical moment, has just been renewed having been in the clutches of a neofascist administration. The country is still deeply divided and despairing, riven with racist police shootings and white supremacist internecine violence after the outcome of the 2020 election, notwithstanding the new adminstration's rush to normalize and correct much in our America.

This wrenching story of Willowbrook is a harbinger of the most crucial and vital social policy reality funded out-of-home placement that must first be systemically ended. The public must understand and stop the public financing of obligatory out-of-home placement at its fount. We are at a historical political crossroads where the existing sprawling institutional system of smaller Willowbrooks everywhere in our society are our common destination for us as we age! It is essential to appreciate this with alarm.

Willowbrook is *every* institution that deals in dehumanization, big or small. The sixty-year-old political strategy of making removal from home and community the major precondition of getting essential support services is a bankrupt legislated policy that does not serve us! Though we started in the nineteenth century with the most extraordinary "special" population around whom it is relatively easy to forge a public consensus that institutionalization (congregate, segregated domicile) was thought to be the best thing to do, we are clearly in an era where that places all of us, by virtue of aging, in the chute to that end. Though the Willowbrook story had its unique personalities, twists, and turns, the basic stakeholders—the institutionalized themselves, their families, facilities workers, professionals, administrators, politicians, financiers, civic volunteers, community activists, corporate leaders, and media people—are the same constellation of folks that continue to struggle, each in self-interest.

The New York developmental disability bureaucracy, the plastic mass of public workers, is in constant flux with regular reorganizations, the metronome of cosmetic change that allows business as usual to continue despite the change in political rhetoric, titles, jurisdictions, and advocacy challenges. Now, in lieu of the monolithic New York Department of Mental Hygiene stand six separate "offices" that circumscribe the policy obligations and public revenue pools to serve people with developmental disabilities, mental health, office of aging, child and family services, and quality management, a maze of operations arbitrarily divided to control and assure no one really understands or can simply solve any significant problem of life. Identical in form, though the details are endlessly shuffled, each state invents its own facade of how to stream funds, power, control, and collaborate with the overriding agenda of preserving privilege for the few and token resources with mind-numbing barriers to living life for the majority of people intentionally kept poor, divided, confused, compliant, and worst, monetized.

To be sure, the thousands of souls in the federal Willowbrook class were, slowly but surely, decentralized. This was done, in many instances, under the ongoing iron surveillance of the federal court monitor's office that administered the court-ordered changes, who found individual or small (six-bed) facilities across New York to replace the death camp where people who were previously held. The sixty institutions that were the extent of New York's hundreds of billions of misspent dollar fortresses for its members with intellectual disabilities and mental illness no longer operate at the center of care, and languish in a variety of states of vacancy or repurposing, absent their original legitimacy and enormous revenue (ransom) attraction. The governor of New York, Andrew Cuomo, set 2015 as their terminus when all must be closed from their original purpose, an unkept promise.

From no community services for people with disabilities in New York when our great struggle began, the bureaucracy now administers a massive constellation of alternative living arrangements that arose with the new river of Medicaid funding, too numerous to accurately track, supported by the mix of federal and state subsidies to keep these services at the low edge of a dedicated ability to elevate quality of life for their still-labeled inhabitants.

In the midst of all these public storms, a strategic set of nationwide system reforms, established in the political wake of the anti-institutional court decisions and public outcry, has come into being. This stream of law and litigation grounded in human rights preceded interim landmark steps forward. Here, the maturing awareness of effective family constituency organizations (intellectual disability, autism, cerebral palsy, learning disabilities, spina bifida, and twenty other diagnostic defense groups) struck the rock, over and over, through mobilizations, litigation, and new laws to force what in essence is a slow redistribution of vital resources, power, and policies that have altered the topography of human services.

These steps include:

- Precedent policies came into being under Lyndon Johnson's Great Society— War on Poverty, reforms after Medicare and Medicaid in 1964. This was the Older Americans Act of 1965. Its "stated" purpose was to ensure equal opportunity to the fair and free enjoyment of adequate income in retirement; the best possible physical and mental health services without regard to economic status; suitable housing; restorative and long-term care; opportunity for employment; retirement in health, honor, and dignity; civic, cultural, educational, and recreational participation and contribution; efficient community services; immediate benefit from proven research knowledge; freedom, independence, and the exercise of self-determination; and protection against abuse, neglect, and exploitation. The Older Americans Act began a mosaic of change as it defined conditions and design of service among all of us in long life. Though this act had been established in 1965, prior to the Willowbrook trial, its relevance to mindless institutionalization and its contemporary aftermath was still to come.

- In 1975, a decade afterward, the Education for All Handicapped Children's Act (PL 94-142) exploded into law when the direction, clearly taken by state and federal courts, was spurred by the landmark *Pennsylvania Association for Retarded Children (PARC) v. Commonwealth of Pennsylvania* 1971 lawsuit for right to education for children with special needs including those at Pennhurst State School, Pennsylvania's Willowbrook. In 1972, the Willowbrook class action suit, *New York State Association for Retarded Children and Parisi v. State of New York*, was first filed on the initial finding of violations of the Eighth Amendment against cruel and unusual punishment.

- The PARC suit was followed by the 1972 *Mills v. State Board of Education* to establish the right to education in the Washington, DC, public school system. The systemic and astounding data of the Children's Defense Fund found two million children out of school in 1974 due to outrageous excuses due to poverty, language, disability, all driven by arbitrary and callous nationwide education system exclusionary practices. This paradigm shift legislation turned nineteenth-century industrial education on its head and stated for the first time that all children with developmental disabilities (defined as those with intellectual disability, autism, cerebral palsy, epilepsy, and some learning disabilities occurring prior to age twenty-one) had a "right to education" and that there was an affirmative obligation for schools to fit and fund the needs of the individual child and not vice versa. So uniformly extensive was school exclusion in America associated with the label of mental retardation / intellectual disability that tens of thousands of families were drowned with basic day-in-and-day-out caring requirements of the indifferent and discriminatory education system everywhere. The new law required that children be taught in the "least restrictive environment." This meant in fully integrated classrooms with other typical-age peers with whatever special teaching support that implied. Parents would participate in determining their child's mandated annual individual education program (IEP) and had strong due process protections to challenge school restrictions and imposed barriers.

• In 1981, the Medicaid Home and Community Based Services Waiver Program was established based on pressures on policy makers that institutional payments for intermediate care for developmental disability services and nursing care were consuming the lion's share of Medicaid resources despite the public's preference for home and community care. This waiver program, offered to states by amendments to Section 1915(c) of the Social Security Act, sought to invite states to identify cost-effective alternatives to institutional care to obtain sanctions that would allow implementation to those home-and community-based medical care solutions. In its first decade from 1990 to 2000, expenditures grew from $1.2 billion to $13.7 billion.

• After decades of organizing and fierce demonstrations by the broad disability rights movement, the Americans with Disabilities Act (ADA) was written in 1988 and passed on July 26, 1990, establishing a guarantee to full respect and human rights recognition, thorough physical access and inclusion, despite some specific exclusions, in all aspects of American life for people with every kind of disability.

• In 1999, the Supreme Court accepted an appeal from a suit, *Olmstead v. L. C.* filed in Georgia on behalf of two institutionalized young women that made full constitutional guarantees and right to service in the most individual and socially integrated way, by all states human services for people with special needs. This ruling, written by Justice Ruth Bader Ginsberg, imposed a single progressive principle and standard of care that confronted all the states in planning and implementing what must be provided, notwithstanding their prior sovereign residential institutions operations. The Olmstead ruling clearly stated that institutionalization was discriminatory and violated the Americans with Disabilities Act. Every state was mandated to establish its own plan for compliance that extended across all developmental and mental disabilities populations. The Supreme Court based its ruling on two evident judgments. First, "institutional placement of persons who can handle and benefit from community settings perpetuates unwarranted assumptions that persons so isolated are incapable of or unworthy of participating in community life." Second, "confinement in an institution severely diminishes the everyday life activities of individuals, including family relations, social contacts, work options, economic independence, educational advancement, and cultural enrichment."

• Beginning in 2008, the Obama administration battled to establish the Affordable Care Act, moving toward a solution that provided medical coverage to most Americans through a massive standards-based tax subsidy provided to the private insurance system and coordination with a partial Medicaid expansion. Here, the intention to reach toward an access and a mandate for uncovered Americans is exactly in the wrong direction, further pouring 780 billion public dollars into the hands of the industry profiteers with no measures to control cost and that leave more than 30 million of us without health-care coverage. And as could be expected, the river of out-of-home placement and its callous partner, unremunerated indulgence on forcing family and friends to eat the cost of keeping dependent loved ones at home, continued unchanged.

Back to the Heart of the Matter so as to address the message of this book is the policy advocacy of making expanded and improved Medicare for All the solution to America's rightful health care coverage and social justice needs. That is of central concern to us. We see over and over the policy opposition to one of the few actions that can actually effect profound system change. It is this universal, rightful, single payer health care system that America needs as a national priority, especially given the ferocious and unremitting hostility of the billionaire class, the Republican oligarchy, numerous 'Top 500 corporations' and the destructive power of Citizen's United "*dark money*". This cabal cannot allow any government, pubic tax funded program to be credited or credible, trusted or successful."

Universal, rightful single tier of care Medicare for All was denied and never even allowed to be debated in Congress. Even its diversionary payer health system "public option," buying into Medicare and Medicaid without outlawing private insurance, was completely blocked. Thus, what would have created a policy sea change, qualitatively transforming America's body politic through assuring 100 percent public rightful coverage for all health and prevention services to all Americans, never saw the light of day. This "single-payer" solution would essentially outlaw private medical insurance and bring the entirety of the chaotic and heterogeneous medical delivery system into public focus and democratic reconstruction. It would replace medical management for profit with a "health-care system" that currently does not exist in America. As an initial step, notwithstanding that 70 percent of every medical dollar comes from public taxes, it would leave the existing fee for service delivery system intact and accessible to everyone.

It is this oligarchy-rejected entitlement that would finally bring the general public into the power to once and for all eliminate the devastating equation between health and wealth. It would liberate all working Americans from the tyranny of bondage to the lowest benefit work to preserve any modicum of health coverage, and gird the ability to challenge the inflationary and Big Pharma cartel set costs of all medicines, durable medical equipment, and hospital care. It would match and exceed the incentives for out-of-home placement and profoundly reduce the need for the massive US charity industry (a second form of cloying taxation on Americans) that has compensated for the lack of rightful health care and prevention. The irony of such a simple system being seen as pie in the sky when the rest of the industrialized world possesses some form of national health-care financing speaks to the cruel power of the forces of opposition to such an essential need.

We are the inheritors of a 170-year-old well-established segregated institutional system of handling our dependent members in society. The established order has fought to keep resources, control, and definitional power in their hands for which the general public always pays deeply and consistently suffers. This is nowhere clearer than in the continuation of the immensely unaffordable Long-Term Care system that is the channel for all community institutionalization.

Faced with the massive transition of the population toward elder status with its inherent dependencies, one can be absolutely sure that all the public democratic solutions to respond to that evolution threaten the very core of corporate moneymaking and population control that maintains the basic status quo.

The bias for dislocating those in need, dismantling families, especially when they have declining resources, or no money to buy out from the slide downward, dominates public policy and law. Title XIX of the Social Security Act is the law of the land despite the growing struggle to force states to opt out of traditional out-of-home placement support requirements where change is slowly coming. States may apply to the federal government to obtain permission to alter the rigid funding model (obtaining a Title XIX waiver), but face prodigious difficulties and delays in doing so. These delays are invariably directed by executive bureaucrats who, in large majority, seek to save their economic skins. The motivation to change the social structure toward more democratization and enfranchisement inherent in approaches that fund individuals and families to deliver quality of life support is sadly terribly rare and a strategic threat to the corporate power structure.

The importance of telling the story of public hostage as people with special needs become less and less the object of categorical funding and solutions, and as the larger identical needs, population of people who are aging, represent a tsunami of demographic demand, the two devalued populations are converging as a connected profit center opportunity to the policy makers of America. The story of Willowbrook is so easy to extrapolate to the experience that we will all have with our aging relatives—grandparents, parents, aunts, and uncles who must have individualized support to maintain maximum independence and autonomy, lifetime care.

Lifetime care must do away with:

- a nation of segregated, congregate, deviant facilities;

- an underpaid and devalued shift staff, paraprofessional workforce;

- a profit-, greed-, and bureaucratic-based administration system whose norm are abuses; and

- billions of dollars of lost wages and imposed time upon often desperate unremunerated family and friends that are forced to become indentured caring community for their loved ones with special needs across all ages.

Care must maximize community inclusion, security, liberty, health and wellness, social and personal productivity, financial and economic stability.

"Long-Term Care" is inconsistent with health care as a human right both in its gravely antisocial and anti-family applications and in its staggering, escalating unaffordable costs as a categorical and distinct expenditure model.

As universal, expanded, and improved single-payer Medicare for All policy is detailed nationally in the 2019 federally authored Pramila Jayapal's HR 1384 and Bernie Sanders's S 1129, and in increasing numbers of state models (New York, California, Oregon, Washington, Hawaii, Vermont, Illinois, Massachusetts, Rhode Island, Colorado, Pennsylvania, etc.) the "inclusion" of long-term care is a profound challenge given its currently defined segregated wealth extraction and non-normalized model and cost. Here, the comprehensive continuum of social to health to habilitation to medical services needed to genuinely address the needs of the twentieth-century long-term care patient community (birth to death), and given the definition of desired outcomes, cannot be rationally separated from the continuum of Lifetime Care as a fluid and integrated twenty-first-century model delivered to achieve individual and community health goals, outcomes, and personal freedoms.

The principle of "health care as a human right" must thoroughly embrace life-time care and reject Medicaid's long-term care as an inconsistent policy and program framework. The former must clearly define, structure, and integrate individualized family and neighborhood comprehensive human services, independent of any segregated facility, whose goal is to maximize inclusion, liberty, health and wellness, social and personal productivity, and community and financial and economic stability. Only with this progressive and commonsense policy adoption can we responsibly establish the most ethical and just bond among the disability, elder, economically suffering, special needs, and our labor allied sectors.

The interruption in our largely self-absorbed work lives, the major time demands, the punishing array of barriers, alienated professionals, absurd and self-serving bureaucratic rules and regulations appear in every step of the effort to solve service needs. The norm, stunning expenses and lack of long-term care cost coverage available in the insurance market, the obligatory pressures to surrender our family member to a professional out-of-home operation, the savage policy to spend down all saved wealth to obtain eligibility for the final American solution—Medicaid subsidized out-of-home placement, at the point of utter penury—combine into a gigantic money squeeze that destroys everyone in its process to strengthen the grip of a corporate, totalitarian America.

Nearly fifty years have passed since the federal class action suit against Willowbrook, the New York Department of Mental Hygiene, and the governor, for human rights violations, was litigated. Nevertheless, there is no true paradigm shift that would allow the spectrum of real change to alter the experience we all share, in large part, alone, guilt ridden, sad, and anger riven as we either provide the care or become the object of institutionalization itself. There can be no more awful experience than losing one's unique identity, peers, mobility, memory, familiar and decorated personal space, daily living skills, choice, pride, wellness, strength, continence, and spirit of life that should be part and parcel of our end of life. As long as profit drives most care, out-of-home (long-term care) placement and obligatory impoverishment are still mandated. It is not acceptable for us and our loved ones to opt for even the best segregated high-end residential institution. We cannot be consigned in a system branded for persons who are labeled disabled, aging, increasingly isolated in our dog-eat-dog, competitive culture that crushes true human differentness, instills insecurity and fearfulness, and is shadowed by our death-making culture.

The door to thinking and looking at the big picture of how to establish intimate neighborhood relations, a functional "village," and the assistance to support and maintain life in one's home is the challenge. This must include contributing roles for all, mealtimes and food security, transportation, and access to cultural events. Care and support funding should funnel through the person and not through institutional intermediaries. This will maximize choice and customize support a reform that is fundamental but unconditionally opposed by institutional culture. We must close the quality gap among poor and older people in what they receive in services so that ethnicity, race, sexual orientation, or religion do not result in any stigmatizing or resource disparities. Services must be designed to uplift those most in need.

We need a comprehensive national strategy to compensate the forty-two million individuals who now provide unremunerated supportive care, each day for family and friends, at incalculable personal cost. We must steer those resources through individual and home funding instead of out-of-home placement and integrate health care and social services. This means building the civic infrastructure to maximize independence, and ensure that people have resources to pay for their health and inclusion needs without requiring impoverishment.

We must anticipate the needs in our own lives and examine our final journey of dependency. Will it be dignified? Seven out of ten of us will require assisted and 24/7 personalized care, and that must not mean imposed institutionalization. "Circles of care" able to touch on every aspect of the changes that inevitably come are so obviously lacking in our lives. Individualized and inclusive long-term care, that is to say lifetime care, must be organized and funded as an absolute human right!

This story challenging systematic institutional inhumanity is decades overdue. We must end the assaults on our future autonomy, freedom, and choice in the matter of our own lives and those we love. We now face a historic period where a paradigm shift to universal rightful health care for all—"Everybody in, nobody out"—must be won. Together, we must seize the courage, organization, and discipline to embed this reality in every American's life toward an inspired and democratic society.

CHAPTER 33

Epitaph

THE COVID-19 PANDEMIC IS the hammer blow to our profitable, segregated, congregate, impoverished society. This is the most dramatic evidence of the absolute mortal danger inherent in our institutional culture and ultimate proof of the need for radical policy and structural change called for by the termination of the institutional status quo. The tragedy of the overwhelming deaths that are culling our aged and persons with disabilities (major differentness) members and gravely threaten our poorest human service workers is undeniable. Here is the final statement that demands pro-found transformation and the total shift of how our public and personal monies are assigned to assure the kindest, most skilled, powerful services and creative human care of which we are capable for the foreseeable future.

State lists nursing homes with infections

BY JASON POHL
jpohl@sacbee.com

More than 1,740 nursing home residents and 1,290 employees in California have tested positive for COVID-19, with outbreaks clustered in several major cities and cases confirmed in nearly two-dozen counties, new state data shows.

For the first time, the California Department of Public Health on Friday night published the names of each skilled nursing home with a resident or employee who has tested positive for the disease. Across the country, nursing homes have been devastated with thousands of deaths from the new coronavirus pandemic.

Agencies, including health departments, have been using the coronavirus crisis as a pretext to withhold medical data from the public, The Bee reported last week. Experts, however, say laws such as HIPAA don't apply because there's no realistic way for the public to glean individual patient information from the release of raw numbers for hundreds, if not thousands, of residents, employees and patients.

Results nationally, too, have painted a far more dangerous scenario than government officials have let on.

USA Today surveyed state health departments and found at least 2,300 long-term care facilities in 37 states have reported positive cases. At least 3,000 residents had died. And, on Friday, The New York Times reported at least 6,900 people living in or connected to nursing homes had died because of COVID-19 complications, far higher than previously known.

"They're death pits," said Betsy McCaughey, a former lieutenant governor of New York, told the Times. "These nursing homes are already overwhelmed. They're crowded and they're understaffed. One COVID-positive patient in a nursing home produces carnage."

SUNDAY **APRIL 19** 2020

THE SACRAMENTO BEE

A recent Sacramento Bee review of state and federal records show that California inspectors have cited 18 nursing homes throughout the state for serious violations of infectious disease rules that put residents in "immediate jeopardy." The records review also found approximately 82 percent of the nearly 1,200 nursing homes — 976 separate facilities — in California have been cited with some sort of infection prevention and control violation in the past two years.

CALIFORNIA Forum

Clearly, one of the most dangerous places to be in California in the throes of the COVID-19 pandemic is a nursing facility.

Serving elderly clients, most of whom have underlying health problems, the facilities are hot spots where the coronavirus infects, spreads and kills.

Besides harming the elderly clients, COVID-19 is sickening the workers who staff the facilities. It got so bad at one Riverside facility recently that the workers refused to show up for their shifts, and the patients had to be evacuated to other facilities.

NATIONWIDE PROBLEM

California is not alone in how coronavirus is hitting nursing facilities. More than 3,600 deaths nationwide have been linked to coronavirus outbreaks in nursing homes and long-term care facilities, an alarming rise in just the past two weeks, according to the latest count by The Associated Press.

The latest tally of at least 3,621 deaths is up from about 450 deaths just 10 days ago. But the AP notes that the true toll among the 1 million mostly frail and elderly people who live in such facilities is likely much higher because most state counts don't include those who died without ever being tested for COVID-19.

THE SACRAMENTO BEE

A recent Sacramento Bee review of state and federal records show that California inspectors have cited 18 nursing homes throughout the state for serious violations of infectious disease rules that put residents in "immediate jeopardy." The records review also found approximately 82 percent of the nearly 1,200 nursing homes — 976 separate facilities — in California have been cited with some sort of infection prevention and control violation in the past two years.

THE SACRAMENTO BEE

The Planks' story of isolation, uncertainty, frustration and fear is shared by the families of approximately 400,000 Californians who are cared for each year in licensed long-term care facilities.

Infections were already sickening and killing hundreds of thousands of residents at nursing homes each year — even before COVID-19 hit. Now, the new and catastrophic losses have raised difficult questions about the future of nursing homes and forced a hard look at how the U.S. cares for its elderly residents in their final years.

THE SACRAMENTO BEE

CARE HOMES

More pointedly, has the "warehousing" of senior citizens reached a crisis point that needs urgent correction from the industry, the government, and families?

Most skilled nursing facilities have been locked down for two months to block the new coronavirus from infecting more residents. Because the elderly are disproportionately harmed by COVID-19, nursing homes were some of the first facilities officials closed to outsiders and will likely be the last to re-open.

Experts say it could be at least a year and a half before a vaccine is developed, and some fear nursing home lockdowns could last until the population is fully vaccinated.

After the first major coronavirus outbreak in the United States ravaged a nursing home in Kirkland, Wash., in March, killing more than 40 people, the virus has since infected thousands of residents and employees in nursing homes and assisted-living facilities in California.

As many as 1.3 million Americans live in nursing homes. Despite the shutdown orders, unofficial tallies indicate more than 6,700 skilled nursing home residents have died from the virus nationwide. The World Health Organization says up to half of all coronavirus deaths in Europe are in long-term care facilities.

The U.S. population continues to gray, particularly in California. There will likely be an increased demand for nursing home beds in the near future, despite the headline-grabbing horrors afflicting some places today, said Sergio Landeros, program manager with the state's Long-term Care Ombudsman Program, which acts as an official advocate for people in nursing homes.

"They're not going away," Landeros said of nursing homes and other long-term care facilities. "After this pandemic, there's going to be a much greater need."

Researchers, employees and the state's powerful nursing home lobby mostly agree. Children and grandchildren are simply not equipped to provide complicated, time-intensive medical care for aging or sick family members, said Craig Cornett, CEO of the California Association of Health Facilities.

"I think we have to be a little careful to read too much into this," he said, "because, God help us, hopefully, this is a once-in-a-lifetime kind of pandemic."

Yet nursing home reform advocates say now, more than ever, the coronavirus pandemic should force policymakers to rethink a culture of "warehousing" the elderly.

"This should cause some reflection on how we do long-term care in this country generally," said Tony Chicotel, staff attorney for the California Advocates for Nursing Home Reform. "Putting people in large facilities, and in some cases, warehousing them, in large facilities where there's not a lot of connection to the outside world is just the wrong model."

THE SACRAMENTO BEE

ARE SENIOR FACILITIES ADEQUATELY FUNDED?

Institutions that house the elderly have existed in some form in America since colonial times.

English colonists imported the idea of almshouses for the elderly, mentally ill and orphans. They continued to operate in some form into the Great Depression, when ghastly reports of overwhelmed and unsafe conditions led to reforms.

The modern nursing home model began to take shape after World War II as eldercare became subsidized with federal dollars. By 1954 there were 9,000 skilled nursing facilities in the U.S. More taxpayer money led to increased scrutiny and renewed worry about staffing shortages and lagging standards.

Years of oversight demands and calls to tighten standards culminated in 1965 with the passage of the Medicare and Medicaid acts, which unleashed even more money and spurred the decades-long, back-and-forth debate about the funding, oversight and role of nursing homes in the U.S.

In the years since, skilled nursing homes and assisted living facilities have morphed into an industry that takes in tens of billions of dollars each year, much of it from federal and state tax dollars. In addition to the 1.3 million residents of nursing homes, another 800,000 live in assisted living facilities, and 75,000 are in intermediate care facilities, according to the Kaiser Family Foundation. Three million people work in the eldercare industry.

The Sacramento Bee

Nearly 40% of state's virus deaths from senior facilities

BY JASON POHL
jpohl@sacbee.com

Residents of long-term care homes in California make up nearly 40 percent of the CO-VID-19 deaths in the state, new public health data shows, making skilled nursing and assisted living facilities by far the deadliest hotspots in the coronavirus pandemic.

At least 578 nursing home residents in California have died of complications caused by the new coronavirus, according to state health department data published Tuesday morning, approximately one-third of all confirmed COVID-19 deaths in the state.

Tuesday was the first time California officials had released any numbers about deaths at nursing homes from COVID-19.

More virus cases at Yolo nursing home; U.S. death toll grows

BY MICHAEL MCGOUGH
AND ALEXANDRA
YOON-HENDRICKS
mmcgough@sacbee.com

At least 1,939 Californians have died from the coronavirus as of Wednesday afternoon, according to a Sacramento Bee survey of individual counties' public health departments. More than 48,328 have tested positive for COVID-19, the disease caused by the highly contagious virus.

In data released over the weekend and updated Wednesday, the state reported that more than 600 of those deaths have been residents of skilled nursing facilities, plus 19 staff members at those facilities. As of last Friday, another nearly 150 deaths were patients at assisted living facilities, which cater to the elderly but do not provide the same level of medical care as nursing home, according to the California Department of Social Services. In total, senior care homes have made up about 40 percent of the state's coronavirus deaths so far.

By Friday, at least 144 residents in California assisted living facilities, which cater to the elderly but do not provide the same level of medical care as nursing homes, had died of COVID-19 complications, according to the most recent report from the California Department of Social Services.

Fewer than 11 employees at nursing homes have also died, according to the data. The state did not provide a precise number of employee deaths, only saying that the number was less than 11. The state also is not yet providing the number of fatalities linked to specific facilities.

To date, slightly more than 1,800 Californians have died from COVID-19. The dramatic death numbers for long-term care facilities puts California's eldercare facilities alongside other large states and Western Europe as the deadliest places to live.

Despite state-at-home orders across the country, unofficial tallies indicate more than 6,700 skilled nursing home residents have died from the virus nationwide. The World Health Organization says up to half of all coronavirus deaths in Europe are in long-term care facilities.

Nursing homes have to meet standards set by the Centers for Medicare and Medicaid Services (CMS) in order to receive Medicare and Medicaid funding. So far, the agency has issued guidance telling nursing homes to adhere to usual disinfection guidance, limiting non-essential staff and requiring the use of personal protective equipment such as face masks.

On April 19, the agency required nursing homes to report positive cases of COVID-19 to all residents and their families, as well as the Centers for Disease Control and Prevention.

More than 16,000 of the nearly 70,000 COVID-19 deaths in the U.S. have been residents or employees of nursing facilities, according to a USA Today compiling of state agencies.

In California, at least 644 of more than 2,100 coronavirus deaths have been related to nursing homes, according to the California Department of Public Health.

At a nursing home in Harder's district, Turlock Nursing and Rehabilitation Center, at least 94 people tested positive for the novel coronavirus and five people have died of the virus.

"The (President Donald) Trump Administration's own estimates indicate the number of daily deaths will double between today and the proposed date for convening your commission. If that estimate is accurate, older Americans — especially those in nursing homes — will continue to become sick and die at shocking, disproportionate rates," Harder wrote to Verma. "It's clear that drastic and immediate action must be taken to ensure the safety of seniors in long-term care facilities.

FRIDAY **JULY 3** 2020
SATURDAY **JULY 4** 2020

THE SACRAMENTO BEE

Nursing homes had inside access to state regulators

All of this came while Cornett and a host of industry officials were asking Gov. Gavin Newsom to grant nursing homes immunity from criminal prosecution and make it harder to sue when residents get sick or die. (Newsom has yet to endorse or reject the idea.)

The largely for-profit nursing home industry has been long criticized for cutting staff and benefits to save costs, which, according to experts, can allow for dangerous infections to spread.

And over the past four months, nursing homes have suffered the brunt of the pandemic across the country. In California, at least 2,480 residents and 92 nursing home employees have died because of COVID-19 — about 42 percent of the pandemic death toll, according to state data.

More than 40 percent of all coronavirus deaths in the United States have been tied to nursing homes, according to a New York Times analysis, which found that the virus had infected 316,000 people at 14,000 facilities as of July 15. The virus has been particularly lethal to those in their 60s and older, more so for those in poor health, and it can rapidly spread through buildings where residents live in close quarters and workers move from room to room.

"The federal response to protect one of the most vulnerable populations in the country has been a dismal failure," said Tamara Konetzka, a health economist at the University of Chicago who has been studying the pandemic's outsize impact on nursing home residents.

ACKNOWLEDGMENTS

THROUGHOUT THE THREE YEARS I was inside Willowbrook, a single person shared these days with me providing the support, the counsel, the tenderness to unravel the knot that came home night after night. My ex-wife, Kathleen Bronston, was a constant source of judgment and restraint. Without her continuous participation in all my decisions, another human being so close, so moved by the whole drama, so understandingly assaulted by my moods at day's end, I would have been overwhelmed on dozens of occasions.

Other dear friends shared the struggle of finishing this project in its first telling. Deborah Coleman, who was the first to really take hold the first draft with me and criticize and remold it into a whole. Mary Jane Boswell, executive director of the Youth Association of Retarded Citizens, with whom I completed, added, and rewrote major sections of the book before it was ready to submit for publication. Howard Blatt took the majority of the timeless photographs and lent his political convictions, comradeship, and whose support gave this document a special life and role in the literature of protest and social action. Colleen Wieck, the executive director of the Minnesota Governor's Advisory Committee on Developmental Disabilities who constructed the most brilliant historical and political website anywhere in the field, brought her genius counsel and detailed technical help to getting me and the manuscript ready for completion. Ed Goldman, Pennsylvania's Commissioner of Mental Retardation, who has been by my side for decades. Merlin Chowkwanyon, a peerless faculty member and researcher in the field of progressive health service politics at Columbia University, intensely worked over the manuscript to detail ways to strengthen and aim its message for maximum impact. David Goode, a New York City University senior faculty member and writer in the field, and Co-author of *The History and Sociology of Willowbrook State School* had for the last decade pressed me to record much of my work for his students and continually guided and encouraged me. Peter D'Anna, the retired chief of the Social Security office in Sacramento, California, brought me the most important facts and data to help connect "Public Hostage" to the contemporary realities of long-term care realities and the deeper history and politics of public law and policy related to the growing elder and poor populations of America. For each of these extraordinary people, each motivated with a deep sense of importance of the issues and a devotion to a better life for all people, I am indebted in a way that can never really be repaid. The support, love, and confidence that these profound friends invested in this lifetime project have assured its debut and significance.

Another deep bond during the struggle at Willowbrook came from Mark Marcario, a parent of a youngster, Robbie, with Down syndrome who headed a rare community Down syndrome organization whose families refused to surrender their children to institutionalization. Mark shared much of the daily travail and trauma and would pick me up at least once a week for lunch where we drove across the bridge for hamburgers to New Jersey. Our laughter and friendship were a routine healing hour and soulful reminder of one of the shared rewards of ending the evil that was Willowbrook. This book is filled with my love, devotion, and gratitude for so many heroic family leaders who really were the resolute driver for this change we all sought.

The intimate and poignant photos throughout this book where taken, and the majority compiled for submission to the US Federal Court in the course of this struggle as evidence of the realities the Court grappled to adjudicate and correct. The artistry and power of these images starkly multiply the narrative and bring the wretched reality and suffering of the residents of Willowbrook to a terrible crescendo where words may fail. They were were shot by Hans Jung, Bob Parsons, John Setzer, Howard Blatt and myself.

INDEX

ABOUT THE AUTHOR

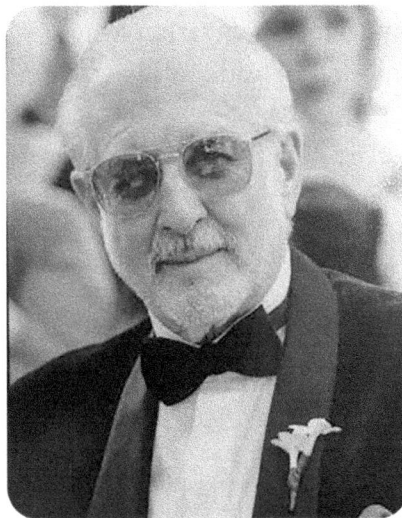

BORN AND EDUCATED IN Los Angeles, CA, William Bronston received his MD at the University of Southern CA School of Medicine, completed his internship in Pediatrics at *Children's Hospital of Los Angeles,* and was a resident in psychiatry at Menningers School of Psychiatry in Topeka, Kansas.

While a senior in Medical School, Bronston founded the Student Health Organization in 1964, a nationwide graduate health science student movement dedicated to promoting universal health care as a human right, overcoming racism, sexism, war, poverty and physician elitism in the health system as the greatest challenges facing society. In 1968 after organizing the American Federation of State, County and Medical Employees mental health worker union in Topeka, Bronston moved to New York where he was a leader in a range of human rights and labor issues in the health care field, a career pursuit continued to the present day.

Deeply concern about the plight of children with developmental special needs while in New York, Bronston spent 3 years as a staff physician in the infamous Willowbrook State School in Staten Island. As a public advocate he helped architect the 1971 Federal Class Action Law Suit against New York State for Constitutional violations of due process, right to treatment and decent care aimed to close and replace its state institutions with individualized family and community services. After a 2 year post doctoral fellowship at Syracuse University in Human Service policy, Bronston returned to

California where he was appointed as the senior consultant to the Director of the CA State Health Department in the field of Developmental Disabilities, then served as medical consultant to the Secretary of Health and Welfare and finally as the Medical Director of the State Department of Rehabilitation where he served till retirement in 2006.

Starting with the 1981, United Nations International Year of Disabled Persons, Bronston organized a 6-year, state-wide model, *Project Interdependence*, to integrate hundreds of multicultural teen youth, with and without disabilities, toward career futures in fields of science, sport, recreation and the arts. In 1997, he established the non profit *Tower of Youth* to promote digital media arts and technology as a system wide reform in the CA Education system, producing 37 bi-annual regional and North American-wide, teen youth film festivals.

Returning to his central and life long devotion of advocating US and CA health care as a right, Bronston again became a major voice in the Physicians for a National Health Program, 30,000 strong, nationwide, progressive physician organization where his harbinger experience in ending institutionalization in New York inexorably leads to his strategic engagement advancing Medicare for All, Single Payer Health Care in America.

www.ingramcontent.com/pod-product-compliance
Lightning Source LLC
Chambersburg PA
CBHW080416030426

42335CB00020B/2471